KT-545-080

Trust Library
Clinical Skills Centre
Queen Elizabeth Hospital
Tel: 0191 445 2935
email: medical.library@ghnt.nhs.uk

Clinics Review Articles

ELSEVIER

EARN MORE CREDITS IN LESS TIME

with **Radiologic Clinics CME**

As a current Radiologic Clinics subscriber, you can take advantage of the companion CME program to earn **90 AMA category 1 credits per year.** Each test is based on the Radiologic Clinics issue of that same topic. Earn **15 credits per single issue!**

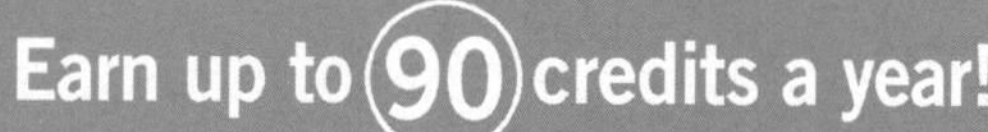

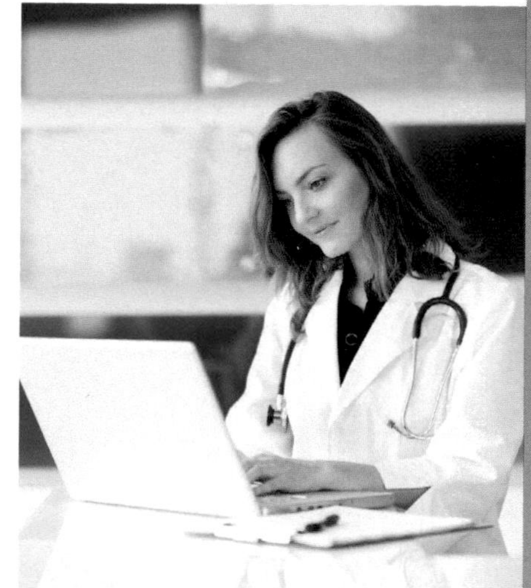

Other benefits of subscribing to the Radiologic Clinics CME program include:

- Convenience and ease of taking and scoring each test online at your own pace
- Immediate receipt of your CME certificate

VISIT: **www.radiologic.theclinics.com/cme/home**
to start earning all the credits you need in one place!

Skull Base Imaging

Editor

NAFI AYGUN

RADIOLOGIC CLINICS OF NORTH AMERICA

www.radiologic.theclinics.com

Consulting Editor
FRANK H. MILLER

January 2017 • Volume 55 • Number 1

ELSEVIER

1600 John F. Kennedy Boulevard • Suite 1800 • Philadelphia, Pennsylvania, 19103-2899

http://www.theclinics.com

RADIOLOGIC CLINICS OF NORTH AMERICA Volume 55, Number 1
January 2017 ISSN 0033-8389, ISBN 13: 978-0-323-48270-7

Editor: John Vassallo (j.vassallo@elsevier.com)
Developmental Editor: Donald Mumford

© **2017 Elsevier Inc. All rights reserved.**

This periodical and the individual contributions contained in it are protected under copyright by Elsevier, and the following terms and conditions apply to their use:

Photocopying
Single photocopies of single articles may be made for personal use as allowed by national copyright laws. Permission of the Publisher and payment of a fee is required for all other photocopying, including multiple or systematic copying, copying for advertising or promotional purposes, resale, and all forms of document delivery. Special rates are available for educational institutions that wish to make photocopies for non-profit educational classroom use. For information on how to seek permission visit www.elsevier.com/permissions or call: (+44) 1865 843830 (UK)/(+1) 215 239 3804 (USA).

Derivative Works
Subscribers may reproduce tables of contents or prepare lists of articles including abstracts for internal circulation within their institutions. Permission of the Publisher is required for resale or distribution outside the institution. Permission of the Publisher is required for all other derivative works, including compilations and translations (please consult www.elsevier.com/permissions).

Electronic Storage or Usage
Permission of the Publisher is required to store or use electronically any material contained in this periodical, including any article or part of an article (please consult www.elsevier.com/permissions). Except as outlined above, no part of this publication may be reproduced, stored in a retrieval system or transmitted in any form or by any means, electronic, mechanical, photocopying, recording or otherwise, without prior written permission of the Publisher.

Notice
No responsibility is assumed by the Publisher for any injury and/or damage to persons or property as a matter of products liability, negligence or otherwise, or from any use or operation of any methods, products, instructions or ideas contained in the material herein. Because of rapid advances in the medical sciences, in particular, independent verification of diagnoses and drug dosages should be made.

Although all advertising material is expected to conform to ethical (medical) standards, inclusion in this publication does not constitute a guarantee or endorsement of the quality or value of such product or of the claims made of it by its manufacturer.

Radiologic Clinics of North America (ISSN 0033-8389) is published bimonthly by Elsevier Inc., 360 Park Avenue South, New York, NY 10010-1710. Months of issue are January, March, May, July, September, and November. Periodicals postage paid at New York, NY and additional mailing offices. Subscription prices are USD 474 per year for US individuals, USD 831 per year for US institutions, USD 100 per year for US students and residents, USD 551 per year for Canadian individuals, USD 1062 per year for Canadian institutions, USD 680 per year for international individuals, USD 1062 per year for international institutions, and USD 315 per year for Canadian and international students/residents. To receive student and resident rate, orders must be accompanied by name of affiliated institution, date of term and the signature of program/residency coordinatior on institution letterhead. Orders will be billed at individual rate until proof of status is received. Foreign air speed delivery is included in all *Clinics* subscription prices. All prices are subject to change without notice. **POSTMASTER:** Send address changes to *Radiologic Clinics of North America*, Elsevier Health Sciences Division, Subscription Customer Service, 3251 Riverport Lane, Maryland Heights, MO63043. **Customer Service: Telephone: 1-800-654-2452** (U.S. and Canada); **1-314-447-8871** (outside U.S. and Canada). **Fax: 1-314-447-8029. E-mail: journalscustomerservice-usa@elsevier.com (for print support); journalsonlinesupport-usa@elsevier.com (for online support)**.

Reprints. For copies of 100 or more of articles in this publication, please contact the Commercial Reprints Department, Elsevier Inc., 360 Park Avenue South, New York, New York 10010-1710. Tel.: +1-212-633-3874; Fax: +1-212-633-3820; E-mail: reprints@elsevier.com.

Radiologic Clinics of North America also published in Greek Paschalidis Medical Publications, Athens, Greece.

Radiologic Clinics of North America is covered in *MEDLINE/PubMed (Index Medicus), EMBASE/Excerpta Medica, Current Contents/Life Sciences, Current Contents/Clinical Medicine, RSNA Index to Imaging Literature, BIOSIS, Science Citation Index,* and *ISI/BIOMED*.

Printed in the United States of America.

Contributors

CONSULTING EDITOR

FRANK H. MILLER, MD
Chief, Body Imaging Section and Fellowship Program; Medical Director of MRI; Professor, Department of Radiology, Northwestern University Feinberg School of Medicine, Chicago, Illinois

EDITOR

NAFI AYGUN, MD
Associate Professor of Radiology, Division of Neuroradiology, Russel H. Morgan Department of Radiology and Radiological Science, Johns Hopkins Hospital, Johns Hopkins University School of Medicine, Baltimore, Maryland

AUTHORS

YOSHIMI ANZAI, MD, MPH
Professor; Associate Chief Medical Quality Officer, Department of Radiology, University of Utah Health Sciences Center, Salt Lake City, Utah

NAFI AYGUN, MD
Associate Professor of Radiology, Division of Neuroradiology, Russel H. Morgan Department of Radiology and Radiological Science, Johns Hopkins Hospital, Johns Hopkins University School of Medicine, Baltimore, Maryland

DAVID BADGER, MD
Division of Neuroradiology, Johns Hopkins University School of Medicine, Baltimore, Maryland

KRISTEN BAUGNON, MD
Assistant Professor, Department of Radiology and Imaging Sciences, Emory University School of Medicine, Atlanta, Georgia

KAREN BLACK, MD
Director, Department of Radiology, North Shore University Hospital, Northwell Health, Manhasset, New York

ARI MEIR BLITZ, MD
Assistant Professor, Division of Neuroradiology, Department of Radiology and Radiological Science, Johns Hopkins Hospital, Baltimore, Maryland

BARTON F. BRANSTETTER IV, MD, FACR
Chief of Neuroradiology, Department of Radiology, University of Pittsburgh Medical Center, University of Pittsburgh, Pittsburgh, Pennsylvania

LINDSEY M. CONLEY, MD
Department of Radiology, Weill Cornell Medical College, NewYork-Presbyterian Hospital, New York, New York

ELLIOT DICKERSON, MD
Resident, Department of Radiology, University of Michigan Health System, Ann Arbor, Michigan

JOSEPH H. DONAHUE, MD
Assistant Professor, Department of Radiology and Medical Imaging, University of Virginia Health System, Charlottesville, Virginia

GARY L. GALLIA, MD, PhD
Associate Professor, Department of Neurosurgery, Johns Hopkins Hospital, Baltimore, Maryland

DHEERAJ GANDHI, MD
Professor of Radiology, Neurosurgery, and Neurology, Department of Radiology, University of Maryland Medical Center, Baltimore, Maryland

JOHN L. GO, MD
Assistant Professor of Radiology, Division of Neuroradiology, Department of Radiology, Keck School of Medicine, University of Southern California, Los Angeles, California

DANIEL A. HERZKA, PhD
Assistant Professor, Department of Biomedical Engineering, Johns Hopkins Hospital, Johns Hopkins University, Baltimore, Maryland

ESTUSHI IIDA, MD
Department of Radiology, Yamaguchi University Graduate School of Medicine, Ube, Yamaguchi, Japan

MASARU ISHII, MD, PhD
Associate Professor, Department of Otolaryngology – Head and Neck Surgery, Johns Hopkins Hospital, Baltimore, Maryland

GAURAV JINDAL, MD
Assistant Professor of Radiology, Neurosurgery, and Neurology, Department of Radiology, University of Maryland Medical Center, Baltimore, Maryland

JOICI JOB, MD
Department of Radiology, University of Pittsburgh Medical Center, University of Pittsburgh, Pittsburgh, Pennsylvania

CLAUDIA F.E. KIRSCH, MD
Division Chief, Neuroradiology; Associate Professor of Neuroradiology and Otolaryngology, Department of Radiology, North Shore University Hospital, Long Island Jewish Medical Center, Northwell Health, Hofstra Northwell School of Medicine, Manhasset, New York

TIMOTHY MILLER, MD
Assistant Professor of Radiology, Department of Radiology, University of Maryland Medical Center, Baltimore, Maryland

SUGOTO MUKHERJEE, MD
Associate Professor of Radiology, Department of Radiology and Medical Imaging, University of Virginia Health System, Charlottesville, Virginia

DAVID A. ORNAN, MD
Assistant Professor, Department of Radiology and Medical Imaging, University of Virginia Health System, Charlottesville, Virginia

C. DOUGLAS PHILLIPS, MD
Director of Head and Neck Imaging, Department of Radiology, Weill Cornell Medical College, NewYork-Presbyterian Hospital, New York, New York

PRASHANT RAGHAVAN, MD
Associate Professor of Radiology, Department of Radiology, University of Maryland Medical Center, Baltimore, Maryland

ANANDH G. RAJAMOHAN, MD
Assistant Professor of Radiology, Division of Neuroradiology, Department of Radiology, Keck School of Medicine, University of Southern California, Los Angeles, California

MAHATI REDDY, MD
Emory University Hospital, Atlanta, Georgia

DOUGLAS D. REH, MD
Associate Professor, Department of Otolaryngology – Head and Neck Surgery, Johns Hopkins Hospital, Baltimore, Maryland

CHRISTOPHER R. ROXBURY, MD
Resident, Department of Otolaryngology – Head and Neck Surgery, Johns Hopkins Hospital, Baltimore, Maryland

ASHOK SRINIVASAN, MBBS
Associate Professor, Department of Radiology, University of Michigan Health System, Ann Arbor, Michigan

Contents

Preface: Skull Base Imaging in the Era of Minimal Access Surgery xiii

Nafi Aygun

Expanded Endonasal Endoscopic Approaches to the Skull Base for the Radiologist 1

Christopher R. Roxbury, Masaru Ishii, Ari Meir Blitz, Douglas D. Reh, and Gary L. Gallia

The cranial base is a complex 3-D region that contains critical neurovascular structures. Pathologies affecting this region represent some of the most challenging lesions to manage due to difficulty with access and risk of significant postoperative morbidity. With the development of expanded endonasal endoscopic approaches, skull base surgeons use the nose and paranasal sinuses as a corridor to access selected ventral skull base lesions. This review discusses high-resolution imaging in the evaluation of patients with skull base lesions considered for endonasal endoscopic surgery, summarizes various expanded endonasal endoscopic approaches, and provides examples of commonly used expanded endonasal endoscopic procedures.

High Resolution Three-Dimensional MR Imaging of the Skull Base: Compartments, Boundaries, and Critical Structures 17

Ari Meir Blitz, Nafi Aygun, Daniel A. Herzka, Masaru Ishii, and Gary L. Gallia

High-resolution 3D MRI of the skull base allows for a more detailed and accurate assessment of normal anatomic structures as well as the location and extent of skull base pathologies than has previously been possible. This article describes the techniques employed for high-resolution skull base MRI including pre- and post-contrast constructive interference in the steady state (CISS) imaging and their utility for evaluation of the many small structures of the skull base, focusing on those regions and concepts most pertinent to localization of cranial nerve palsies and in providing preoperative guidance and post-operative assessment. The concept of skull base compartments as a means of conceptualizing the various layers of the skull base and their importance in assessment of masses of the skull base is discussed.

Imaging of Paranasal Sinuses and Anterior Skull Base and Relevant Anatomic Variations 31

Estushi Iida and Yoshimi Anzai

This article reviews the normal anatomy and variants of the anterior skull base and sinonasal cavities that are relevant to endoscopic sinus and skull base surgery. Radiologists should be aware of sinonasal anatomy that can be impediments to surgical access and increase risk of vascular or cranial nerve injury during surgery. Imaging features of the paranasal sinuses and anterior skull base pathologies are also discussed.

Imaging of the Central Skull Base 53

Lindsey M. Conley and C. Douglas Phillips

The skull base is a complex bony and soft tissue interface that is divided anatomically into compartments. This article will focus specifically on the central skull

base, which has a complex embryologic development and anatomy. Multiple entities from notochord remnants, neoplasm, infection, and other abnormalities may occur, and imaging is critical for depicting skull base pathology.

Diplopia: What to Double Check in Radiographic Imaging of Double Vision 69

Claudia F.E. Kirsch and Karen Black

When patients see double with both eyes open, known as "binocular diplopia," this may be a harbinger of underlying life-threatening causes. This article presents pertinent anatomy, critical abnormality, and radiographic features that should be double checked for in diplopia. Key areas requiring a double check using the acronym VISION include Vascular, Infectious and Inflammatory, the Scalp for giant cell arteritis, Sphenoid and Skull base in trauma, Increased intracranial pressure (pseudotumor cerebri), Onset of new headaches or psychosis, and Neoplasm. This article reviews the pertinent abnormalities and radiographic imaging critical to assess in patients with diplopia.

Imaging of the Sella and Parasellar Region 83

John L. Go and Anandh G. Rajamohan

The sella and parasellar region, found between the anterior and central skull base, represents the central aspect of the skull base. Given the location of the pituitary gland in this location, small lesions in this location may have major physiologic effects on the human body. This article reviews the anatomy, development, and pathologic processes that may involve this region.

Imaging of the Posterior Skull Base 103

Joici Job and Barton F. Branstetter IV

The posterior skull base can be involved by a variety of pathologic processes. They can be broadly classified as: traumatic, neoplastic, vascular, and inflammatory. Pathology in the posterior skull base usually involves the lower cranial nerves, either as a source of pathology or a secondary source of symptoms. This review will categorize pathology arising in the posterior skull base and describe how it affects the skull base itself and surrounding structures.

Imaging of Vascular Compression Syndromes 123

Joseph H. Donahue, David A. Ornan, and Sugoto Mukherjee

Trigeminal neuralgia, hemifacial spasm, vestibulocochlear neuralgia and glossopharyngeal neuralgia represent the most common neurovascular compression syndromes. Repeated vascular pulsations at the vulnerable transitional zone of the individual cranial nerves lead to focal axonal injury and demyelination. High-resolution 3-D T2-weighted MR imaging is essential in detecting and mapping neurovascular compression for directed therapy. Knowledge of the specific nerve root exit, the transitional zones, and the adjacent vasculature is critical in proper management. Treatment options for these neurovascular compressions syndromes run the gamut from medical therapy to stereotactic radiosurgery to botulinum injections and to surgical decompression.

Imaging of Perineural Spread in Head and Neck Cancer 139

David Badger and Nafi Aygun

Perineural spread (PNS) of tumor is a recognized pattern of metastasis occurring in the head and neck. Imaging plays a critical role in identifying PNS for adequate

PROGRAM OBJECTIVE

The objective of the *Radiologic Clinics of North America* is to keep practicing radiologists and radiology residents up to date with current clinical practice in radiology by providing timely articles reviewing the state of the art in patient care.

TARGET AUDIENCE

Practicing radiologists, radiology residents, and other health care professionals who provide patient care utilizing radiologic findings.

LEARNING OBJECTIVES

Upon completion of this activity, participants will be able to:

1. Review approaches for imaging various regions of the skill base.
2. Discuss imaging of vascular lesions, diplopia, and CSF rhinorrhea and ororrhea at the skull base.
3. Recognize advanced imaging techniques for the skull base.

ACCREDITATION

The Elsevier Office of Continuing Medical Education (EOCME) is accredited by the Accreditation Council for Continuing Medical Education (ACCME) to provide continuing medical education for physicians.

The EOCME designates this enduring material for a maximum of 15 *AMA PRA Category 1 Credit*(s)™. Physicians should claim only the credit commensurate with the extent of their participation in the activity.

All other health care professionals requesting continuing education credit for this enduring material will be issued a certificate of participation.

DISCLOSURE OF CONFLICTS OF INTEREST

The EOCME assesses conflict of interest with its instructors, faculty, planners, and other individuals who are in a position to control the content of CME activities. All relevant conflicts of interest that are identified are thoroughly vetted by EOCME for fair balance, scientific objectivity, and patient care recommendations. EOCME is committed to providing its learners with CME activities that promote improvements or quality in healthcare and not a specific proprietary business or a commercial interest.

The planning committee, staff, authors and editors listed below have identified no financial relationships or relationships to products or devices they or their spouse/life partner have with commercial interest related to the content of this CME activity:

Yoshimi Anzai, MD, MPH; Nafi Aygun, MD; David Badger, MD; Kristen Baugnon, MD; Karen Black, MD; Barton F. Branstetter IV, MD, FACR; Lindsey M. Conley, MD; Elliot Dickerson, MD; Joseph H. Donahue, MD; Anjali Fortna; Gary L. Gallia, MD, PhD; Dheeraj Gandhi, MD; John L. Go, MD; Daniel A. Herzka, PhD; Etsushi Iida, MD; Masaru Ishii, MD, PhD; Joici Job, MD; Timothy Miller, MD; Sugoto Mukherjee, MD; David A. Ornan, MD; C. Douglas Philips, MD; Prashant Raghavan, MD; Anandh G. Rajamohan, MD; Mahati Reddy, MD; Douglas D. Reh, MD; Christopher R. Roxbury, MD; Ashok Srinivasan, MBBS; Karthik Subramaniam; Megan Suermann; John Vassallo.

The planning committee, staff, authors and editors listed below have identified financial relationships or relationships to products or devices they or their spouse/life partner have with commercial interest related to the content of this CME activity:

Ari Meir Blitz, MD is a consultant/advisor for Guerbet, and has research support from Aesculab.

Gaurav Jindal, MD has research support from Stryker; MicroVention; Codman Neurovascular, part of DePuy Synthes Companies of Johnson & Johnson; and Medtronic

Claudia F.E. Kirsch, MD is a consultant/advisor for Primal, part of Pharma Intelligence, with research support from Idiopathic Intracranial Hypertension Foundation and RTOG Foundation Inc.

UNAPPROVED/OFF-LABEL USE DISCLOSURE

The EOCME requires CME faculty to disclose to the participants:

1. When products or procedures being discussed are off-label, unlabelled, experimental, and/or investigational (not US Food and Drug Administration [FDA] approved); and
2. Any limitations on the information presented, such as data that are preliminary or that represent ongoing research, interim analyses, and/or unsupported opinions. Faculty may discuss information about pharmaceutical agents that is outside of FDA-approved labelling. This information is intended solely for CME and is not intended to promote off-label use of these medications. If you have any questions, contact the medical affairs department of the manufacturer for the most recent prescribing information.

TO ENROLL

To enroll in the PET Clinics Continuing Medical Education program, call customer service at 1-800-654-2452 or sign up online at http://www.theclinics.com/home/cme. The CME program is available to subscribers for an additional annual fee of USD $315.

METHOD OF PARTICIPATION

In order to claim credit, participants must complete the following:

1. Complete enrolment as indicated above.
2. Read the activity.
3. Complete the CME Test and Evaluation. Participants must achieve a score of 70% on the test. All CME Tests and Evaluations must be completed online.

CME INQUIRIES/SPECIAL NEEDS

For all CME inquiries or special needs, please contact elsevierCME@elsevier.com.

RADIOLOGIC CLINICS OF NORTH AMERICA

FORTHCOMING ISSUES

March 2017
Genitourinary Imaging
Andrew B. Rosenkrantz, *Editor*

May 2017
Breast Imaging
Sarah M. Friedewald, *Editor*

July 2017
Practical Pediatric Imaging
Edward Y. Lee, *Editor*

RECENT ISSUES

November 2016
Diffuse Lung Disease
Jeffrey P. Kanne, *Editor*

September 2016
Imaging of the Athlete
Adam C. Zoga and Johannes B. Roedl, *Editors*

July 2016
Extranodal Lymphoma from Head to Toe
Mark D. Murphey, *Editor*

ISSUE OF RELATED INTEREST

Magnetic Resonance Imaging Clinics of North America
November 2016 (Vol. 24, Issue 4)
Imaging of Brain Tumors
Rivka R. Colen, *Editor*
Available at: http://www.mri.theclinics.com

THE CLINICS ARE AVAILABLE ONLINE!
Access your subscription at:
www.theclinics.com

Preface
Skull Base Imaging in the Era of Minimal Access Surgery

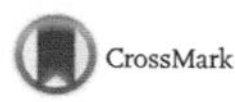

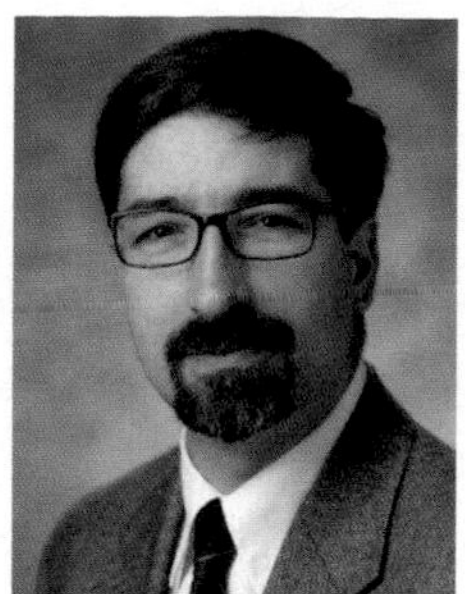

Nafi Aygun, MD
Editor

Ancient Egyptians who extracted the brain through the nose in the process of embalming are to be credited for laying the path for the twentieth century surgeons who used endoscopes to explore the possibilities of surgical treatment of sinonasal pathologies. This is followed by the development of techniques to access the sella turcica via the transnasal route. By the 1990s, transsphenoidal resection of pituitary tumors using endoscope was the standard of care. Experience gained in endoscopic sinonasal and transphenoidal pituitary surgery provided the vision for the expanded endonasal approaches to the skull base pathology. Fueled by the fascinating advances in optical and intraoperative navigational techniques, miniaturization of surgical instruments and radiologic imaging, minimal access skull base surgery is today pushing the limits of resectability while simultaneously decreasing morbidity. Many otolaryngology and neurosurgery training programs are now offering dedicated skull base surgery fellowships that herald the spread of these techniques from academic centers to community practices in the next decade.

The role of the radiologist is also being redefined in the era of minimal access skull base surgery. In addition to the traditional radiologic approach that is mostly concerned about delineating the extent and nature of pathology, we are now asked to address issues related to access and safety. Having at least a basic understanding of potential access routes and hazards is now essential for radiologists to tailor their reads according to the needs of the surgeon. The first article of this issue provides a comprehensive review of surgical approaches. The second article highlights the importance of high-resolution imaging in surgical planning and how high-resolution imaging is reshaping our understanding of anatomy and pathology at the skull base. The following articles, organized based on clinical symptoms and/or scenarios, address lesion detection and characterization using conventional and advanced imaging techniques. One article in this issue covers vascular lesions and their treatment by endovascular means. Cerebrospinal fluid leaks, more common in the era of minimally invasive surgery, are addressed in another article.

I thank all the authors for their outstanding contributions, and I hope that you find the issue as interesting, comprehensive, and educational as it is practical.

Nafi Aygun, MD
Division of Neuroradiology
Russel H. Morgan Department of Radiology
Johns Hopkins University
School of Medicine
600 North Wolfe Street Phipps B112B
Baltimore, MD 21287, USA

E-mail address:
naygun1@jhmi.edu

Radiol Clin N Am 55 (2017) xiii
http://dx.doi.org/10.1016/j.rcl.2016.10.009
0033-8389/17/© 2016 Published by Elsevier Inc.

Expanded Endonasal Endoscopic Approaches to the Skull Base for the Radiologist

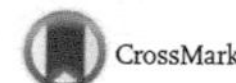

Christopher R. Roxbury, MD[a], Masaru Ishii, MD, PhD[a], Ari Meir Blitz, MD[b], Douglas D. Reh, MD[a], Gary L. Gallia, MD, PhD[c,*]

KEYWORDS

- Endoscopy • Endonasal endoscopic approach • Skull base • Skull base surgery
- Skull base imaging

KEY POINTS

- The development of expanded endonasal endoscopic procedures over the past couple decades has transformed the field of skull base surgery and, together with open techniques, these approaches provide circumferential access to the skull base.
- High-resolution imaging is essential in the surgical evaluation of patients with skull base pathologies.
- There are various approaches or modules to ventral skull base pathologies; these can be defined along the midsagittal and paramedian regions of the skull base.

INTRODUCTION

The skull base is a complex 3-D structure. Traditional approaches to skull base pathologies include open as well as transnasal transsphenoidal microsurgical procedures. Over the past couple decades, endoscopic procedures and in particular expanded endonasal endoscopic approaches (EEAs), have been developed and are increasingly used to treat anterior, middle, and posterior cranial base pathologies.[1–32] These procedures, together with open approaches, provide circumferential access to the skull base. Key developments and the efforts of many pioneers in this field have been expertly reviewed.[33]

Similar to open neurosurgical skull base procedures, EEAs comprise various surgical components. The first component, the surgical approach, creates a working corridor through the nose and paranasal sinuses. The second component involves the resection and definitive surgical management of the pathology. During the third component, the skull base is reconstructed to re-establish an anatomic barrier between the nose and intracranial space to prevent a cerebrospinal fluid leak and associated complications. These components, which are performed collaboratively by otolaryngologists and neurosurgeons, are planned preoperatively. This overview

Disclosure Statement: C.R. Roxbury, M. Ishii, D.D. Reh, and G.L. Gallia have nothing to disclose. A.M. Blitz: Grant support — Aesculab, Medical advisory board — Guerbet.

[a] Department of Otolaryngology – Head and Neck Surgery, Johns Hopkins Hospital, 601 North Caroline Street, Baltimore, MD 21287, USA; [b] Division of Neuroradiology, Department of Radiology and Radiological Science, Johns Hopkins Hospital, 600 North Wolfe Street, Baltimore, MD 21287, USA; [c] Department of Neurosurgery, Johns Hopkins Hospital, 600 North Wolfe Street, Baltimore, MD 21287, USA
* Corresponding author.
E-mail address: ggallia1@jhmi.edu

Radiol Clin N Am 55 (2017) 1–16
http://dx.doi.org/10.1016/j.rcl.2016.09.001
0033-8389/17/© 2016 Elsevier Inc. All rights reserved.

reviews the critical importance of high-resolution imaging in the evaluation of patients with skull base lesions considered for endonasal endoscopic surgery, summarizes EEAs, and provides illustrative examples of commonly used EEAs.

GENERAL PRINCIPLES

As the field of endoscopic cranial base surgery continues to develop, EEAs are applied to increasingly complex pathologies. These approaches are limited by the location of pathology, the extent to which the lesion involves neurovascular structures, and the amount the nasal cavities and paranasal sinuses can be modified to permit sufficient exposure of the lesion and surrounding critical structures. The technical experience and expertise of the skull base team is also important for these procedures; there is a learning curve and proposed incremental training program when performing these procedures.[34–37]

In general, lesions may be accessed endonasally if the pathology is medial and anterior to key neurovascular structures at the skull base. Although vascular structures, including the internal carotid artery, may be mobilized to some degree, cranial nerves (CN) cannot be manipulated without a high risk of creating neurologic deficits.[38] In cases of pathology that is lateral or distal to critical neurovascular structures, open, combined, and multiportal approaches must be considered to achieve the best surgical result and the lowest risk of morbidity (**Fig. 1**). Therefore, the decision as to whether or not a particular case is amenable to an endonasal procedure depends on the knowledge of the extent of the lesion and its relationship with adjacent neurovascular structures. This requires a thorough understanding of skull base anatomy as well as an ability to interpret high-resolution imaging.

High-Resolution Imaging

Preoperative imaging is essential in the surgical evaluation of patients with skull base pathologies. Although the specifics regarding imaging are beyond the scope of this article and are reviewed elsewhere in this issue, patients typically undergo high-resolution CT, including CT angiography (CTA) and MR imaging. Moreover, both CTA and MR imaging are performed with protocols suited for the use of image guidance for intraoperative navigation.

High-resolution CT/CTA is performed to characterize the osseous involvement/extent of the pathology, evaluate the bony sinonasal and skull base anatomy of the planned surgical corridor, detect anatomic variants that have an impact on the surgical approach (**Fig. 2**A–C), and identify

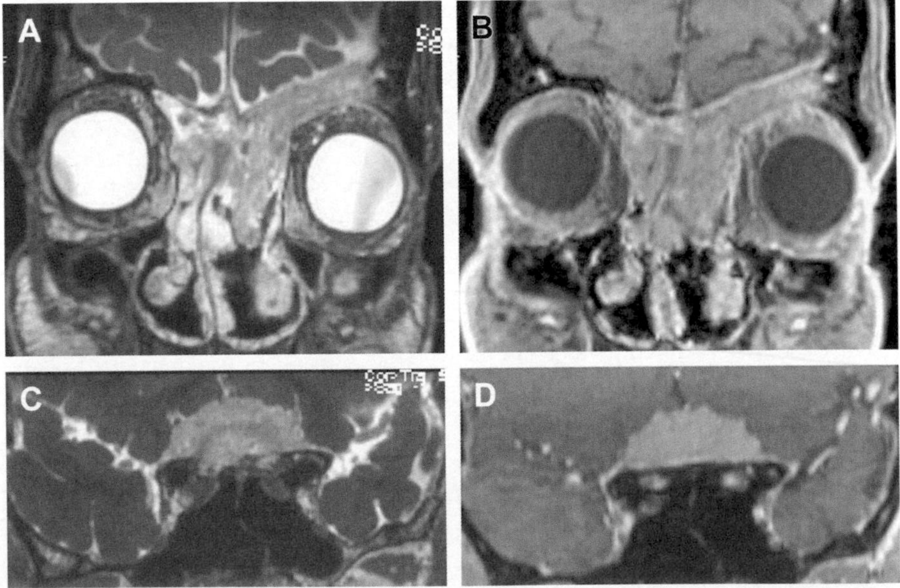

Fig. 1. Illustrative cases of skull base pathologies managed with open surgical procedures. High-resolution constructive interference in steady state (CISS) (*A*) and postcontrast volumetric interpolated breath-hold examination (VIBE) (*B*) sequences in a patient with a sinonasal carcinoma extending above the left orbit. High-resolution CISS (*C*) and postcontrast VIBE (*D*) sequences in a patient with a planum sphenoidale meningioma. Extension above and lateral to both optic nerves is seen. Given the lateral extension of pathology in these cases, both were managed with open procedures.

the location and possible vascular abnormalities of the carotid artery (**Fig. 2**D) and other vessels. Anatomic variants, such as septal deviations and spurs, may require a septoplasty or may make harvest of a nasoseptal flap, which is often used for reconstructing skull base defects where there is a high-flow cerebrospinal fluid leak or an exposed carotid artery in patients who will receive postoperative radiotherapy, more difficult. It is also important to understand the sinonasal anatomy, which can be highly variable in patients.[39–44] A complete understanding of the bony and vascular anatomy is important in preoperative planning and also anticipation of intraoperative findings.

MR imaging is also important in preoperative evaluation. Although thin-slice protocols for sellar and orbital disease exist, imaging of the skull base on most conventional MR studies is confined to the inferior slices on a brain MR scan or the superior slices on a neck or cervical spine study. This lack of detailed information severely limits the presurgical evaluation of patients with skull base pathologies and, to address these limitations, a dedicated high-resolution 3-D skull base MR imaging (HR-SB–MR imaging) protocol was developed at the authors' institution in 2009. This protocol, as described by Blitz and colleagues[45] in this *Radiologic Clinics of North America* issue, incorporates constructive interference in steady state (CISS), volumetric breath-hold examination (VIBE), and short-tau inversion-recovery (STIR) SPACE sequences and is extremely useful for preoperative assessment of patients with skull base pathologies. HR-SB–MR imaging is used to identify pathology not visualized on conventional imaging (**Fig. 3**A), evaluate the segments of the CNs, characterize the differential diagnosis of the pathology in question, and precisely define the extent of disease as well as the relationship to adjacent neurovascular structures (**Fig. 3**B–D). Osseous

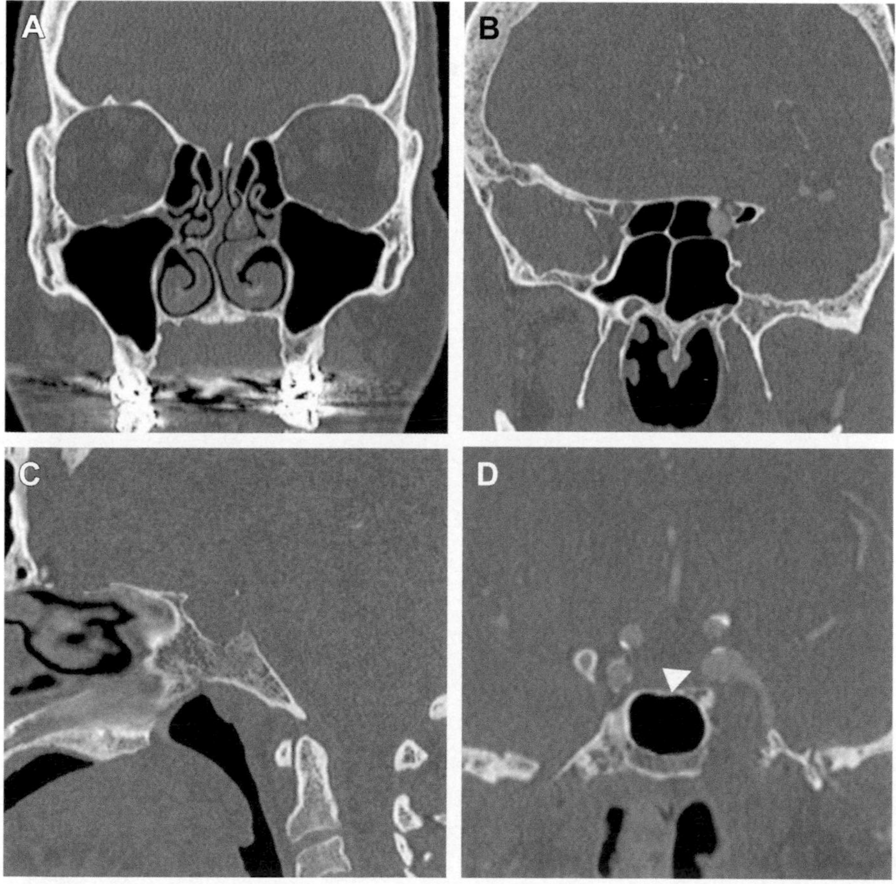

Fig. 2. CTA studies performed in 4 different patients undergoing endoscopic skull base surgery. (*A*) A large right-sided septal spur is visualized. (*B*) Bilateral Onodi cells and a dehiscent left carotid artery are notable. (*C*) A presellar sphenoid sinus is noted in this patient with an enlarged sella secondary to a pituitary adenoma. (*D*) An anterolaterally displaced carotid artery and cavernous carotid artery segment aneurysm (*arrowhead*) are noted in this patient with a chondrosarcoma.

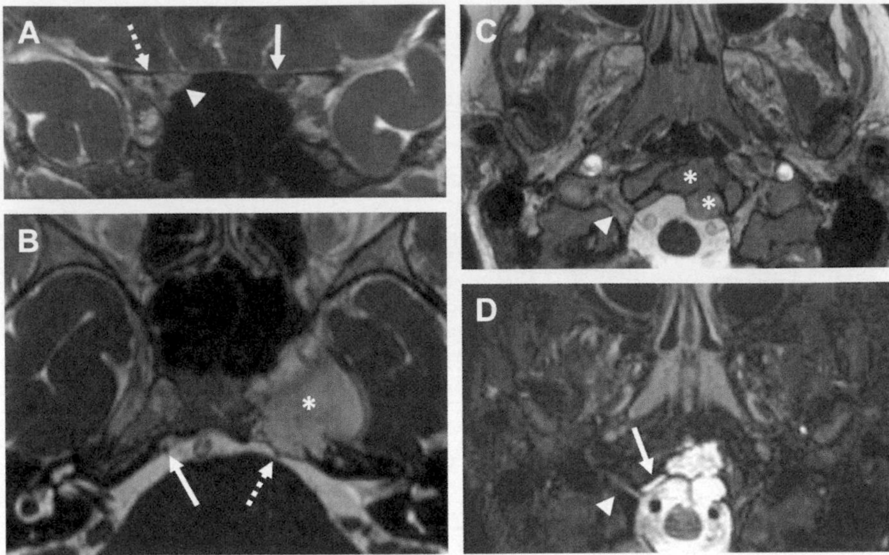

Fig. 3. Examples of HR-SB–MR imaging scans in several patients undergoing endoscopic skull base surgery. (*A*) A medially situated optic canal mass is seen in this patient whose conventional imaging was unremarkable. The right CN II.f (*dotted arrow*) is displaced laterally by the mass (*arrowhead*); the contralateral nerve is noted by the solid white arrow. (*B*) The right CN VI.c/e is seen entering Dorello canal (*solid arrow*). On the left, the nerve (*dotted arrow*) is seen along the posterior aspect of this chondrosarcoma (*asterisk*). (*C*) Postcontrast CISS and (*D*) STIR SPACE sequences demonstrate an interdural component of a chordoma (*white arrow*) extending to the medial aspect of the hypoglossal canal (*arrowheads*). The bulk of the tumor is noted on the left (*asterisks*) and this patient also underwent a right inferolateral clivectomy to access this right lateral extension of tumor.

structures of the skull base are also well visualized on HR-SB–MR imaging and CT should be viewed as a complementary technique in this regard. Because EEAs are best for lesions where critical neurovascular structures are distal to the pathology, a thorough understanding of these relationships, which is possible by HR-SB–MR imaging, is essential in planning the optimal surgical approach and minimizing patient morbidity. Postoperative HR-SB–MR imaging is also performed for postsurgical assessment and serial monitoring.

EXPANDED ENDONASAL ENDOSCOPIC APPROACHES TO THE SKULL BASE

EEAs have been classified into various anatomically based modules to access the ventral skull base.[17,18,20,23,32,46] In this classification scheme, the modules are defined based on their location in sagittal and coronal/parasagittal planes. The approaches to access the median skull base (along the sagittal plane) include transfrontal, transcribriform, transplanum/transtuberculum, transsellar, transclival, and transodontoid (**Box 1**, **Fig. 4**). The modules to access the paramedian skull base (along the coronal plane) are based on their depth from superficial to deep and include

Box 1
Expanded endonasal endoscopic approaches to skull base pathologies

Sagittal plane approaches

Transfrontal

Transcribriform

Transtuberculum/transplanum

Transsellar

Transclival (upper, middle, and lower)

Transodontoid

Coronal plane approaches

Anterior

- Transorbital

Middle

- Transpterygoid
- Infratemporal fossa
- Transpetrous
- Transcavernous

Posterior

- Jugular foramen
- Occipital condyle

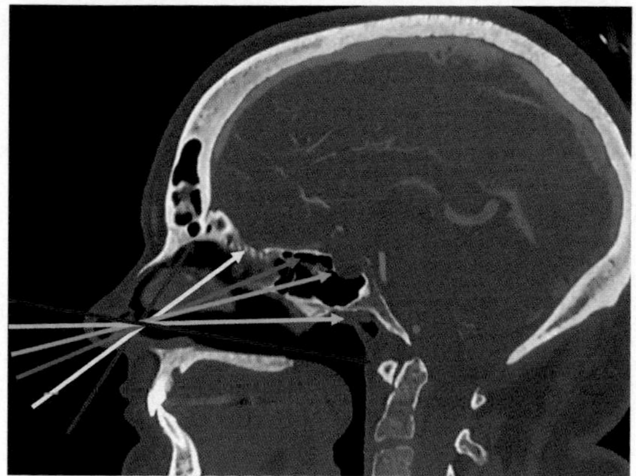

Fig. 4. Midsagittal CT/CTA scan with the various endoscopic trajectories noted by color arrows. The red arrow depicts the transfrontal approach. The yellow arrow depicts the approach to the cribriform. The blue arrow depicts the approach to the planum sphenoidale. The green arrow depicts the approach to the sella. The orange arrow depicts the approach to the clivus. The purple arrow depicts the approach to craniocervical junction, anterior aspect of C1, and odontoid.

anterior, middle, and posterior segments to access the paramedian anterior, middle, and posterior cranial fossae, respectively (see **Box 1**). Each module consists of a defined anatomic target and a nasal/sinonasal corridor to access the particular target. Modules are often combined to address pathologies that span multiple regions. Although the surgical details of each of these procedures are beyond the scope of this overview, the approaches, indications, and limitations of the most common EEAs are reviewed. The location of the carotid artery and CNs is important in each of the modules.[32,47]

MODULES ALONG THE SAGITTAL PLANE

Transfrontal Approach (Endoscopic Modified Lothrop Procedure)

The endoscopic modified Lothrop procedure (EMLP) is an extended frontal sinus approach with the goal of opening the frontal recesses by removing the entire frontal sinus floor.[48–51] The anterior limit of the cavity is the nasal beak, the posterior limit is the posterior table of the frontal sinus, and the lateral limit is the lamina papyracea of the orbits bilaterally. The anterosuperior nasal septum is resected to gain bilateral access for drilling of the nasal beak anteriorly to create a common frontal sinus cavity.

The most common indication for this procedure is failure of previous frontal sinus surgery for chronic sinusitis. This procedure has also been adapted for resection of benign lesions of the frontal sinus, including osteomas, mucoceles (**Fig. 5**), meningoceles, meningoencephaloceles, and fibrous dysplasia. In addition, this is one of the key steps in gaining exposure to the anterior aspect of the anterior skull base in a transcribriform approach.

There are limitations to the EMLP because this approach does not provide access to the entire frontal sinus. The lateral aspects of the frontal sinus often cannot be reached in well-pneumatized frontal sinuses, limiting access to pathologies involving these regions. Such lesions, which extend laterally beyond the meridian of the orbit, may be best approached via an external approach. The anterior to posterior distance of the frontal recess must also be evaluated and is usually done on CT, with a distance less than 1 cm considered a relative contraindication due to lack of working space for drilling.[52]

Transcribriform Approach

The goal of the transcribriform approach is to control the central aspect of the anterior cranial fossa floor, with the anterior limit the posterior table of the frontal sinus, the posterior limit the planum sphenoidale, and the lateral limits the lamina papyracea bilaterally.[16,17,53] To gain exposure, this approach requires bilateral sphenoethmoidectomies, EMLP, and an extended septectomy.

This approach may be used in the management of anterior skull base meningoceles and meningoencephaloceles as well as resection of benign tumors of the anterior cranial fossa and cribriform plate, such as olfactory groove meningiomas.[32,54] **Fig. 6** illustrates a patient with a sinonasal tumor with intracranial extension, which was biopsied and confirmed to be meningioma, who underwent this approach. This approach has also been used for resection of anterior skull base malignancies.[32,55–64] Contraindications to this approach include encasement of the anterior cerebral vasculature,[32,65] extension above the meridian of the orbit that precludes obtaining a lateral dural margin (see **Fig. 1**A, B), and extension of malignancy into the skin and soft tissue of the face. In these situations, a traditional open craniofacial approach or an endoscopic-assisted craniofacial resection, where a craniotomy is combined with an endonasal endoscopic resection, should be considered.

Transplanum/Transtuberculum Approach

The endoscopic transplanum/transtuberculum approach is defined by resection of the planum sphenoidale and tuberculum sellae. The anatomic boundaries of this approach include the posterior ethmoid arteries anteriorly, the anterosuperior

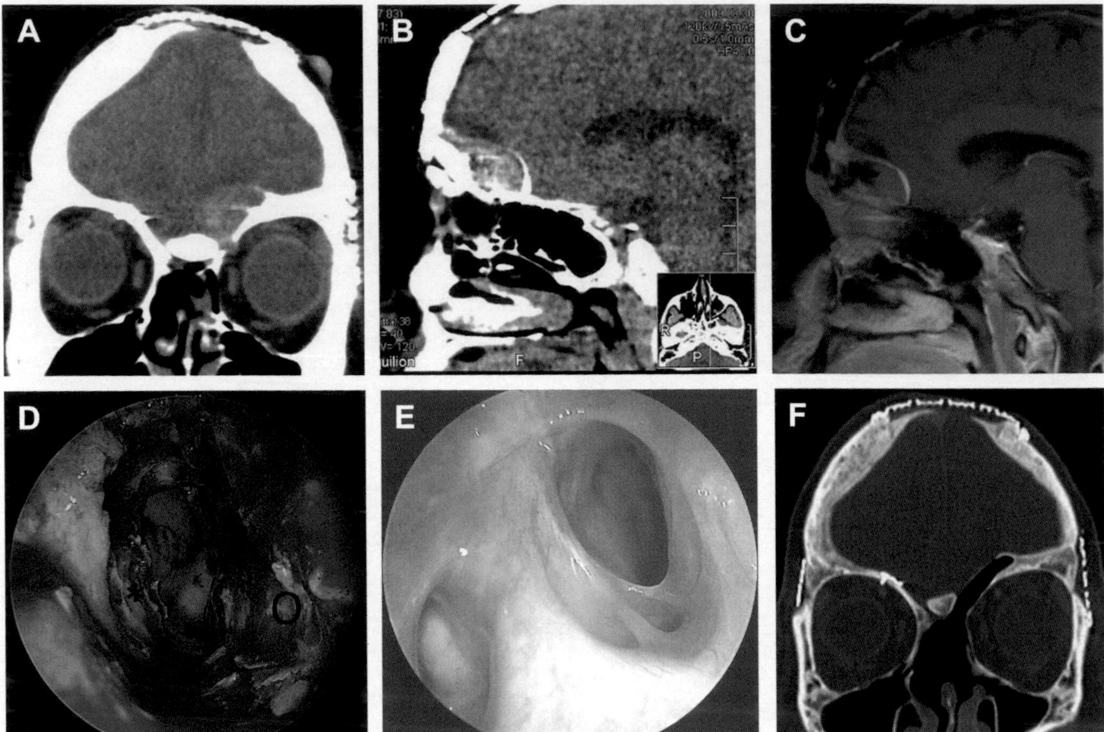

Fig. 5. Illustrative example of an endonasal endoscopic transfrontal approach. Preoperative (*A*) coronal and (*B*) parasagittal (inset noting parasagittal plane) CT and parasagittal MR imaging (*C*) sequences of a patient with a history of a hypothalamic astrocytoma who underwent a craniotomy for tumor resection and subsequent craniofacial excision of a mucocele a decade later who presented with left orbital and frontal swelling, which failed medical therapy. Her preoperative studies demonstrate an extra-axial fluid collection consistent with a mucocele. (*D*) An intraoperative photograph after an endonasal endoscopic transfrontal approach. The cut edge of the bone graft used in the previous reconstruction of her skull base is seen (*asterisk*) with a wide opening into the mucocele cavity. (*E*) An in office postoperative photograph demonstrating a patent outflow tract. (*F*) Coronal CT scan 4 years after her endoscopic procedure confirming patency. O, orbit.

sella posteriorly, and the medial opticocarotid recesses, cavernous sinuses, and paraclinoid carotid arteries laterally.[16,17,66,67]

Indications for this approach include pathologies of the planum sphenoidale and tuberculum sellae, most commonly meningiomas (**Fig. 7**). Other pathologies that often require a transplanum/transtuberculum approach of varying degrees include sellar lesions that have significant suprasellar extension, such as large/giant pituitary adenomas and craniopharyngiomas. Lesions that completely encase the carotid artery are unable to be completely resected via this approach. Other limitations to this approach include cavernous sinus invasion, encasement of the anterior cerebral vasculature, and extension above the roof of the optic canal (see **Fig. 1**C, D).

Transsellar Approach

The first purely endoscopic pituitary tumor resections were performed in the 1990s.[1–8] This module is the central and most commonly used EEA. With this approach, access from the inferior aspect of the tuberculum sellae superiorly, the cavernous sinuses laterally, and the sellar floor inferiorly is achieved. There are various modifications of this approach depending on surgeon preference and the size of the lesion. For example, the approach may be performed transnasally with lateralization of the turbinates or transethmoidally with or without resection of the middle turbinate. Wide bilateral sphenoidotomies and a posterior septectomy are typically performed.

The transsellar approach is used for sellar pathology, including pituitary adenomas, Rathke cleft cysts, craniopharyngiomas, and other lesions centered in the sella. This central approach can be combined with a transtuberculum/transplanar approach for sellar lesions with suprasellar extension, a transclival approach for sellar pathologies that extend inferiorly into the clivus (**Fig. 8**), or clival pathologies that extend superiorly into or behind the sella or require mobilization of the pituitary

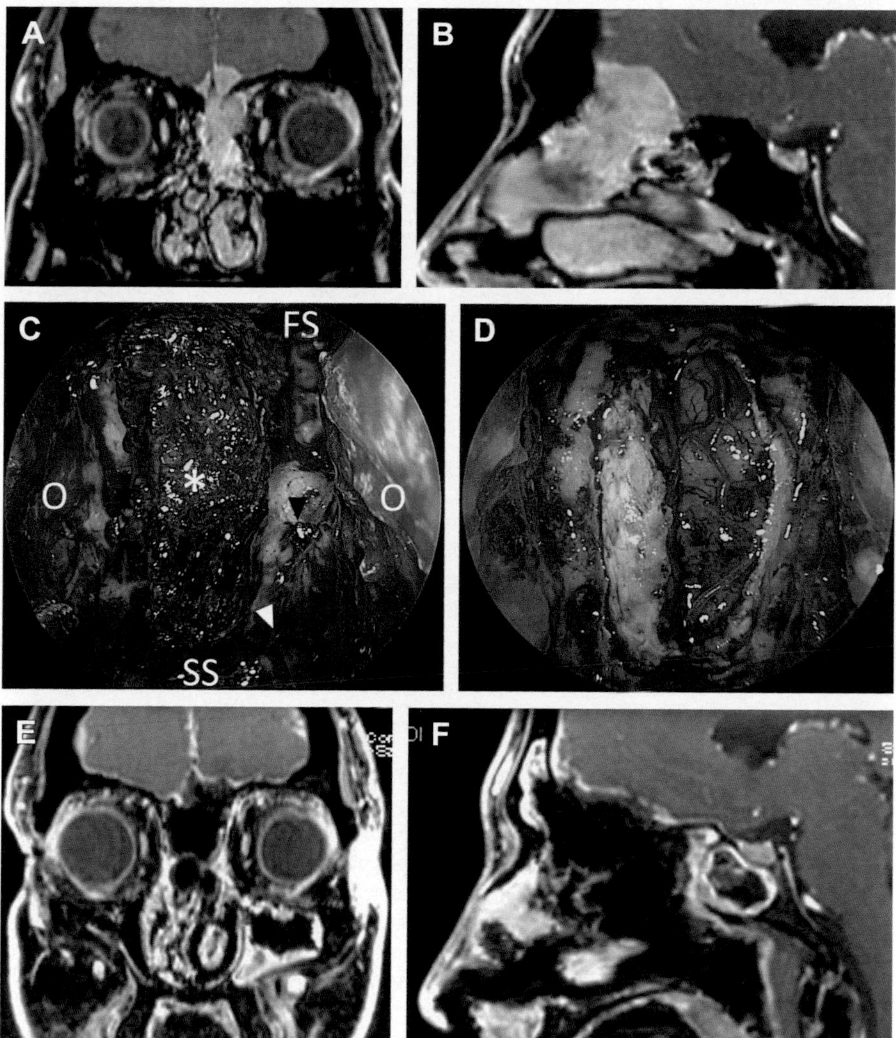

Fig. 6. Illustrative case of an expanded endonasal endoscopic transcribriform approach. Preoperative (*A*) coronal and (*B*) sagittal postcontrast VIBE sequences of a patient with a biopsy-proved meningioma. (*C*) An intraoperative photograph demonstrating the EEA and exposure of the tumor (*asterisk*) at the skull base extending intracranially. The anterior and posterior ethmoidal arteries are noted by the black and white arrowheads, respectively. (*D*) An intraoperative photograph after resection of the tumor; the cut edge of dura and inferior aspect of the frontal lobes are seen. Postoperative (*E*) coronal and (*F*) sagittal postcontrast VIBE sequences demonstrating a gross total resection. FS, frontal sinus; O, orbit; SS, sphenoid sinus.

gland for retrodorsal access.[68–70] Paramedian approaches can also be added to address pathologies with lateral extension.

Transclival Approach

The clivus is comprised of portions of the sphenoid and occipital bones and lies anterior to the brainstem and posterior fossa. There are many classification schemes for the clivus. With respect to EEAs, the clivus is divided into upper, middle, and lower thirds. The upper third extends from the dorsum sellae and posterior clinoid to Dorello canal; the middle third extends from Dorello canal to foramen lacerum; and the lower third extends from foramen lacerum through the basion.[32] Exposure of the clivus itself varies depending on the location and extent of the tumor being resected and typically requires unilateral or bilateral ethmoidectomies and wide bilateral sphenoidotomies, depending on the size of the lesion to be addressed and the endonasal access required.[14,18,24,71] Neurovascular structures important at surgery are location dependent.[32]

The superior clivus may be accessed via a pituitary transposition approach,[68,69] with the most

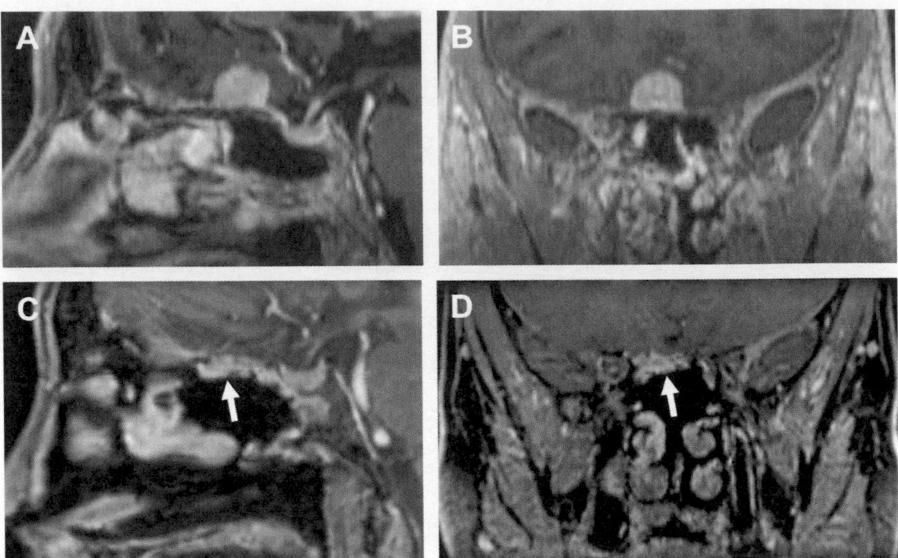

Fig. 7. Illustrative case of an expanded endonasal endoscopic transplanar approach. Preoperative (*A*) sagittal and (*B*) coronal postcontrast VIBE sequences demonstrating a planum sphenoidale meningioma. Postoperative (*C*) sagittal and (*D*) coronal sequences demonstrating gross total resection of the tumor, which was resected via an expanded endonasal endoscopic transplanum approach. The enhancing soft tissue seen below the skull base is the vascularized nasoseptal flap used for reconstruction of the skull base (*arrows*).

important landmarks the pituitary gland and stalk, the dorsum sellae, posterior clinoid processes, and the inferior and superior hypophyseal arteries. An extradural approach has also been described, which allows for exposure of the posterior clinoid processes with preservation of the sellar dura.[70] The middle and lower thirds of the clivus require extensive bony removal extending from the floor of the sella superiorly to the foramen magnum inferiorly, with the lateral borders of dissection the paraclival carotid arteries.

Transclival approaches are applied for resection of benign and malignant tumors of the clivus, including meningiomas, chordomas (**Fig. 9**), and chondrosarcomas. Clival pathologies that extend posterior to the carotid artery can be addressed with some mobilization of the vessel. Pathologies with significant lateral extension, for example, petroclival meningiomas, may require an open or combination approach. Tumors that originate lateral to the carotid artery and CNs and displace these structures medially into the surgical corridor should be considered for an open approach.

Transodontoid Approach

Transcervical or transoral approaches are the traditional management options for pathologies of the craniocervical junction.[72–74] The endonasal approach has been developed with the goal of avoiding morbidity associated with these approaches including increased risk of infection and palatal dysfunction.[23,75] The anatomic borders of this approach include the floor of the sphenoid sinus superiorly, the junction of the hard and soft palates inferiorly, and the parapharyngeal carotid arteries and eustachian tubes laterally. In many cases, the approach requires a posterior septectomy, wide bilateral sphenoidotomies with removal of the sphenoid floor, and resection of the nasopharyngeal mucosa, buccopharyngeal fascia, and paraspinous musculature. The anterior aspect of C1 is removed to access the odontoid. Numerous investigators have described methods that may be used to define the inferior extent of the approach.[76–78] For lesions that extend inferior to these boundaries, multiportal surgery may be indicated.[79–81]

Pathology that may be managed with this approach includes pannus formation in rheumatoid arthritis as well as cranial settling and basilar invagination. Tumors that typically occur in this region, such as chordomas, meningiomas, and nasopharyngeal carcinomas, may also be accessed through this approach. Contraindications to this approach include pathology that extends inferior to the nasopalatine line that may be better accessed through a transpalatal, transoral, or multiportal approach, medially ectatic parapharyngeal carotid arteries that lie in the surgical corridor, and situations where a posterolateral approach mitigates the need for

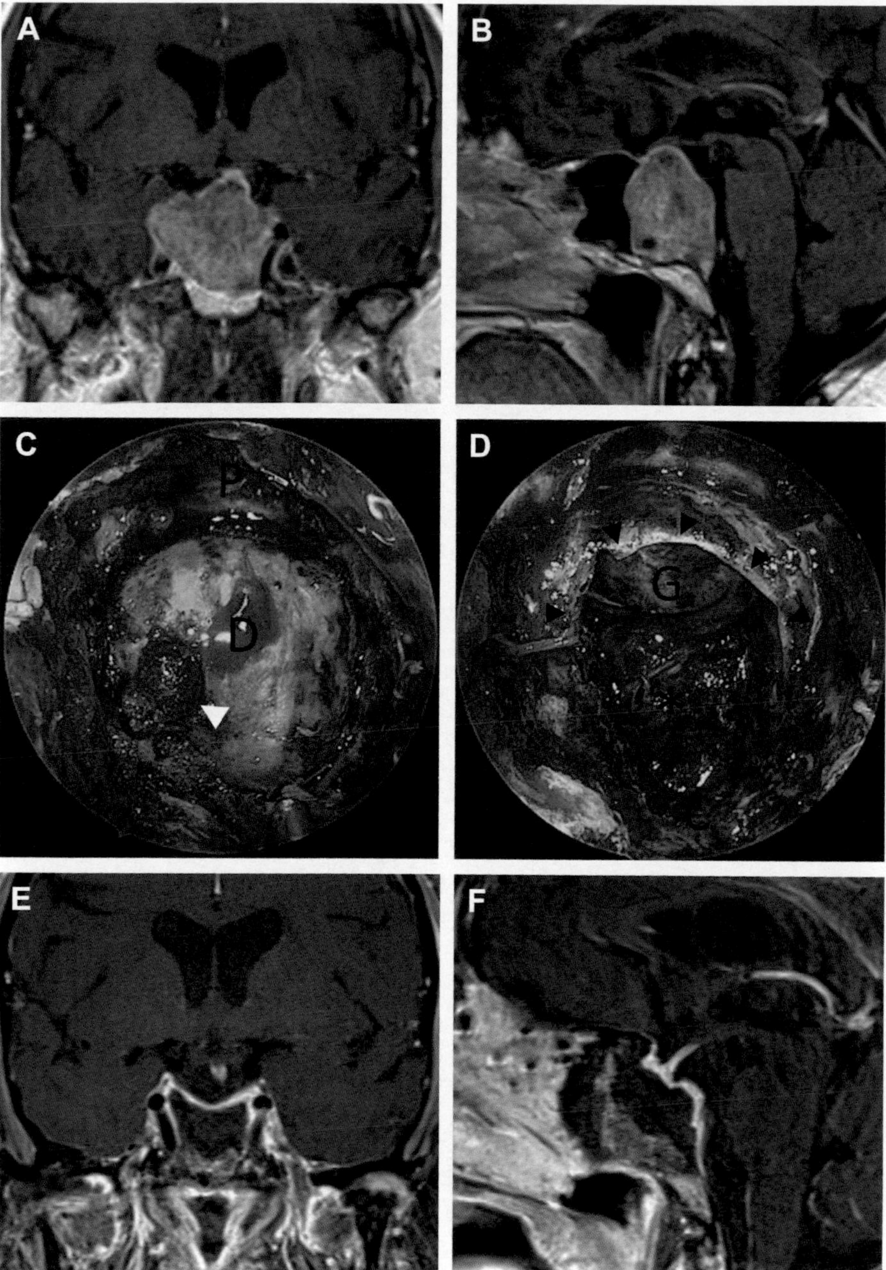

Fig. 8. Illustrative case of an expanded endonasal endoscopic transsellar approach. Preoperative (*A*) coronal and (*B*) sagittal postcontrast MR imaging scans in an octogenarian who developed difficulty opening her eyes and double vision. On neuro-ophthalmological evaluation, she had a bitemporal hemianopsia, a partial right CN III palsy, and a right Horner syndrome. On endocrinological evaluation, the patient had central hypothyroidism and this lesion was determined to be nonfunctional. Her preoperative imaging studies demonstrate a large sellar and suprasellar mass associated with elevation of the optic apparatus and cavernous sinus invasion. Retroclival extension is also seen. (*C*) An intraoperative photograph following the approach, the sellar dura (D) is exposed craniocaudally from the anterior intercavernous sinus superiorly to the caudal extent of the tumor, which in this case required removal of the superior aspect of the clivus. On the left side, bone is removed to the medial aspect of the cavernous sinus; on the right, the cavernous sinus is exposed given tumor extension in this region. The arrowhead marks focal epidural extension of tumor. (*D*) The resection cavity (*asterisk*) is seen after removal of the tumor. The gland (G) is nicely seen descending inferiorly. The cut edge of the dura (*arrowheads*) and (C) clivus are noted. The large surgical cavity was filled with pieces of absorbable gelatin sponge and the skull base reconstructed in a multilayered fashion. Postoperative (*E*) coronal and (*F*) sagittal postcontrast MR imaging sequences demonstrate a gross total resection of this tumor, including the disease in the cavernous sinus and behind the clivus. The gland and infundibulum are nicely visualized. Reconstructive packing material is also seen. P, planum sphenoidale.

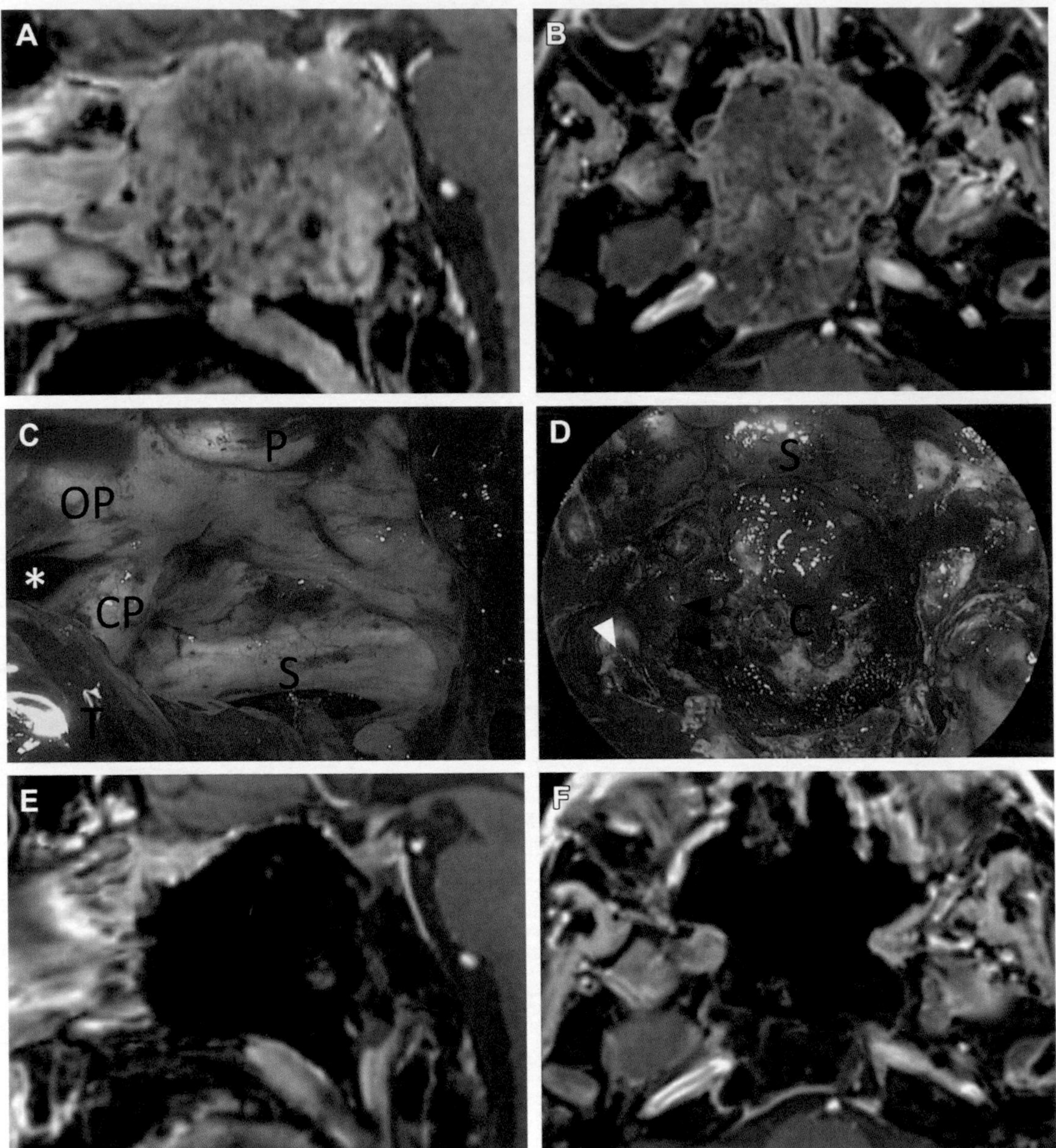

Fig. 9. Illustrative case of an expanded endonasal endoscopic transclival approach. Preoperative (*A*) sagittal and (*B*) axial postcontrast VIBE sequences demonstrating a clival chordoma extending up to the anterior skull base and inferiorly into the nasopharynx. Partial encasement of the right petrous and paraclival carotid artery is seen. (*C*) Intraoperative photograph after the approach and initial debulking of the tumor (T). Various skull base landmarks are nicely visualized, including the optic protuberance (OP), carotid protuberance (CP), lateral opticocarotid recess (*asterisk*), planum sphenoidale (P), and sella turcica (S). (*D*) Intraoperative photograph after the resection. The large resection cavity is seen below the sella. A right transpterygoid transpetrous approach was performed to address the tumor around the right petrous and paraclival (*black arrowheads*) segments of the carotid artery. The white arrowhead notes the cut vidian artery. Postoperative (*E*) sagittal and (*F*) axial postcontrast VIBE sequences demonstrate a gross total resection.

occipitocervical stabilization secondary to craniocervical destabilization from an EEA.

MODULES ALONG THE CORONAL PLANE

The coronal plane represents the paramedian extension of EEAs, lateral to the plane of the paraclival carotid artery, to address pathology of the orbit, pterygopalatine fossa, infratemporal fossa, middle cranial fossa, and inferolateral aspects of the clivus and foramen magnum. These approaches have been classified into anterior, middle, and posterior segments. Approaches in the anterior coronal plane are used to access pathology in the inferior and medial orbit; those in the middle coronal plane are used to access pathology in the pterygopalatine fossa, infratemporal fossa, and middle cranial fossa; and those in the posterior coronal plane are used to access pathology in the jugular foramen and occipital condyles[20,32,46,82] (see **Box 1**). Although the specifics of approaches to these complex anatomic regions are beyond the scope of this review, the most often used EEAs to approach pathology in these regions are highlighted.

Transorbital Approach

There is one approach in the anterior coronal plane, the transorbital approach.[32,82–85] This approach includes removal of the lamina papyracea and bone of the orbital floor. The most important anatomic landmarks are the optic nerve and ophthalmic artery, which generally runs in a plane inferolateral to the nerve. The position of the anterior and posterior ethmoid arteries and medial and inferior recti muscles is also important. The approach requires a total sphenoethmoidectomy and maxillary antrostomy to control the lamina papyracea and orbital floor, respectively. Transorbital procedures can be used for orbital decompression and intraconal tumors, such as meningiomas and hemangiomas. In intraconal approaches, a plane between the medial and inferior rectus muscles is formed. Although there is some controversy regarding the management of orbital disease in sinonasal malignancies, these approaches are also used in these situations when on high-resolution imaging there is erosion of the lamina and no frank invasion through the periorbita into orbital fat. Lesions that are superior and lateral to the optic nerve are an absolute contraindication to this approach. A medial ophthalmic artery may be considered a relative contraindication.

Transpterygoid and Infratemporal Fossa Approaches

Transpterygoid and infratemporal fossa approaches provide access to the corresponding fossae.[19,20,86] These approaches require a large maxillary antrostomy that may be extended to include a medial maxillectomy inferiorly. More lateral access may require an endoscopic transmaxillary approach or decompression of the lacrimal apparatus anteriorly.[87,88] These approaches may be used to access benign tumors of the pterygopalatine fossa, such as juvenile nasopharyngeal angiofibroma (**Fig. 10**), inverting papilloma, and schwannoma. Limitations include involvement of the parapharyngeal space with internal carotid artery encasement and extension of the tumor into the orbit superiorly or palate inferiorly. There is emerging experience with malignancies in this region.[89–91]

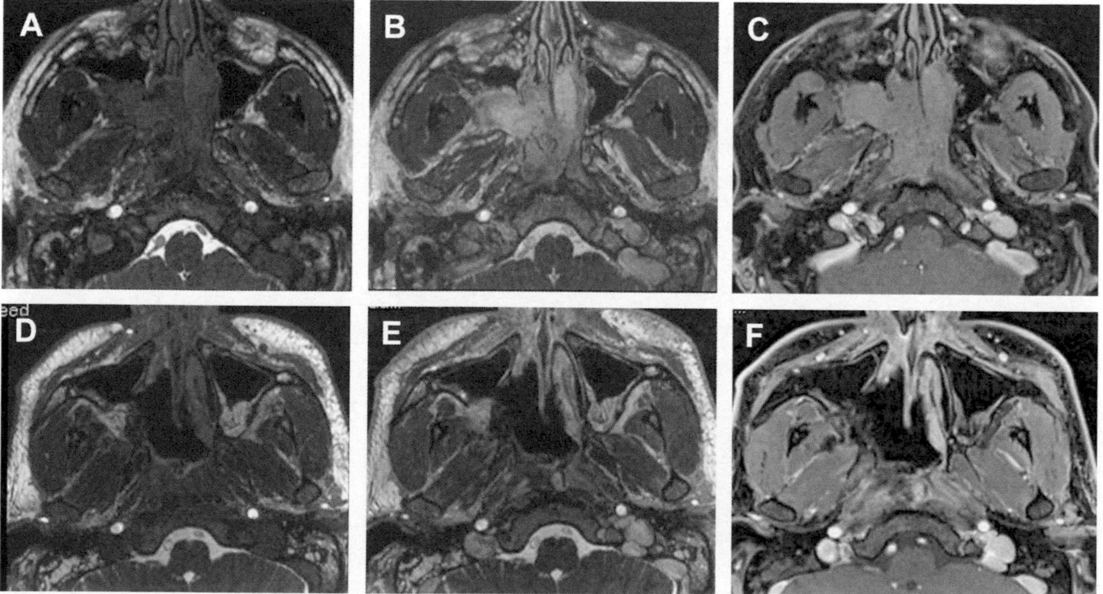

Fig. 10. (*A–C*) Preoperative and (*D–F*) postoperative (*A, D*) precontrast and (*B, E*) postcontrast CISS and (*C, F*) VIBE sequences in a young male patient with a large sinonasal and skull base mass consistent with a juvenile nasopharyngeal angiofibroma. A transpterygoid/infratemporal fossa approach was required for resection of the lateral components of the tumor. A gross total resection was achieved.

Transpetrous Approaches

Transpetrous approaches may be classified by the zone of the petrous temporal bone addressed and include the petrous apex, infrapetrous, and suprapetrous approaches.[20,32,46,82] These approaches are a lateral extension of the approaches to the middle and inferior thirds of the clivus and thus require a sphenoethmoidectomy and removal of the floor of the sphenoid sinus. The most important anatomic structure is the paraclival and petrous carotid artery. Other structures of importance are the vidian neurovascular bundle, CN V.1 to V.3, CN VI, and the eustachian tube.[46,92]

The petrous apex may be approached with or without lateralization of the internal carotid artery.[93] The infrapetrous approach combines the approach to the petrous apex with the transpterygoid approach, with the medial limit of dissection the vidian nerve and the medial pterygoid plate. The lateral extent is the foramen rotundum and CN V.3, which is anterior to the petrous carotid artery. The suprapetrous approach is an extension of dissection superior to the petrous carotid artery and can be used to access Meckel's cave and the middle cranial fossa.[20,82,94] This dissection is bordered by the paraclival carotid artery medially, CN VI in the cavernous sinus superiorly, petrous carotid inferiorly, and CN V.2 laterally.[94]

The transpetrous approaches may be used to access pathology, such as petrous apex cholesterol granulomas, chordomas, chondrosarcomas (**Fig. 11**), and trigeminal schwannomas. Contraindications include encasement of the carotid artery and origination of the lesion posteriorly or laterally, with displacement of important neurovascular structures medially into the operative corridor.

Transcavernous Approaches

Transcavernous approaches are most commonly used to address cavernous sinus invasion by pituitary adenomas (see **Fig. 8**) and may also be used to manage primary cavernous sinus pathology.[32,95,96] The critical anatomic structures in this approach include the cavernous internal carotid artery and CNs III, IV, V.1 to V.3, and VI.

Inferolateral Approaches

Approaches to the inferolateral skull base are contained in the posterior coronal plane. These approaches, which access the occipital condyle and jugular foramen, represent advanced skull base procedures.[20,82,97,98] The key anatomic landmark in these approaches is the parapharyngeal internal carotid artery. Other landmarks of importance are the occipital condyle, the jugular foramen and its contents (internal jugular vein and CNs IX, X, and IX), and the hypoglossal canal and nerve (CN XII). Approaches to the occipital condyle and jugular foramen may be used to manage pathology of the posterolateral skull base, including petroclival meningiomas, chordomas, chondrosarcomas, and tumors of the jugular foramen, such as paragangliomas. Limitations to this approach, similar to that of other approaches in the coronal plane, include encasement of the carotid artery and significant lateral extension deep to critical nervous structures.

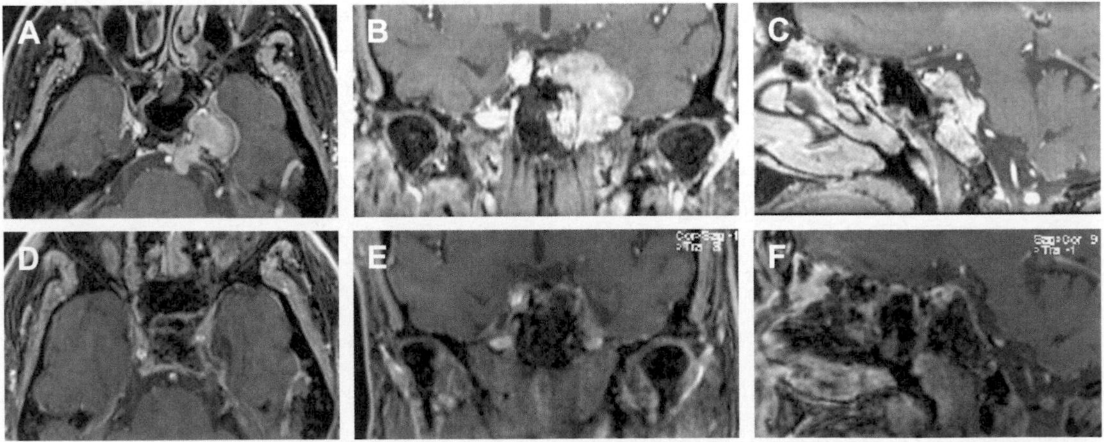

Fig. 11. Preoperative (*A*) axial, (*B*) coronal, and (*C*) parasagittal postcontrast VIBE sequences in a patient with a left CN VI palsy demonstrate a petroclival lesion with sellar, cavernous sinus, and intradural extension. A gross total resection was achieved via an expanded endonasal endoscopic transsellar, transcavernous, and transpetrous approach. Postoperative (*D*) axial, (*E*) coronal, and (*F*) parasagittal postcontrast VIBE sequences demonstrate complete tumor removal.

RECONSTRUCTION

The goal of reconstruction of the skull base is separation of the intracranial and sinonasal compartments and this is achieved by a multilayered watertight closure. There are numerous techniques and materials available for reconstruction of the skull base, including allografts, autografts, and vascularized flaps.[22,26,99] From an imaging perspective, vascularized flaps, such as the nasoseptal flap, often enhance on postoperative MR scans[100] (see **Fig. 7**C, D).

SUMMARY

EEAs have been tranformative in skull base surgery. These approaches provide access to a wide variety of extradural and intradural cranial base lesions and complement open surgical procedures in the contemporary management of skull base pathologies. HR-SB-MR imaging precisely determines the extent of disease as well as the relationship to adjacent neurovascular structures and is critical in the preoperative surgical evaluation of patients being considered for open and endoscopic skull base procedures. The limits of expanded endonasal endoscopic procedures are continuing to be defined in this evolving field.

REFERENCES

1. Jankowski R, Auque J, Simon C, et al. Endoscopic pituitary tumor surgery. Laryngoscope 1992;102:198–202.
2. Shikani AH, Kelly JH. Endoscopic debulking of a pituitary tumor. Am J Otolaryngol 1993;14:254–6.
3. Sethi DS, Pillay PK. Endoscopic management of lesions of the sella turcica. J Laryngol Otol 1995;109:956–62.
4. Rodziewicz GS, Kelley RT, Kellman RM, et al. Transnasal endoscopic surgery of the pituitary gland: technical note. Neurosurgery 1996;39:189–92 [discussion: 192–3].
5. Jho JD, Carrau RL, Ko Y, et al. Endoscopic pituitary surgery: an early experience. Surg Neurol 1997;47:213–22.
6. Jho HD, Carrau RL. Endoscopic endonasal transsphenoidal surgery: experience with 50 patients. J Neurosurg 1997;87:44–51.
7. Cappabianca P, Alfieri A, de Divitiis E. Endoscopic endonasal transsphenoidal approach to the sella: towards functional endoscopic pituitary surgery (FEPS). Minim Invasive Neurosurg 1998;41:66–73.
8. Sheehan MT, Atkinson JL, Kasperbauer JL, et al. Preliminary comparison of the endoscopic transnasal vs the sublabial transseptal approach for clinically nonfunctioning pituitary macroadenomas. Mayo Clin Proc 1999;74:661–70.
9. Locatelli D, Castelnuovo P, Santi L, et al. Endoscopic approaches to the cranial base: perspectives and realities. Childs Nerv Syst 2000;16:686–91.
10. Cappabianca P, Cavallo LM, Colao A, et al. Endoscopic endonasal transsphenoidal appraoch: outcome analysis of 100 consecutive procedures. Minim Invas Neurosurg 2002;45:193–200.
11. De Divitiis E, Cappabianca P, Cavallo LM. Endoscopic transsphenoidal approach: adaptability of the procedure to different sellar lesions. Neurosurgery 2002;51:699–705.
12. Jho HD, Ha HG. Endoscopic endonasal skull base surgery: Part 1—The midline anterior fossa skull base. Minim Invasive Neurosurg 2004;47:1–8.
13. Jho HD, Ha HG. Endoscopic endonasal skull base surgery: Part 2—The cavernous sinus. Minim Invasive Neurosurg 2004;47:9–15.
14. Jho HD, Ha HG. Endoscopic endonasal skull base surgery: Part 3—The clivus and posterior fossa. Minim Invasive Neurosurg 2004;47:16–23.
15. Maroon JC. Skull base surgery: past, present, and future trends. Neurosurg Focus 2005;19:1E1.
16. Cavallo LM, Messina A, Cappabianca P, et al. Endoscopic endonasal surgery of the midline skull base: anatomical study and clinical considerations. Neurosurg Focus 2005;19:E2.
17. Kassam AB, Synderman CH, Mintz A, et al. Expanded endonasal approach: the rostrocaudal axis. Part I. Crista galli to the sella turcica. Neurosurg Focus 2005;19:E3.
18. Kassam AB, Snyderman CH, Mintz A, et al. Expanded endonasal approach: the rostrocaudal axis. Part II. Posterior clinoids to foramen magnum. Neurosurg Focus 2005;19:E4.
19. Cavallo LM, Messina A, Gardner P, et al. Extended endoscopic endonasal approach to the pterygopalatine fossa: anatomical study and clinical considerations. Neurosurg Focus 2005;19:E5.
20. Kassam AB, Gardner PA, Snyderman CH, et al. Expanded endonasal approach: fully endoscopic, completely transnasal approach to the middle third of the clivus, petrous bone, middle cranial fossa, and infratemporal fossa. Neurosurg Focus 2005;19:E6.
21. Kassam A, Snyderman CH, Carrau RL, et al. Endoneurosurgical hemostasis techniques: lessons learned from 400 cases. Neurosurg Focus 2005;19:E7.
22. Kassam A, Carrau RL, Snyderman CH, et al. Evolution of reconstructive techniques following endoscopic expanded endonasal approaches. Neurosurg Focus 2005;19:E8.
23. Kassam AB, Snyderman C, Gardner P, et al. The expanded endonasal approach: a fully endoscopic transnasal approach and resection of the odontoid process: technical case report. Neurosurgery 2005;57:E213.

24. Stamm AC, Pignatari SS, Vellutini E. Transnasal endoscopic surgical approaches to the clivus. Otolaryngol Clin North Am 2006;39:639–56.
25. Frank G, Pasquini E, Doglietto F, et al. The endoscopic extended transsphenoidal approach for craniopharyngiomas. Neurosurgery 2006;59(1 Suppl 1):ONS75–83.
26. Hadad G, Bassagasteguy L, Carrau RL, et al. A novel reconstructive technique after expanded endonasal approaches: vascular pedicle nasoseptal flap. Laryngoscope 2006;116:1882–6.
27. Kassam A, Thomas AJ, Snyderman C, et al. Fully endoscopic expanded endonasal approach treating skull base lesions in pediatric patients. J Neurosurg 2007;106:75–86.
28. Laufer I, Anand VK, Schwartz TH. Endoscopic, endonasal extended transsphenoidal, transplanum transtuberculum approach for resection of suprasellar lesions. J Neurosurg 2007;106:400–6.
29. Cavallo LM, Cappabianca P, Messina A, et al. The extended endoscopic endonasal approach to the clivus and cranio-vertebral junction: anatomical study. Childs Nerv Syst 2007;23:665–71.
30. Schwartz TH, Fraser JF, Brown S, et al. Endoscopic cranial base surgery: classification of operative approaches. Neurosurgery 2008;62:991–1002.
31. Snyderman CH, Pant H, Carrau RL, et al. What are the limits of endoscopic sinus surgery? : the expanded endonasal approach to the skull base. Keio J Med 2009;58:152–60.
32. Kassam AB, Prevedello DM, Carrau RL, et al. Endoscopic endonasal skull base surgery: analysis of complications in the authors' initial 800 patients. A review. J Neurosurg 2011;114:1544–68.
33. Prevedello DM, Doglietto F, Jane JA, et al. History of endoscopic skull base surgery: its evolution and current reality. J Neurosurg 2007;107:206–13.
34. Snyderman C, Kassam A, Carrau R, et al. Acquisition of skills for endonasal skull base surgery: a training program. Laryngoscope 2007;117:699–705.
35. Leach P, Abou-Zeid AH, Kearney T, et al. Endoscopic transsphenoidal pituitary surgery: evidence of an operative learning curve. Neurosurg 2010; 67(5):1205–12.
36. Snyderman CH, Fernandez-Miranda JC, Gardner PA. Training in neurorhinology: the impact of case volume on the learning curve. Otolaryngol Clin North Am 2011;44:1223–8.
37. Dedhia RC, Lord CA, Pinheiro-Neto CD, et al. Endoscopic endonasal pituitary surgery:impact of surgical education on operation length and patient morbidity. J Neurol Surg B Skull Base 2012; 73:405–9.
38. Kassam AB, Snyderman CH, Carrau RL, et al. The Expanded endonasal approach to the ventral skull base: sagittal plane. Tuttlingen (Germany): Endo-Press; 2007.
39. Campero A, Emmerich J, Socolovsky M, et al. Microsurgical anatomy of the sphenoid ostia. J Clin Neurosci 2010;17:1298–300.
40. Peris-Celda M, Kucukyuruk B, Monroy-Sosa A, et al. The recesses of the sellar wall of the sphenoid sinus and their intracranial relationships. Neurosurgery 2013;73(2 Suppl Operative):ons117–31.
41. Hwang SH, Joo YH, Seo JH, et al. Analysis of sphenoid sinus in the operative plane of endoscopic transsphenoidal surgery using computed tomography. Eur Arch Otorhinolaryngol 2014;271: 2219–25.
42. Kaplanoglu H, Kaplanoglu V, Dilli A, et al. An analysis of the anatomic variations of the paranasal sinuses and ethmoid roof using computed tomography. Eurasian J Med 2013;45:115–25.
43. Tomovic S, Esmaeili A, Chan N, et al. High-resolution computed tomography analysis of the prevalence of onodi cells. Laryngoscope 2012;122: 1470–3.
44. Fernandez-Miranda JC, Prevedello DM, Madhok R, et al. Sphenoid septations and their relationship with internal carotid arteries: anatomical and radiological study. Laryngoscope 2009;119:1893–6.
45. Blitz AM, Aygun N, Herzka DA, et al. High-resolution three-dimensional MR imaging approach to the skull base: compartments, boundaries, and critical structures. Radiol Clin N Am 2017. [Epub ahead of print].
46. Kassam AB, Vescan AD, Carrau RL, et al. Expanded endonasal approach: vidian canal as a landmark to the petrous internal carotid artery. J Neurosurg 2008;108:177–83.
47. Labib MA, Prevedello DM, Carrau RL, et al. A road map to the internal carotid artery in expanded endoscopic endonasal approaches to the ventral cranial base. Neurosurgery 2014;10:448–71.
48. Gross WE, Gross CW, Becker D, et al. Modified tranasal endoscopic Lothrop procedure as an alternative to frontal sinus obliteration. Otolaryngol Head Neck Surg 1995;113:427–34.
49. Becker DG, Moore D, Lindsey WH, et al. Modified transnasal endoscopic Lothrop procedure: further considerations. Laryngoscope 1995;105:1161–6.
50. Wormald PJ, Ananda A, Nair S. The modified endoscopic Lothrop procedure in the treatment of complicated chronic frontal sinusitis. Clin Otolaryngol Allied Sci 2003;28:215–20.
51. Wormald PJ, Ananda A, Nair S. Modified endoscopic Lothrop as a salvage for the failed osteoplastic flap with obliteration. Laryngoscope 2003; 113:1988–92.
52. Chiu AG, Schipor I, Cohen NA, et al. Surgical decisions in the management of frontal sinus osteomas. Am J Rhinol 2005;19:191–7.
53. Greenfield JP, Anand VK, Kacker A, et al. Endoscopic endonasal transethmoidal transcribriform

transfovea ethmoidalis approach to the anterior cranial fossa and skull base. Neurosurgery 2010; 66:883–92.
54. Gardner PA, Kassam AB, Thomas A, et al. Endoscopic endonasal resection of anterior cranial base meningiomas. Neurosurgery 2008;63: 36–52.
55. Casiano RR, Numa WA, Falquez AM. Endoscopic resection of esthesioneuroblastoma. Am J Rhinol 2001;15:271–9.
56. Carrau RL, Kassam AB, Snyderman CH, et al. Endoscopic transnasal anterior skull base resection for the treatment of sinonasal malignancies. Oper Tech Otolaryngol 2006;17:102–10.
57. Nicolai P, Battaglia P, Bignami M, et al. Endoscopic surgery for tumors of the sinonasal tract and adjacent skull base: a 10 year experience. Am J Rhinol 2008;22:308–16.
58. Hanna E, DeMonte F, Ibrahim S, et al. Endoscopic resection of sinonasal cancers with and without craniotomy: oncologic results. Arch Otolaryngol Head Neck Surg 2009;135:1219–34.
59. Lund VJ, Stammberger H, Nicolai P, et al. European position paper on endoscopic management of tumors of the nose, paranasal sinuses and skull base. Rhinol Suppl 2010;22:1–143.
60. Nicolai P, Castelnuovo P, Villaret AB. Endoscopic resection of sinonasal malignancies. Curr Oncol Rep 2011;13:138–44.
61. Castelnuovo P, Battaglia P, Turri-Zanoni M, et al. Endoscopic endonasal surgery for malignancies of the anterior cranial base. World Neurosurg 2014;82(6 Suppl):S22–31.
62. Gallia GL, Reh DD, Salmasi V, et al. Endonasal endoscopic resection of esthesioneuroblastoma: the Johns Hopkins Hospital experience and review of the literature. Neurosurg Rev 2011;34:465–75.
63. Roxbury CR, Ishii M, Richmon JD, et al. Endonasal endoscopic surgery in the management of sinonasal and anterior skull base malignancies. Head Neck Pathol 2016;10:13–22.
64. Moya-Plana A, Bresson D, Temam F, et al. Development of minimally invasive surgery for sinonasal malignancy. Eur Ann Otorhinolaryngol Head Neck Dis 2016. [Epub ahead of print].
65. Khan OH, Anand VK, Schwartz TH. Endoscopic endonasal resection of skull base meningiomas: The significance of a "cortical cuff" and brain edema compared with careful case selection and surgical experience in predicting morbidity and extent of resection. Neurosurg Focus 2014; 37:E7.
66. De Divitiis E, Cappabianca P, Cavallo LM, et al. Extended endoscopic transsphenoidal approach for extrasellar craniopharyngiomas. Neurosurgery 2007;61(5 Suppl 2):E239–40.
67. Cavallo LM, De Divitiis O, Aydin S, et al. Extended endoscopic endonasal transsphenoidal approach suprasellar area: anatomic considerations—part 1. Neurosurgery 2008;62(6 Suppl 3):1202–12.
68. Kassam AB, Prevedello DM, Thomas A, et al. Endoscopic endonasal pituitary transposition for a transdorsum sellae approach to the interpeduncular cistern. Neurosurgery 2008;62:57–72.
69. Fernandez-Miranda JC, Gardner PA, Rastelli MM, et al. Endoscopic endonasal transcavernous posterior clinoidectomy with interdural pituitary transposition. Technical note. J Neurosurg 2014;121: 91–9.
70. Silva D, Attia M, Kandasamy J, et al. Endoscopic endonasal posterior clinoidectomy. Surg Neurol Int 2012;3:64.
71. Stippler M, Gardner PA, Snyderman CH, et al. Endoscopic endonasal approach for clival chordomas. Neurosurgery 2009;64:268–77.
72. Apuzzo ML, Weiss MH, Heiden JS. Transoral exposure of the atlantoaxial region. Neurosurgery 1978; 3:201–7.
73. Demonte F, Diaz E, Callender D, et al. Transmandibular, circumglossal, retropharyngeal approach for chordomas of the clivus and upper cervical spine. Neurosurg Focus 2001;10:E10.
74. Menezes AH. Surgical approaches: postoperative care and complications "transoral-transpalatopharyngeal approach to the craniocervical junction." Childs Nerv Syst 2008;24:1187–93.
75. Nayak JV, Gardner PA, Vescan AD, et al. Experience with the expanded endonasal approach for resection of the odontoid process in rheumatoid disease. Am J Rhinol 2007;21:601–6.
76. De Almeida JR, Zanation AM, Snyderman CH, et al. Defining the nasopalatine line: the limit for endonasal surgery of the spine. Laryngoscope 2009; 119:239–44.
77. Aldana PR, Naseri I, La Corte E. The naso-axial line: a new method of accurately predicting the inferior limit of the endoscopic endonasal approach to the craniovertebral junction. Neurosurgery 2012;71:308–14.
78. La Corte E, Aldana PR, Ferroli P, et al. The rhinopalatine line as a reliable predictor of the inferior extent of endonasal odontoidectomies. Neurosurg Focus 2015;38:E16.
79. El-Sayed IH, Wu JC, Ames CP, et al. Combined transnasal and transoral endoscopic approaches to the craniovertebral junction. J Craniovertebr Junction Spine 2010;1:44–8.
80. Dallan I, Castelnuovo P, Montevecchi F, et al. Combined transoral transnasal robotic-assisted nasopharyngectomy: a cadaveric feasibility study. Eur Arch Otorhinolaryngol 2012;269:235–9.
81. Turri-Zanoni M, Battaglia P, Dallan I, et al. Multiportal combined transnasal transoral transpharyngeal

endoscopic approach for selected skull base cancers. Head Neck 2016;38:2440–5.
82. De Lara D, Ditzel Filho LF, Prevedello DM, et al. Endoscopic endonasal approaches to the paramedian skull base. World Neurosurg 2014;82(6 Suppl):S121–9.
83. Castelnuovo P, Dallan I, Locatelli D, et al. Endoscopic transnasal intraorbital surgery: our experience with 16 cases. Eur Arch Otorhinolaryngol 2012;269:1929–35.
84. Castelnuovo P, Turri-Zanoni M, Battaglia P, et al. Endoscopic endonasal management of orbital pathologies. Neurosurg Clin N Am 2015;26:463–72.
85. Yao WC, Bleier BS. Endoscopic management of orbital tumors. Curr Opin Otolaryngol Head Neck Surg 2016;24:57–62.
86. Bolger WE. Endoscopic transpterygoid approach to the lateral sphenoid recess: surgical approach and clinical experience. Otolaryngol Head Neck Surg 2005;133:20–6.
87. Kasemsiri P, Solares A, Carrau RL, et al. Endoscopic endonasal transpterygoid approaches: anatomical landmarks for planning the surgical corridor. Laryngoscope 2013;123:811–5.
88. Hosseini SM, Razfar A, Carrau RL, et al. Endonasal transpterygoid approach to the infratemporal fossa: correlation of endoscopic and multiplanar CT anatomy. Head Neck 2012;34:313–20.
89. Yoshizaki T, Wakisaka N, Murono S, et al. Endoscopic nasopharyngectomy for patients with recurrent nasopharyngeal carcinoma at the primary site. Laryngoscope 2005;115:1517–9.
90. Hosseini SM, McLaughlin N, Carrau RL, et al. Endoscopic transpterygoid nasopharyngectomy: correlation of surgical anatomy with multiplanar CT. Head Neck 2013;35:704–14.
91. Wong EH, Liew YT, Abu Baker MZ, et al. A preliminary report on the role of endoscopic endonasal nasopharyngectomy in recurrent rT3 and rT4 nasopharyngeal carcinoma. Eur Arch Otorhinolaryngol 2016. [Epub ahead of print].
92. Liu J, Pinheiro-Neto CD, Fernandez-Miranda JC, et al. Eustachian tube and internal carotid artery in skull base surgery: an anatomical study. Laryngoscope 2014;124:2655–64.
93. Zanation AM, Snyderman CH, Carrau RL, et al. Endoscopic endonasal surgery for petrous apex lesions. Laryngoscope 2009;119:19–25.
94. Kassam AB, Prevedello DM, Carrau RL, et al. The front door to Meckel's cave: an anteromedial corridor via expanded endoscopic endonasal approach - technical considerations and clinical series. Neurosurg 2009;64:71–82.
95. Patrona A, Patel KS, Bander ED, et al. Endoscopic endonasal surgery for nonadenomatous, nonmeningeal pathology involving the cavernous sinus. J Neurosurg 2016;29:1–9.
96. Ferreli F, Turri-Zanoni M, Canevari FR. Endoscopic endonasal management of non-functioning pituitary adenomas with cavernous sinus invasion: a 10-year experience. Rhinology 2015;53:308–16.
97. Lee DL, McCoul ED, Anand VK, et al. Endoscopic endonasal access to the jugular foramen: defining the surgical approach. J Neurol Surg B Skull Base 2012;73:342–51.
98. Dallan I, Bignami M, Battaglia P, et al. Fully endoscopic transnasal approach to the jugular foramen: anatomic study and clinical considerations. Neurosurgery 2010;67(3 Suppl Operative):1–8.
99. Klatt-Cromwell CN, Thorp BD, Del Signore AG, et al. Reconstruction of skull base defects. Otolaryngol Clin North Am 2016;49:107–17.
100. Kang MD, Escott E, Thomas AJ, et al. The MR imaging appearance of the vascular pedicle nasoseptal flap. AJNR Am J Neuroradiol 2009;30:781–6.

High Resolution Three-Dimensional MR Imaging of the Skull Base

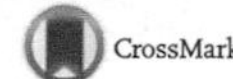

Compartments, Boundaries, and Critical Structures

Ari Meir Blitz, MD[a,*], Nafi Aygun, MD[a], Daniel A. Herzka, PhD[b], Masaru Ishii, MD, PhD[c], Gary L. Gallia, MD, PhD[d,*]

KEYWORDS

• High-resolution 3D MR imaging • Skull base MR imaging • Cranial nerves
• Skull base compartments • CISS

KEY POINTS

- High-resolution 3D skull base protocol MR imaging provides a means of assessing the cranial nerves from their points of apparent origin in the cisterns and as they pass through the skull base.
- High-resolution 3D skull base protocol MR imaging allows for an accurate and precise depiction of the skull base compartments and their boundaries.
- High-resolution 3D skull base MR imaging, by precisely defining the extent of skull base pathologies and their relationship with surrounding neurovascular structures, aids the surgeon in preoperative planning and defining operative risks.

INTRODUCTION

High-resolution three-dimensional (3D) MR imaging of the skull base (HR-SB-MR imaging) allows for a more detailed and accurate assessment of normal anatomic structures and the location and extent of skull base pathologies. This article describes the techniques used for HR-SB-MR imaging at our institution and their utility for evaluation of the many small structures of the skull base, focusing on those regions and concepts most pertinent to localization of cranial nerve (CN) palsies and in providing preoperative guidance and postoperative assessment. We introduce the concept of skull base compartments as a useful means of conceptualizing the various layers of the skull base and emphasize their importance in assessment of masses of the skull base.

TECHNICAL CONSIDERATIONS FOR HIGH-RESOLUTION SKULL BASE MR IMAGING

Two-Dimensional Versus Three-Dimensional

Two-dimensional (2D) imaging protocols of the skull base and CNs are limited by the necessity of optimizing the acquisition for the structure of

Grant support Aesculab (PI = Daniele Rigamonti, MD), Medical advisory board, Guerbet (A.M. Blitz). Nothing to disclose (N. Aygun, D. Herzka, M. Ishii, G.L. Gallia).
[a] Division of Neuroradiology, Department of Radiology and Radiological Science, Johns Hopkins Hospital, 600 North Wolfe Street, Baltimore, MD 21287, USA; [b] Department of Biomedical Engineering, Johns Hopkins Hospital, Johns Hopkins University, 600 North Wolfe Street, Baltimore, MD 21287, USA; [c] Department of Otolaryngology, Johns Hopkins Hospital, 600 North Wolfe Street, Baltimore, MD 21287, USA; [d] Department of Neurosurgery, Johns Hopkins Hospital, 600 North Wolfe Street, Baltimore, MD 21287, USA
* Corresponding author.
E-mail addresses: ablitz1@jhmi.edu; ggallia1@jhmi.edu

Radiol Clin N Am 55 (2017) 17–30
http://dx.doi.org/10.1016/j.rcl.2016.08.011
0033-8389/17/© 2016 Elsevier Inc. All rights reserved.

interest in a single plane or performing multiple acquisitions in varying planes. 2D imaging requires altering sequence parameters and attention to the angle of acquisition and slice placement to ensure that the region of the CN in question is appropriately visualized.[1,2] The 2D approach is limited not just by the multiple protocols it necessitates, but also by the potential of encountering abnormalities unexpected at the time the study was ordered or the necessity of compromising visualization of one aspect of a CN or mass for another. Instead of 2D imaging of the skull base we advocate acquisition of a 3D volume to encompass the entire region of interest, with isotropic imaging in the constructive interference in steady-state (CISS) sequence, which is performed with the highest spatial resolution, from which reformatted images are reconstructed in any arbitrary plane post hoc (**Fig. 1**).

Magnet Field Strength

Higher field strength MR imaging magnets generally return images with improved tissue discrimination compared with lower field strength units,[3] although there are few direct comparisons between imaging at different field strengths in the general field of brain imaging.[4] In the region of the skull base 3-T images have been shown to be superior to those at 1.5 T for imaging of the CNs,[5] among the most critical structures requiring evaluation at the skull base. Individual cases have also demonstrated improvements in detection of small pathologic changes, such as perineural spread of tumor.[6]

Although images are achieved of equal spatial resolution and signal-to-noise ratio at 1.5 T as at 3 T, the lower field strength 1.5-T technique requires longer acquisition times to match those at 3 T. With prolonged acquisition times it has been our experience (in excess of a thousand HR-SB-MR imaging examinations over 8 years) that the likelihood of patient movement increases significantly for acquisition times longer than approximately 6 minutes. Because even small movements may potentially negate the benefits of the intended high spatial resolution evaluation and require repeat acquisitions further prolonging the evaluation, we prefer to perform HR-SB-MR imaging a 3 T when possible, although diagnostic images may be obtained at either field strength.

Multiple air-tissue interfaces in the region of the skull base introduce magnetic field inhomogeneity, which in turn may limit the evaluation at increasing field strength. With some exceptions, however, we have found the field inhomogeneity artifacts at 3 T do not limit the clinical utility of imaging and are more than offset by improvements in image clarity when compared with 1.5 T. Attempts at imaging of masses at 7 T have been reported for research purposes. Significant field inhomogeneity limits the applicability of current ultrahigh-field MR imaging techniques in the region of the skull base.[7]

Sequence Selection

Evaluation of the skull base and adjoining structures requires assessment of a wide variety of anatomic contexts ranging from the fluid-filled subarachnoid space to the various soft tissues in

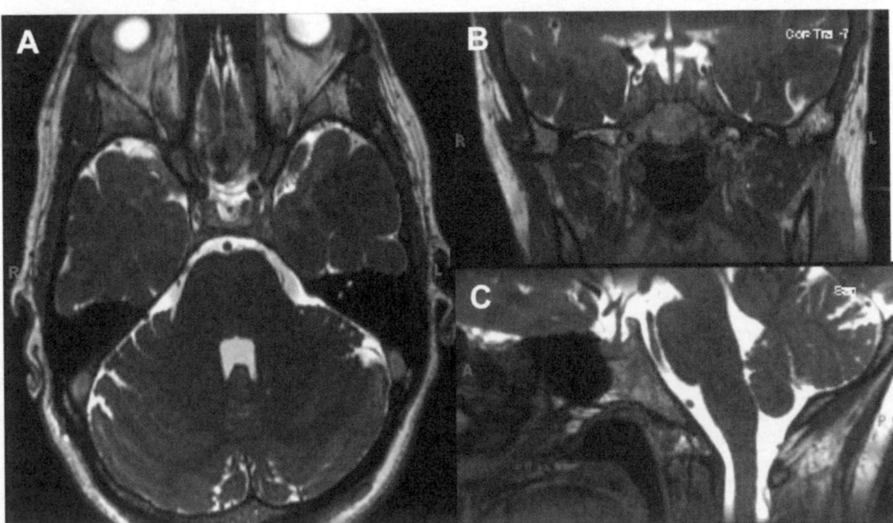

Fig. 1. (*A*) Axial isotropic 3D CISS acquisition through the skull base is readily reformatted in any plane post hoc. (*B*) Coronal and (*C*) sagittal reformatted images from the original acquisition are shown. (*From* Blitz AM, Choudhri AF, Chonka ZD, et al. Anatomic considerations, nomenclature, and advanced cross-sectional imaging techniques for visualization of the cranial nerve segments by MR imaging. Neuroimaging Clin N Am 2014;24(1):1–15; with permission.)

the extracranial space. The CNs, important in and of themselves, serve as an excellent example of structures that traverse the skull base. We have previously described a generic nomenclature for the imaging segments of the CNs based on their anatomic context (discussed later).[8] Skull base imaging should optimally provide sufficient spatial resolution to visualize the CNs and maximize the extent to which the CNs are visualized in each segment by accounting for the various tissue types encountered. Likewise, evaluation of mass lesions of the skull base may also traverse the various skull base layers and similarly calls for an approach that provides for evaluation of signal characteristics and extent through a variety of anatomic contexts.

To this end we prefer a protocol that incorporates T1- and T2-weighted images, postcontrast-T1-weighted images, and high-resolution balanced steady-state free precession imaging before and after contrast (**Fig. 2**, **Table 1**). 3D T1-weighted images before contrast without fat saturation allow for the assessment of the presence or absence of intrinsic T1 hyperintensity including fat signal, such as within the medullary space, extracranial space, and lesion (if present). Sequences should be chosen to provide signal intensity similar to that of standard spin echo sequences. Additionally, a 3D T2-weighted sequence with signal properties similar to that of spin echo T2-weighted images with fat saturation allows for evaluation of intrinsic T2 signal and significantly increases the conspicuity of T2 hyperintense abnormalities. After contrast, 3D T1-weighted images are performed with fat saturation to provide high conspicuity for enhancement and also to allow for confident characterization of precontrast T1 hyperintensity because of fat. Casselman and colleagues[9] described the use of balanced steady-state free precession images for evaluation of the CNs surrounded by cerebrospinal fluid (CSF) in the subarachnoid space. Balanced steady-state free precession images have the advantage of high

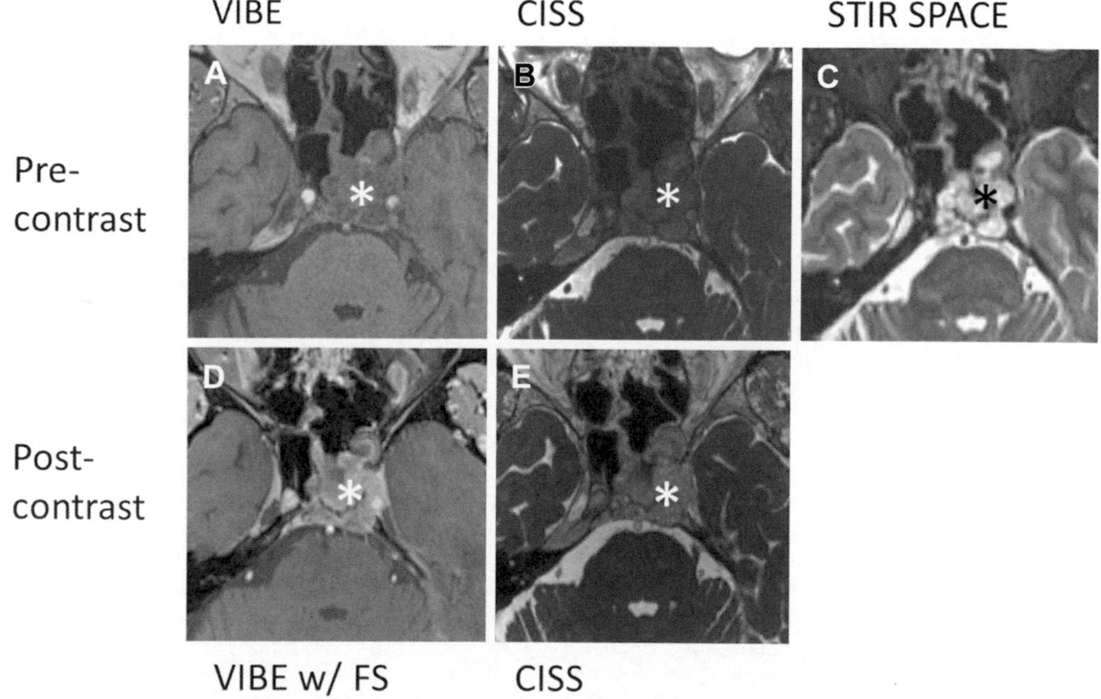

Fig. 2. Components of the HR-SB-MR imaging protocol (images have been cropped to highlight the evaluation of a mass lesion, *asterisk*). (*A*) Precontrast 3D T1-weighted VIBE demonstrates a hypointense mass in the region of the clivus. The mass demonstrates T2 hyperintensity on 3D STIR SPACE imaging (*C*) and enhancement on postcontrast 3D T1-weighted VIBE with fat saturation (FS) (*D*). The intensity of the mass on 3D CISS, a balanced steady-state free precession sequence, is different from that on standard imaging with mixed T2/T1 weighting, but allows for high spatial resolution, high signal-to-noise evaluation of the detailed anatomy of the skull base, and assessment for the presence or absence of enhancement (*B*, *E*). This T2-hyperintense mass with enhancement was proven to be a chordoma at surgery.

Table 1
Parameters of the HR-SB-MR imaging protocol at the authors' institution[a]

	TR (ms)	TE (ms)	TI (ms)	Flip Angle (deg)	Field of View (mm)	Slices	Voxel Size (mm)[b]	Averages	Time of Acquisition
STIR SPACE	3000	256	220	—	256	88	1.0 × 1.0 × 1.0	1.4	5:23
VIBE	4.93	2.46		9	210	112	0.78 × 0.78 × 0.8	3	4:38
CISS[c]	5.46	2.43		42	152	112	0.6 × 0.6 × 0.6	1	5:17
Intravenous contrast									
CISS	5.46	2.43		42	152	112	0.6 × 0.6 × 0.6	1	5:17
VIBE with SPAIR FS	11.6	4.3		10.5	210	112	0.73 × 0.73 × 0.8	1	4:16

[a] Please note that standard pre-contrast imaging through the head is typically performed prior to the high resolution skull base examination and standard post-contrast imaging of the head is generally performed following the high resolution sequences listed.
[b] Reconstructed voxel size.
[c] Acquired and reconstructed voxel size are identical.

signal-to-noise ratio[10] allowing for high spatial resolution and high signal-to-noise ratio in a clinically reasonable acquisition time. Yagi and colleagues[11] described the use of CISS imaging, a form of balanced steady-state free precession imaging, with intravenous contrast for evaluation of the CNs outside of the subarachnoid space within the cavernous sinus, the result of mixed T2/T1 weighting and therefore visualization of venous and other enhancement.[10] CISS imaging allows for a high spatial resolution acquisition with excellent signal-to-noise ratio in a clinically acceptable time period and allowing for the assessment of contrast enhancement. CISS imaging forms the core of the HR-SB-MR imaging protocol and its application to skull base imaging is the principal focus of this article.

Coverage and Positioning

Typically, slabs are positioned at an angle parallel to the floor of the anterior cranial fossa with the superior extent covering the orbitofrontal region and caudal extent including the hard palate. Posteriorly, imaging typically extends to the ventral aspect of the forth ventricle and anteriorly an attempt is made to cover the tip of the nose. In most patients this approach allows for imaging of the skull base from the frontal sinus through the craniocervical junction. Inline subtracted images may be created but have not proven to be of great utility. Techniques are modified in real time when necessary to tailor the study to the requirements of the care of the patient at hand. In particular the technologist and supervising radiologist may modify the placement of the imaging slabs to cover the superior- and inferior-most extent of skull base masses. Additionally, although the spatial resolution of the HR-SB-MR imaging protocol as described is adequate for visualization of most of the relevant skull base structures, an even higher spatial resolution is often used, such as when assessing CN IV.[8,12]

Coil Choice

Use of a variety of different coils has been advocated for evaluation of the CNs.[13] However, for most applications in the region of the skull base including CN imaging we have found standard phased array head or head and neck coils provide excellent images.

CRANIAL NERVES

The 12 pairs of CNs arise directly from the surface of the brain (with the exception of CN XI, which arises from the rostral cervical spine) and (with the exception of CN VIII, which terminates in the structures of the inner ear within the temporal bone) must traverse the skull base before exiting the head. The varying anatomic context of the CNs presents a challenge for imaging because the contrast with surrounding tissues varies greatly. We have previously suggested the use of a generic segmental nomenclature for imaging of the CNs (**Fig. 3**)[8] (the remainder of this article uses this naming convention; eg, CN IIIc is written to refer to the cisternal segment of the oculomotor nerve).

The cisternal segment of the CNs begins at their apparent origin from the brainstem and extends through CSF to the porus, the entrance to the dural cave segment. In the dural cave segment the CN comes into proximity with the inner layer of dura mater but remains surrounded by CSF. For the purposes of imaging, once the CN is no longer surrounded by visible CSF it is said to be in the interdural segment,[8] between the visible aspects of the

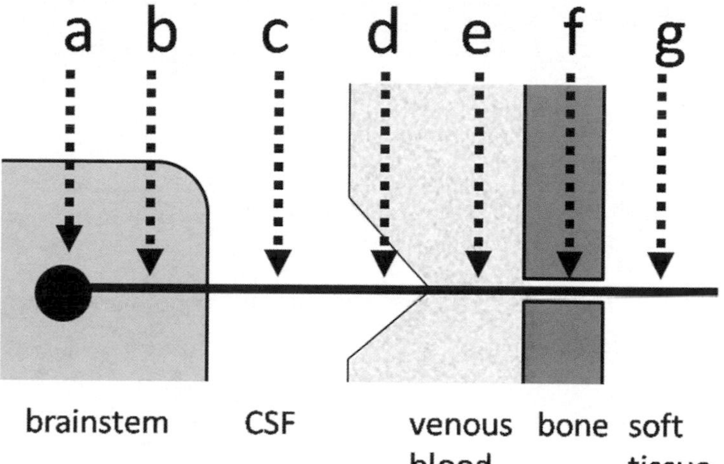

Fig. 3. Anatomic segments of the CNs with surrounding tissue (a, nuclear; b, parenchymal fascicular; c, cisternal; d, dural cave; e, interdural; f, foraminal; g, extraforaminal). (*Data from* Blitz AM, Choudhri AF, Chonka ZD, et al. Anatomic considerations, nomenclature, and advanced cross-sectional imaging techniques for visualization of the cranial nerve segments by MR imaging. Neuroimaging Clin N Am 2014;24(1):3; with permission.)

inner and outer layer of the dura mater, although from a histologic standpoint the inner layer of dura is continuous with the epineurium beyond the neural foramen.[14] The interdural space is occupied in some locations by venous blood. As the CNs pass through the foramina they are surrounded by bone and, also to a variable degree, venous blood before exiting from the skull.

The CNs are visualized most easily on T2-weighted images in the cisternal and dural cave segments because of the intrinsic contrast between the CNs, which are dark, and the surrounding CSF, which is bright.[13] With the exception of the ganglia the CNs do not ordinarily demonstrate significant contrast enhancement. The protocol described previously allows for evaluation of the CNs beyond the subarachnoid space because of enhancement of the surrounding venous blood surrounding the interdural segment (**Fig. 4**) (and often within the foraminal segment).

HIGH-RESOLUTION SKULL BASE MR IMAGING FOR NEUROLOGIC LOCALIZATION

HR-SB-MR imaging has become the standard at our institution for the evaluation of CN palsies. The technique is particularly useful when the neurologic evaluation suggests localization outside of the parenchyma or subarachnoid space and in the setting of unremarkable convention imaging.[15,16] HR-SB-MR imaging allows for depiction of smaller regions of thickening or enhancement of the CNs than is typically possible[8,16] and decreases the likelihood that the radiologist will mistake a similarly located vein for the CN in question.[12] The technique allows for visualization of the various segments of the CN that are not typically well visualized on conventional imaging including and in particular the interdural segment. Pathologic enhancement of the CNs beyond the subarachnoid space may be evident based on

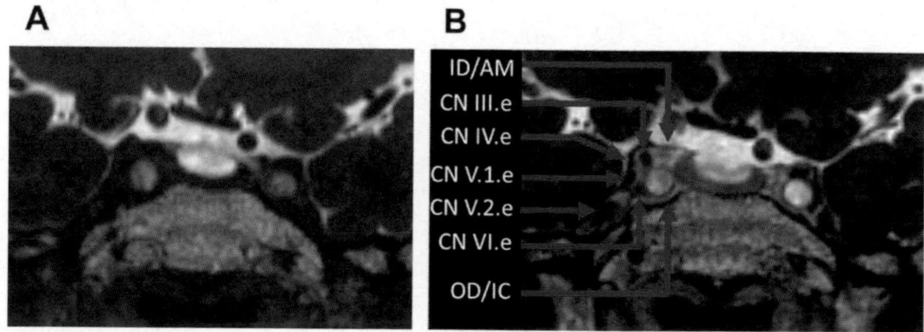

Fig. 4. (*A*) The interdural segments of the CNs are not visualized on coronal reconstructed CISS without contrast through the level of the cavernous sinus. (*B*) After the administration of intravenous contrast the interdural segments of the CNs within the cavernous sinus are visualized in the interdural compartment between the boundaries of the inner layer of dura/outer arachnoid membrane (ID/AM) and the outer layer of dura/inner cortex (OD/IC).

decreased visualization of an enhancing CN surrounded by enhancing venous plexus (**Fig. 5**).

ROLE OF HIGH-RESOLUTION SKULL BASE IMAGING IN THE EVALUATION OF MASSES

HR-SB-MR imaging is particularly helpful in the evaluation of skull base masses. The technique is used to determine the likely cause of masses, whether the mass is amenable to biopsy or resection and via which surgical approach, and the anticipated intraoperative findings (**Box 1**). The results of HR-SB-MR imaging are essential in preoperative surgical planning and counseling of patients regarding surgical morbidity.

Characterization of Mass Lesions

HR-SB-MR imaging has significant advantages over computed tomography (CT) for evaluation of masses and for surgical planning in the region of the skull base because of improved soft tissue discrimination generally and because the soft tissue characteristics of mass lesions are more fully characterized (eg, **Fig. 2**). Improved spatial resolution and 3D technique may allow the radiologist to clarify the region of anatomic origin of masses (**Fig. 6**).

Definition of the Extent of Disease

HR-SB-MR imaging is used for surgical planning when masses are encountered and is an important tool for determining (often with submillimeter precision) the extent of disease (**Fig. 7**).[8,17] At our institution, this technique has been used extensively in particular for planning endoscopic approaches to the skull base since 2009. Surgical decision making with respect to whether or not a lesion can be resected endoscopically depends on the experience and expertise of the surgical team and a thorough three-dimensional understanding of the extent of the pathology and surrounding neurovascular structures. High spatial resolution imaging can better define the extent of

Box 1
Goals of high-resolution skull base MR imaging in the evaluation of masses and in preoperative planning

1. Characterize the pathology in question
2. Define precisely the extent of disease in each dimension to aid in selection of the appropriate surgical approach
3. Define the relationship of the mass to the adjacent segments of the cranial nerves, brain and brainstem, and critical vascular structures
4. Describe the relationship of the mass to the compartments and boundaries of the skull base

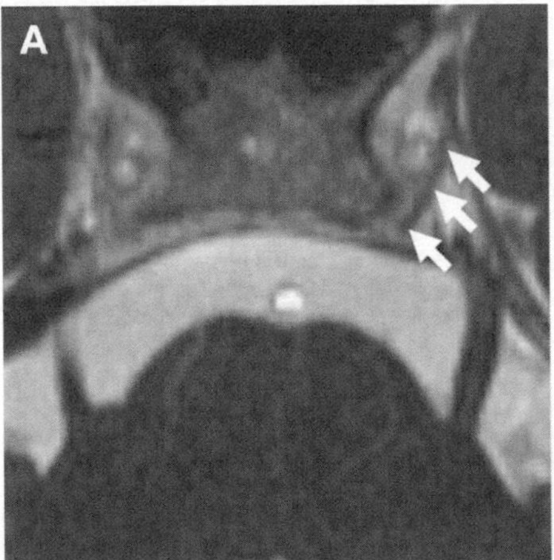

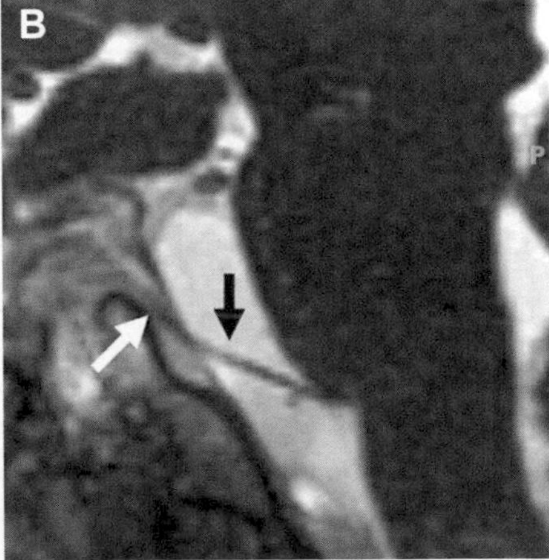

Fig. 5. Several-day history of abducens palsy on the right. Standard protocol MR imaging unremarkable. Postcontrast isotropic CISS. (*A*) Axial image. The left CN VIe (*arrows*) is well visualized extending through Dorello canal into the cavernous sinus. The right abducens nerve is not visualized in the cavernous region because of pathologic enhancement. (*B*) In sagittal oblique reformatted views, CN VIc (*black arrow*) and the proximal CN VIe segment are seen with an abrupt transition to the region of pathologic enhancement (*white arrow*). Tolosa-Hunt syndrome was suggested. No significant CN VId segment was present in this individual, a feature of significant variation between patients. (*From* Blitz AM, Macedo LL, Chonka ZD, et al. High-resolution CISS MR imaging with and without contrast for evaluation of the upper cranial nerves: segmental anatomy and selected pathologic conditions of the cisternal through extraforaminal segments. Neuroimaging Clin N Am 2014;24(1):17–34; with permission.)

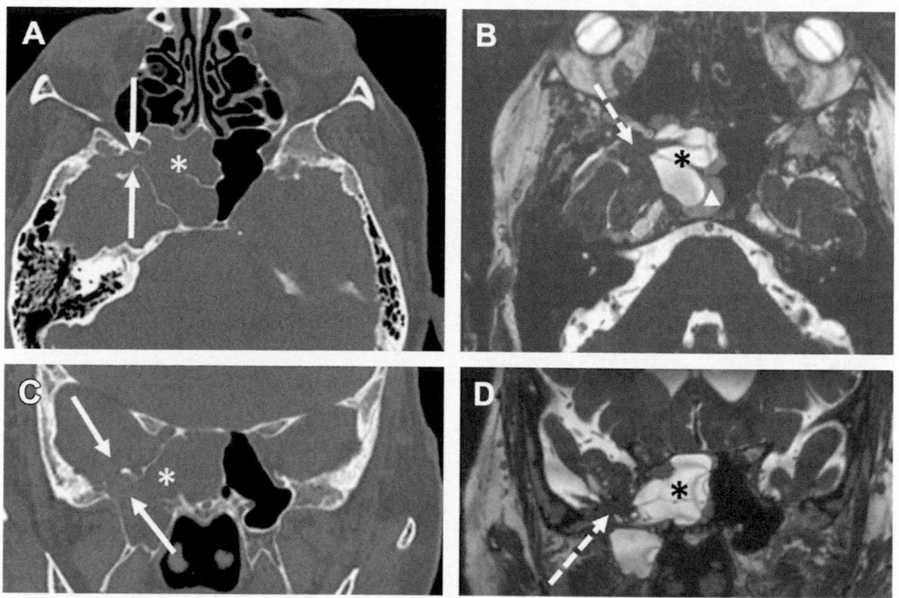

Fig. 6. Axial CT (*A*) and CISS MR imaging (*B*) and coronal CT (*C*) and CISS (*D*) demonstrate a mass lesion (*asterisk*) occupying the right sphenoid sinus. Defect along the floor of the right middle cranial fossa (*arrows*) suggests that this mass may reflect a cephalocele. HR-SB-MR imaging confirms communication with the intracranial compartment with herniation of a component of the right temporal lobe through the skull base defect and fluid with signal equivalent to that within the subarachnoid space, findings compatible with a meningocephalocele. A small amount of postobstructive secretions (*arrowhead*) are distinguished from the meningoencephalocele (*B*) on MR imaging.

the mass in question and aids surgeons in determining if a particular lesion is amenable to a purely endoscopic approach or requires an open or combination approach.[18]

Defining the extent of disease is essential for preoperative planning. However, clinical decision making depends not just on disease extent but also the nature of pathology. For example, as with open surgery the goal of endoscopic oncologic surgery at the skull base for sinonasal malignancies is to achieve negative margin resection.[18,19] For other malignancies, such as

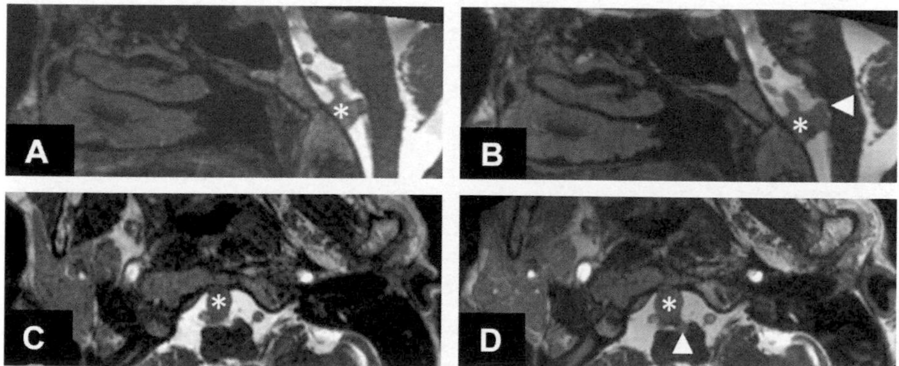

Fig. 7. The small changes detectable over time on HR-SB-MR imaging demonstrate the precision with which extent of disease is ascertained on HR-SB-MR imaging. (*A, C*) Sagittal and the axial appearance, respectively, of a skull base mass (*asterisk*), presumed to be a chordoma, on CISS imaging in 2011. In the axial plane (*C*) a thin cleft of CSF in the subarachnoid space separates the mass from the medulla at its left and posterolateral margin. The patient declined treatment and underwent multiple follow-up examinations to assess for change. When the 2016 evaluation (*B, D*) is compared to that of 5 years prior the mass (*asterisk*) is unchanged except for a 3-mm projection along its posterior and superior margin (*arrowhead*) now directly abutting the ventral medulla where CSF was previously visible.

chordoma it is known that gross total resection, when compared with partial resection, significantly improves patient survival.[20] In both instances surgically removing all visible disease has important clinical consequences and is aided by precisely defining disease extent on HR-SB-MR imaging.

The concept of gross total resection itself is in some sense not precisely defined; one study of endoscopic macroadenoma resection found that the surgical impression of extent of resection was only correct in 65% of cases when compared with high-resolution intraoperative MR imaging.[21] The surgical impression of removal of all visible tumor may vary from the appearance on imaging and the sensitivity of imaging would be expected to vary with technique. The same macroadenoma study found that the extent of resection increased with MR imaging guidance, demonstrating the power of imaging to guide the surgeon to regions of disease unexpected even with direct endoscopic inspection at surgery.

Our experience has been that HR-SB-MR imaging allows for submillimetric definition of the extent of skull base disease and that small projections of tumor into surrounding tissue that might otherwise be missed intraoperatively (**Fig. 8**) are often resected with the use of HR-SB-MR imaging registered to the patient for intraoperative navigation. Likewise, postoperative HR-SB-MR imaging when compared with identical imaging preoperatively often aids the radiologist in identifying the

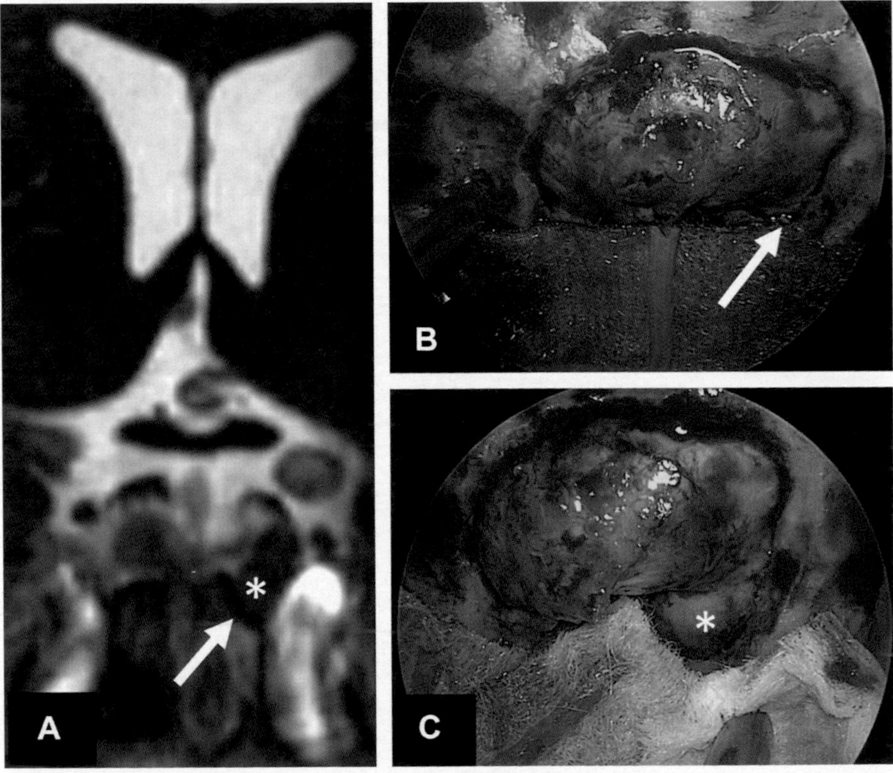

Fig. 8. MR imaging performed for localization of recurrent Cushing disease status post resection of a macroadenoma via a sublabial transsphenoidal approach. (*A*) Coronal reformatted postcontrast CISS demonstrates a hypoenhancing mass (*asterisk*) compatible with recurrent pituitary adenoma along the left lateral aspect of the sella turcica. Note that a component of the mass extends inferior to the floor of the sella turcica with the inner cortex of the adjacent clivus intact (*arrow*), which was not identified on 2D protocol outside institution imaging. (*B*) Endoscopic view at the time of surgery demonstrates the extent of the standard endoscopic transsphenoidal approach with removal of the sellar floor revealing the outer dural layer with a small region of central scarring from prior surgery. Although the superior intercavernous sinus and medial aspect of the left cavernous sinus are exposed, the left inferolateral extent of the exposure (*arrow*) is insufficient to reveal the full extent of the tumor. (*C*) Subsequent extension of the standard surgical exposure with a focal left superior clivectomy demonstrates the component of the mass below the plane of the sellar floor (*asterisk*). The entirety of the recurrent mass was resected and the patient experienced immediate postoperative biochemical remission of disease.

exact extent of the surgical cavity. It remains to be seen whether or to what extent resection of small projections of tumor into surrounding tissues visible on HR-SB-MR imaging might further reduce neoplastic recurrence rates.

High-Resolution Skull Base MR Imaging Defines the Relationship of Mass Lesions to the Cranial Nerves, Vascular Structures, Brain, and Brainstem

One of the primary tasks for the radiologist in aiding in surgical planning in the region of the skull base is the necessity of identifying the relationship of mass lesions to critical neurovascular structures. Reporting the relationship of the mass to vascular and neural structures is essential in determining the approach to effectively address certain pathologies. Defining the relationship of a mass lesion to the internal carotid artery is essential to avoid vascular injury. Although the surgeon may be able to temporarily mobilize vascular structures (eg the cavernous internal carotid artery) to reach disease, the CNs are not mobile and if significantly displaced may be damaged resulting in CN palsy.

One of the primary tasks of the radiologist faced with preoperative evaluation of a skull base mass is to aid the surgeon in avoiding creating CN palsies inadvertently and in avoiding damage to critical vascular structures. This requires an accurate and detailed assessment of the relationship of the lesion to each of the adjacent CNs and vessels. In this task HR-SB-MR imaging has a distinct advantage over CT evaluation in that the soft tissue structures including the CNs are visible, whereas on CT the radiologist must rely on osseous erosion or other indirect signs. Further evaluation of the CN segments adjacent to the lesion in question is more readily accomplished on HR-SB-MR imaging (**Figs. 9** and **10**) than on conventional MR imaging, because the CNs are followed in continuity from their apparent origin through the layers of the skull base.

COMPARTMENTS AND BOUNDARIES OF THE SKULL BASE

The anatomy of the skull base is complex with multiple layers, as described previously. The layers of the skull base (**Fig. 11**) separate the skull base into different compartments and present a barrier to the spread of disease processes and the description of the extent of disease with respect to the layers of the skull base is critical for understanding patterns of spread of disease. This section reviews the anatomy of the layers of the skull base in greater detail with illustrative cases demonstrating the utility of this concept. The layers of the skull base follow the segments of the CNs with the addition that the potential spaces between compartments may be occupied and expanded or disrupted by mass lesions. The compartments of the skull base are described next.

Subarachnoid Space

Briefly, when viewed from the inner surface of the skull base the subarachnoid space is first encountered. The subarachnoid space extends from the pial surface of the brainstem to the outer arachnoidal layer and contains CSF, arteries, veins, and the cisternal and dural cave segments of the CNs.

Interdural Space

Next, the interdural space is encountered. The dura mater is composed of an inner and outer layer[22,23] enclosing the interdural space.[24] The inner layer of the dura mater, often named the meningeal layer, is closely applied to the outer layer of the arachnoid membrane with the subdural space, a potential space, between.

The dura mater is principally composed of collagenous fibers and the outer layer is mostly firmly attached to the inner table of the skull until the age of 10 and is more easily separated from the bone after that age.[22] Interestingly, the dural layers contain a complex vascular network. The

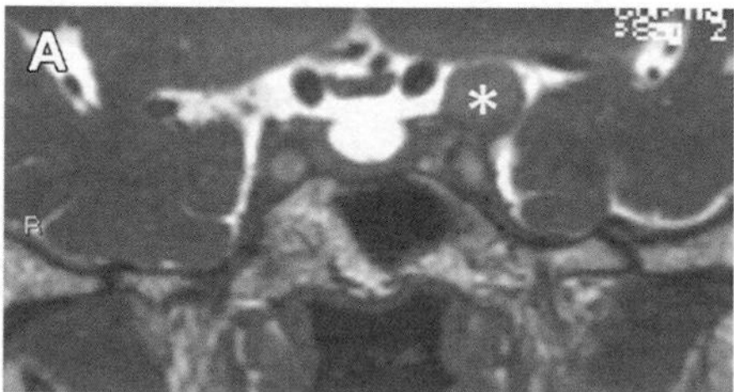

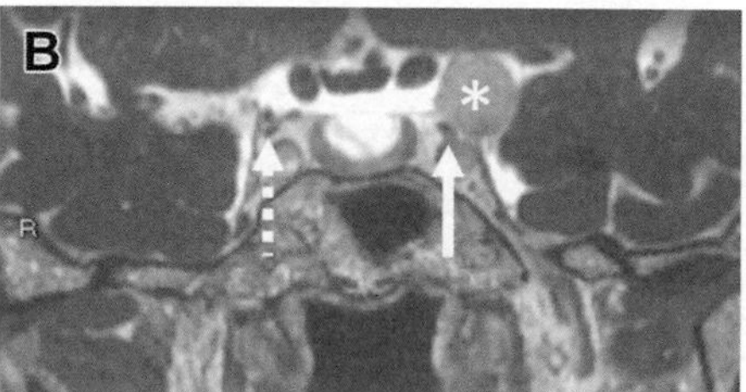

Fig. 9. (*A*) Coronal reconstructed CISS without contrast demonstrates a meningioma (*asterisk*) arising from the anterior clinoid process (not pictured). The relationship of the mass to CN III is not visible. (*B*) After the administration of intravenous contrast enhancement of the mass is noted (*asterisk*). The left CN IIIe is visible at the medial and inferior aspect of the mass (*solid arrow*) without pathologic enhancement. The contralateral CN IIIe is also well seen (*dashed arrow*).

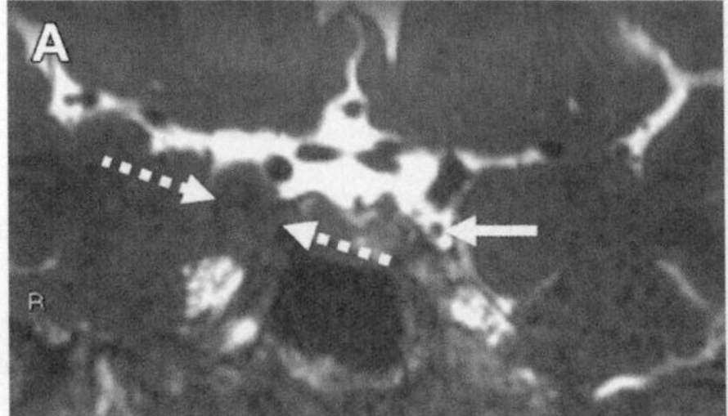

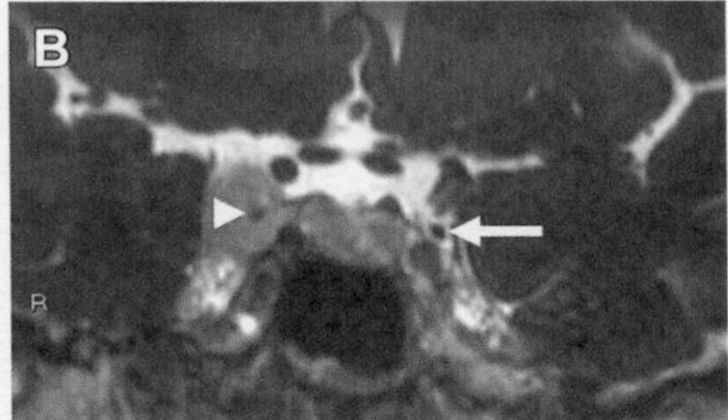

Fig. 10. (*A*) Coronal reformatted CISS image demonstrates the normal left CN IIId (*solid arrow*). A mass, presumed to reflect a meningioma, is noted on the right (between *dashed arrows*). (*B*) Postcontrast CISS demonstrates the right CN III (*arrowhead*) is encased rather than displaced by the mass. The patient did not have a CN III palsy. In general the presence of a portion of a lesion on the opposite side from the perspective of endonasal surgical approach implies that a mass cannot be resected in its entirety endoscopically without injuring the CN in question.

arterial supply to the dura mater is via the meningeal arteries, which are superficial to or partly enmeshed in the outer (periosteal) layer of the dura. There are free anastomoses between the meningeal arteries, which are continuous across the midline.[25] The lumens of the primary meningeal anastomoses measure 0.1 to 0.3 mm[25] and are for this reason below the level of resolution of current clinical skull base evaluation. In addition to giving off additional branches to the skull primary and secondary anastamotic vessels also give rise to small arterioles, which extend into the inner/meningeal layer of the dura, evidently traversing the interdural space, to just above the inner surface of the inner/cerebral layer of the dura matter where they form an "extremely rich capillary network" separated from the arachnoid membrane by only a few microns per Kerber and Newton.[25,26]

The outer and inner layers are directly apposed in most locations, except where they are separated by the venous sinuses.[23] In the region of the skull base the inner and outer dural layers are separated by venous blood with consistency in the cavernous sinus[27] and along the dorsal aspect of the clivus where the more variable basilar venous plexus is found.[28,29] The interdural space is variable in thickness by location along the skull base with some regions containing the interdural venous structures, such as the cavernous sinus, and contains the interdural segments of the CNs. The interdural space, where not occupied by venous blood, serves as a potential space into which tumor can spread (**Fig. 12**). The outer boundary of the interdural space is the outer dural layer, often named the periosteal layer.

Osseous Compartment and Foramina

The inner boundary of the osseous compartment is the inner table of the skull. Between the inner table of the skull and the outer dura mater is another potential space, the epidural space. The compartment is occupied by the medullary space and is limited by the outer and inner cortex along its superficial and deep margins and internally traversed by the foramina. The osseous compartment is variable in thickness by location in the skull base principally because of differences in the thickness of the medullary compartment with the medullary compartment essentially absent in some regions.[1] This variability in thickness has important clinical and radiologic implications with the osseous

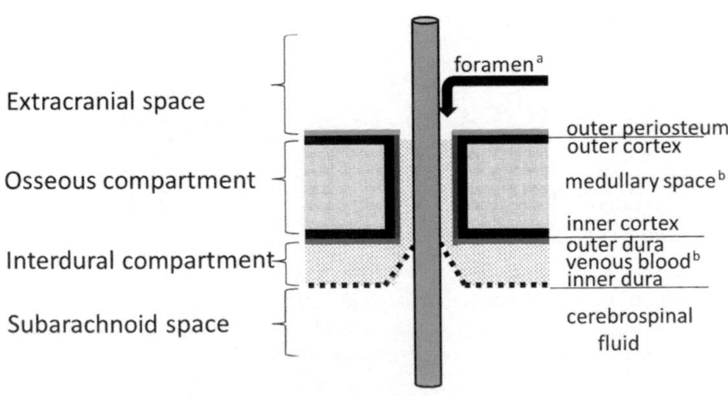

Fig. 11. Diagrammatic representation of the skull base compartments and boundaries. Masses of the skull base may arise from or involve the different layers of the skull base and, unless passing through the foramen (demonstrated with cranial nerve, *gray cylinder*), must traverse the boundaries shown. At the foramina the pericranium (*green*) is continuous with the outer layer of dura (*blue*) via the dural-periosteal sheath (*red*). a, lined by dural-periosteal sheath; b, extent variable by location.

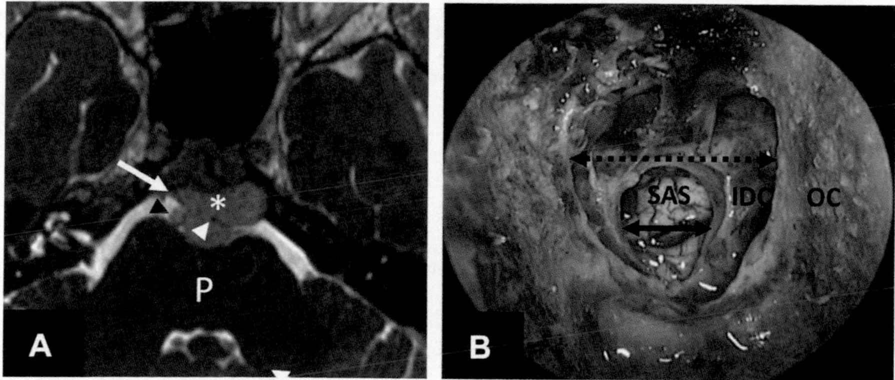

Fig. 12. A 15-year-old boy with clival chordoma. (*A*) Axial preoperative postcontrast CISS demonstrates a mass arising from the dorsal clivus (*asterisk*) primarily occupying the interdural space between the inner table of the skull and associated outer layer of dura mater and the inner layer of the dura mater (plane indicated by *arrow*). Note interruption of the inner layer of dura (left margin demonstrated with *white arrowhead*) and associated outer layer of the arachnoid membrane to extend into the subarachnoid space indenting the pons (P) and minimally displacing the basilar artery (*black arrowhead*). (*B*) Posteriorly directed view following endoscopic resection of the chordoma via a transclival approach. The surgeon has passed through the osseous compartment (OC), performing a clivectomy. The cut margin of the inner clival cortex and associated outer layer of the dura, which represent the inner margins of the osseous compartment and outer margin of the interdural compartment, respectively, are seen (*dashed arrow*). The tumor, which had predominantly extended in the transverse dimension in the interdural compartment (IDC), has been resected. At its depth the tumor had extended through the inner layer of dura and outer layer of the arachnoid membrane (*solid arrow*) to extend into the subarchnoid space (SAS) where the ventral aspect of the pons and overlying vascular structures are seen at the depth of the surgical field.

compartment more easily violated from without by masses or from within by cephaloceles (see **Fig. 5**) in regions where the medullary space is essentially absent or not of significant thickness.

The foramina traverse the osseous compartment and permit the entrance of arteries, veins and the CNs. The foraminal walls are composed of cortical bone, as with the inner and outer cortex easily identified on HR-SB-MR imaging because of the relative lack of water protons and therefore appearing as a dark line (**Fig. 13**). A dural-periosteal sheath that is continuous

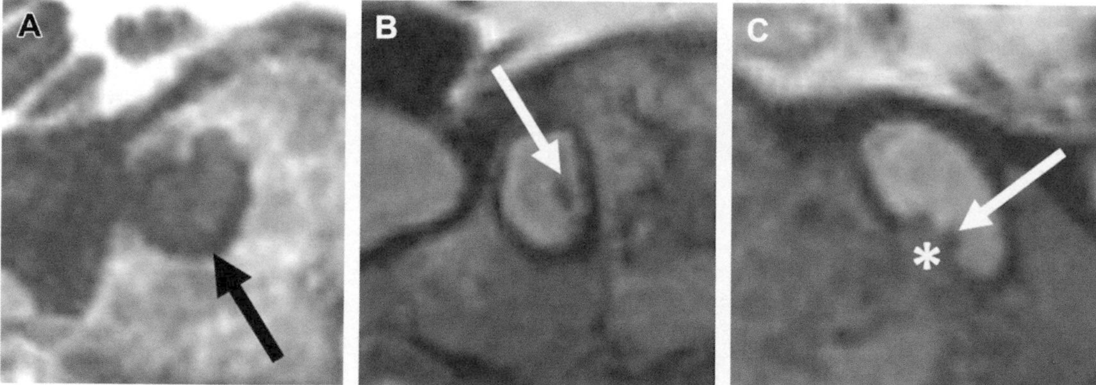

Fig. 13. (*A*) Precontrast CISS in a patient without osseous pathology of the skull base. Multiplanar reformat perpendicular to the hypoglossal canal demonstrating the cortical margin (*arrow*). (*B*) Postcontrast CISS in another patient with a clival chordoma demonstrates CN XIIf (*arrow*) surrounded by enhancement of the venous plexus. The cortical margin and dural-periosteal sheath of the foramen are intact. (*C*) On the contralateral side, a component of the chordoma (*asterisk*) interrupts the cortical margin of the foramen and minimally extends into the hypoglossal canal to abut CN XIIf (*arrow*). The dural-periosteal sheath is not well visualized and likely focally violated. (*From* Blitz AM, Choudhri AF, Chonka ZD, et al. Anatomic considerations, nomenclature, and advanced cross-sectional imaging techniques for visualization of the cranial nerve segments by MR imaging. Neuroimaging Clin N Am 2014;24(1):1–15; with permission.)

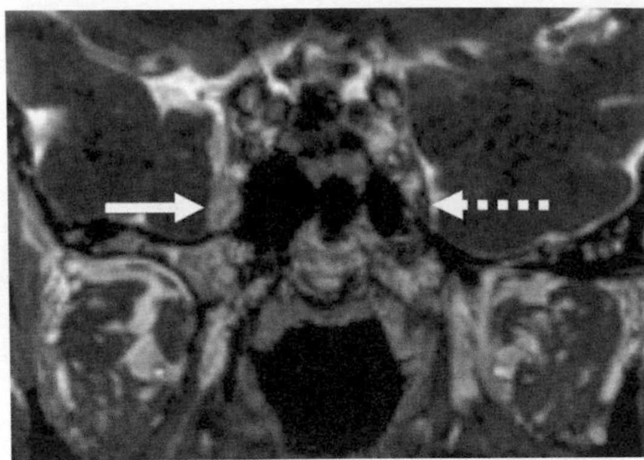

Fig. 14. Trigeminal neuralgia in the setting of perineural spread. Postcontrast coronal CISS images demonstrate the presence of an enhancing soft tissue mass in the inferior aspect of the anterior right cavernous sinus along the expected route of V2e (*solid arrow*). Note the normal appearance of the V2e nerve on the left side, which is surrounded by enhancing venous contrast in the cavernous sinus but without enhancement of the nerve itself (*dashed arrow*). The right cavernous sinus mass was caused by perineural spread from an adenoid cystic carcinoma. (*From* Seeburg DP, Northcutt B, Aygun N, et al. The role of imaging for trigeminal neuralgia: a segmental approach to high-resolution MR imaging. Neurosurg Clin N Am 2016;27(3):315–26; with permission.)

between the dura mater and the pericranium (also known as the external periosteum) lines the skull base foramina.[26] When mass lesions encroach on the foramina the cortical margin may be eroded and the dural-periosteal sheath may be invaded, findings that can allow a mass otherwise confined to the osseous compartment to compromise CNs. Such extension may allow for compression of the applicable CN and present as a CN palsy or, alternatively, might place intact CNs at risk during resection of tumor in the osseous compartment.

The foramina present a potential route of decreased resistance to the spread of neoplastic or infectious inflammatory disease, in some measure bypassing multiple layers of the skull base, which might otherwise present some defense[30] and therefore present a route of entry of extracranial disease into the intracranial compartment or presenting a route by which intracranial disease may spread outside of the head. Because of improved soft tissue discrimination MR imaging is generally superior to CT for detection of perineural spread of neoplasm even on conventional MR imaging[30] because disease does not need to be sufficiently advanced to erode the osseous margins. By extension the CNs themselves are visible

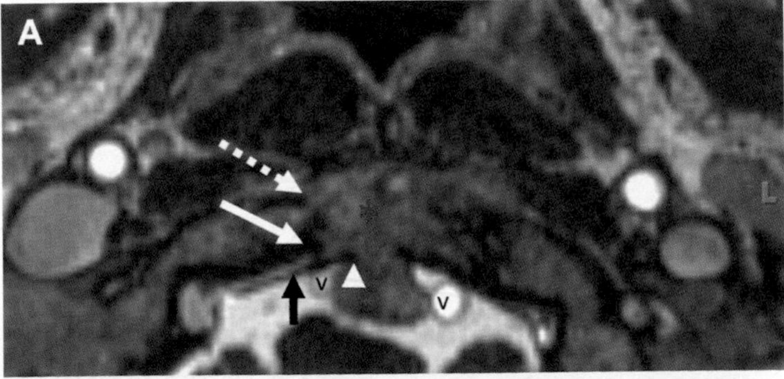

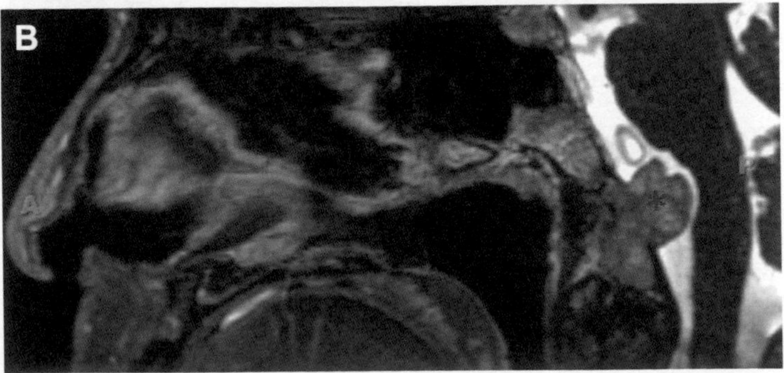

Fig. 15. Demonstration of a mass extending across all of the layers of the skull base. (*A*) Axial postcontrast CISS demonstrates chordoma (*asterisk*) centered in the basiocciput. The mass extends anteriorly through the outer cortex (*dashed arrow*). The mass extends posteriorly through the inner cortex (*solid white arrow*), passing into the inte-dural space, partly contained by the inner layer of dura (*black arrow*), but medially violates the inner dural layer (*arrowhead*) to pass into the subarachnoid space adjacent to the vertebral arteries (V). (*B*) The cranial caudal extent of the mass (*asterisk*) is best visualized on sagittal reformatted images.

on HR-SB-MR imaging permitting evaluation of the nerves for thickening and abnormal enhancement (**Fig. 14**) in a manner that is not as readily evident on conventional MR imaging.

THE LAYERS OF THE SKULL BASE IN PREOPERATIVE ASSESSMENT

Assessment of the extent of involvement of the layers of the skull base is an important task in preoperative planning and is essential in providing appropriate preoperative counseling to the patient. A mass that is confined solely to the osseous compartment may be excised by drilling until normal bone is encountered and the risk of CSF leak is not substantial. When a mass within the osseous compartment extends into one of the skull base foramina, however, the risk of injury to the CN in question increases and special care must be taken to avoid inadvertent injury to the CN. When the mass is seen to extend into the interdural compartment the surgeon must be prepared to address the expected venous bleeding and must take care to avoid injury to the interdural segments of the CNs if they lie in proximity to the expected surgical tract. Because masses may extend laterally through the interdural space, presumably following a path of least resistance, the osteotomy necessary to provide adequate exposure of interdural tumor must be planned appropriately. If an interdural mass abuts the inner layer of dura in some cases whether there has been violation of the inner dural layer may be uncertain, and the possibility of extension into the subarachnoid space with attendant risk of CSF leak should be considered. When masses extend through each of the layers of the skull base into the subarachnoid space the risk of CSF leak increases and assessment of the relationship of the mass to major arterial vascular structures and brainstem itself becomes critical (**Fig. 15**).

SUMMARY

HR-SB-MR imaging including isotropic CISS imaging before and after contrast has several benefits in the radiologic evaluation of the skull base. The technique allows for acquisition of images in a clinically reasonable time period that reveal normal and pathologic anatomic details not readily visualized on standard imaging. The CNs are well visualized with HR-SB-MR imaging, which has the advantage of revealing their course through each of the CN segments. For this reason HR-SB-MR imaging is preferred when referrals are made for CN palsy, particularly when conventional imaging has been unrevealing. When masses of the skull base are encountered HR-SB-MR imaging is used in establishing the appropriate diagnosis or differential diagnosis and is helpful in determining the optimal surgical approach. The technique can demonstrate the extent of masses with precision, aiding the surgeon in achieving optimal resection of the mass and demonstrates the relationship of mass lesions to vascular structures and the CNs, minimizing operative risk to these structures. The skull base is comprised of multiple boundaries separating the skull base compartments including the osseous and interdural compartments. Assessment of the relationship of mass lesions to the compartments and boundaries of the skull base is helpful in surgical planning and counseling the patient with respect to anticipated surgical risks.

REFERENCES

1. Morani AC, Ramani NS, Wesolowski JR. Skull base, orbits, temporal bone, and cranial nerves: anatomy on MR imaging. Magn Reson Imaging Clin N Am 2011;19(3):439–56.
2. Leblanc A. The cranial nerves: anatomy imaging vascularisation. New York: Springer Science & Business Media; 2012.
3. Hart H, Bottomley P, Edelstein W, et al. Nuclear magnetic resonance imaging: contrast-to-noise ratio as a function of strength of magnetic field. Am J Roentgenol 1983;141(6):1195–201.
4. Wardlaw JM, Brindle W, Casado AM, et al. A systematic review of the utility of 1.5 versus 3 Tesla magnetic resonance brain imaging in clinical practice and research. Eur Radiol 2012;22(11):2295–303.
5. Fischbach F, Müller M, Bruhn H. Magnetic resonance imaging of the cranial nerves in the posterior fossa: a comparative study of t2-weighted spin-echo sequences at 1.5 and 3.0 tesla. Acta Radiol 2008;49(3):358–63.
6. Penn R, Abemayor E, Nabili V, et al. Perineural invasion detected by high-field 3.0-T magnetic resonance imaging. Am J Otolaryngol 2010;31(6):482–4.
7. Song SW, Son YD, Cho Z, et al. Experience with 7.0 T MRI in patients with supratentorial meningiomas. J Korean Neurosurg Soc 2016;59(4):405–9.
8. Blitz AM, Choudhri AF, Chonka ZD, et al. Anatomic considerations, nomenclature, and advanced cross-sectional imaging techniques for visualization of the cranial nerve segments by MR imaging. Neuroimaging Clin N Am 2014;24(1):1–15.
9. Casselman J, Kuhweide R, Deimling M, et al. Constructive interference in steady state-3DFT MR imaging of the inner ear and cerebellopontine angle. AJNR Am J Neuroradiol 1993;14(1):47–57.

10. Scheffler K, Lehnhardt S. Principles and applications of balanced SSFP techniques. Eur Radiol 2003;13(11):2409–18.
11. Yagi A, Sato N, Taketomi A, et al. Normal cranial nerves in the cavernous sinuses: contrast-enhanced three-dimensional constructive interference in the steady state MR imaging. AJNR Am J Neuroradiol 2005;26(4):946.
12. Choi B, Kim J, Jung C, et al. High-resolution 3D MR imaging of the trochlear nerve. AJNR Am J Neuroradiol 2010;31(6):1076–9.
13. Casselman J, Mermuys K, Delanote J, et al. MRI of the cranial nerves—more than meets the eye: technical considerations and advanced anatomy. Neuroimaging Clin N Am 2008;18(2):197–231.
14. Warwick R, Williams PL. Gray's anatomy. Edinburgh (United Kingdom): Longman; 1973.
15. Kontzialis M, Choudhri AF, Patel VR, et al. High-resolution 3D magnetic resonance imaging of the sixth cranial nerve: anatomic and pathologic considerations by segment. J Neuroophthalmol 2015;35(4): 412–25.
16. Blitz AM, Macedo LL, Chonka ZD, et al. High-resolution CISS MR imaging with and without contrast for evaluation of the upper cranial nerves: segmental anatomy and selected pathologic conditions of the cisternal through extraforaminal segments. Neuroimaging Clin N Am 2014;24(1):17–34.
17. Hayashi M, Chernov MF, Tamura N, et al. Usefulness of the advanced neuroimaging protocol based on plain and gadolinium-enhanced constructive interference in steady state images for gamma knife radiosurgery and planning microsurgical procedures for skull base tumors. In: Chernov M, Hayashi M, Ganz J, et al, editors. Gamma knife neurosurgery in the management of intracranial disorders. Vienna: Springer; 2013. p. 167–78.
18. Roxbury CR, Ishii M, Richmon JD, et al. Endonasal endoscopic surgery in the management of sinonasal and anterior skull base malignancies. Head Neck Pathol 2016;10(1):13–22.
19. Snyderman CH, Carrau RL, Kassam AB, et al. Endoscopic skull base surgery: principles of endonasal oncological surgery. J Surg Oncol 2008;97(8):658–64.
20. Ahmed R, Sheybani A, Menezes AH, et al. Disease outcomes for skull base and spinal chordomas: a single center experience. Clin Neurol Neurosurg 2015;130:67–73.
21. Zaidi HA, De Los Reyes K, Barkhoudarian G, et al. The utility of high-resolution intraoperative MRI in endoscopic transsphenoidal surgery for pituitary macroadenomas: early experience in the advanced multimodality image guided operating suite. Neurosurg Focus 2016;40(3):E18.
22. Lang J. Skull base and related structures: atlas of clinical anatomy. Stuttgart (Germany): Schattauer Verlag; 2001.
23. Jinkins JR. Atlas of neuroradiologic embryology, anatomy, and variants. Philadelphia: Lippincott Williams & Wilkins; 2000.
24. Ayberk G, Ozveren MF, Aslan S, et al. Subarachnoid, subdural and interdural spaces at the clival region: an anatomical study. Turk Neurosurg 2011; 21(3):372–7.
25. Kerber C, Newton T. The macro and microvasculature of the dura mater. Neuroradiology 1973;6(4): 175–9.
26. Lang J. Clinical anatomy of the posterior cranial fossa and its foramina. New York: Thieme; 1991.
27. Kawase T, van Loveren H, Keller JT, et al. Meningeal architecture of the cavernous sinus: clinical and surgical implications. Neurosurgery 1996;39(3):527–35.
28. Kunicki J, Skadorwa T, Machura W. Microsurgical anatomy of basilar venous plexus in relation to transclival and transsphenoidal approaches to the posterior cranial fossa. Skull Base 2009;19(01):A020.
29. Wanifuchi H, vanLoveren HR, Keller JT, et al. Microanatomy of the clivus: dural architecture and venous pathway. Shimane J Med Sci 2001;19:17–23.
30. Hanna E, Vural E, Prokopakis E, et al. The sensitivity and specificity of high-resolution imaging in evaluating perineural spread of adenoid cystic carcinoma to the skull base. Arch Otolaryngol Head Neck Surg 2007;133(6):541–5.

Imaging of Paranasal Sinuses and Anterior Skull Base and Relevant Anatomic Variations

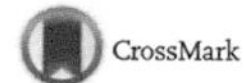

Estushi Iida, MD[a], Yoshimi Anzai, MD, MPH[b,*]

KEYWORDS

• Anterior skull base • Sinonasal cavity • Computed tomography • MR imaging • Neoplasm • Inflammatory disease

KEY POINTS

- The anterior skull base (ASB) is the boundary between the anterior cranial fossa and sinonasal cavities and orbits.
- In addition to the intrinsic ASB lesions, sinonasal lesions extend superiorly to involve ASB and also intracranial lesions extend to ASB.
- CT and MRI play a complementary role in evaluating and characterizing ASB pathologies.
- Radiologists should be familiar with the detailed anatomy, identify dangerous anatomical variations, provide appropriate differential diagnosis, and assess the extent of the lesion for optimal treatment planning.

INTRODUCTION

The anterior skull base (ASB) is the boundary between the anterior cranial fossa and sinonasal cavities and orbit, consisting of the frontal bone, ethmoid bone, and sphenoid bone. ABS pathologic conditions can be divided into 3 major categories: (1) sinonasal lesions extending cranially, (2) intrinsic ASB lesions, and (3) intracranial lesions involving the ASB.

Computed tomography (CT) and MR imaging play important roles in providing a diagnosis or differential diagnosis, assessing the extent of ASB lesions, and guiding treatment decisions and surgical approach.

The recent advances in the endoscopic sinonasal and skull base surgery allow a minimally invasive surgery for a wide variety of pathologic conditions, including congenital and inflammatory diseases, and benign and malignant neoplasms. Because these endoscopic procedures use sinonasal cavity as surgical corridors, the preoperative evaluation of sinonasal cavity is critical to facilitate the safe access to a target lesion. Radiologists should be aware of sinonasal anatomic variants that can create impediments to surgical access, decrease surgical field orientation, and increase risk of vascular or cranial nerve injury during the surgery.

This article briefly addresses CT and MR imaging techniques and reviews the ASB anatomy. In particular, it describes the sinonasal anatomy and its variants pertinent to endoscopic approach to the skull base. Clinical and imaging findings of ASB pathologic conditions are also discussed.

[a] Department of Radiology, Yamaguchi University Graduate School of Medicine, 1-1-1 Minami-Kogushi, Ube, Yamaguchi 755-8505, Japan; [b] Department of Radiology, University of Utah Health Sciences Center, 30 North, 1900 East #1A071, Salt Lake City, UT 84132-2140, USA
* Corresponding author.
E-mail address: Yoshimi.Anzai@hsc.utah.edu

Radiol Clin N Am 55 (2017) 31–52
http://dx.doi.org/10.1016/j.rcl.2016.08.009
0033-8389/17/© 2016 Elsevier Inc. All rights reserved.

IMAGING TECHNIQUE

CT and MR imaging play a complementary role in characterization and determination of the extent of the ASB pathologic condition. CT provides better detail of the bony anatomy and the extent of pneumatization. It also clearly demonstrates presence of calcification, bone remodeling, and destruction, and characterizes fibro-osseous pathologic conditions. MR imaging offers much superior contrast resolution and is useful in delineating the extent of disease and characterizing soft tissue pathologic conditions.

Computed Tomography

Thin axial CT images should be acquired using the multirow detector CT with 0.5 to 0.625 mm collimation to obtain sufficient information about osseous anatomy and pathologic changes in the skull base and sinonasal cavity. Images are reconstructed to axial, coronal, and sagittal planes with high-resolution bone and soft-tissue algorithms.

Noncontrast-enhanced CT is usually sufficient for assessment of fibro-osseous lesion. Contrast-enhanced CT should be considered if there is a clinical concern for extrasinus extension of infection, abscess, venous thrombosis, or neoplasm.

MR Imaging

MR sequences should include T1-weighted images (T1WIs) and T2-weighted images (T2WIs), and contrast-enhanced fat-saturated (CEFS)-T1WI in axial and coronal planes covering the sinonasal cavity to intracranial structures. Thin-slice thickness (2 mm or less) is preferred. T1WI is useful to detect subtle abnormal findings in bone marrow and adipose tissue as well as detection of proteinous secretion, hemorrhage, and melanin. A T1WI with CEFS-T1WI is necessary to delineate an enhancing lesion from intrinsic T1WI hyperintensity due to fat containing lesions. T2WI is useful for distinguishing isointense neoplasm from hyperintense obstructed sinus secretion. Fat suppression allows better contrast between tumor and sinonasal secretion. Coronal CEFS-T1WI is valuable for assessment of perineural spread through the ASB. Sagittal images allow clear delineation of the craniocaudal extension of the ASB lesions.

NORMAL ANATOMY OF THE ANTERIOR SKULL BASE

The ABS consists of the frontal bone (orbital plate), ethmoid bone (cribriform plate, lateral lamella, and fovea ethmoidalis), and sphenoid bone (planum sphenoidale and lesser wing) (**Fig. 1**). The superior surface of the orbital plate forms the lateral parts of the ASB. The planum ethmoidal and sphenoidale are posterior to the cribriform plate, forming the roof of the ethmoid and sphenoid sinuses, respectively. The planum sphenoidale leads laterally to the lesser wing of the sphenoid bone and posteriorly to the prechiasmatic groove and the tuberculum sellae. The anterior clinoid process forms the posteromedial part of the lesser wing. The posterior edge of the lesser wing is the posterior boundary of the anterior cranial fossa.

The crista galli is a bony protuberance in the midline of the cribriform plate. The foramen cecum is between the frontal bone anteriorly and the crista galli posteriorly, and has a variable size. It transmits emissary veins from the nasal mucosa

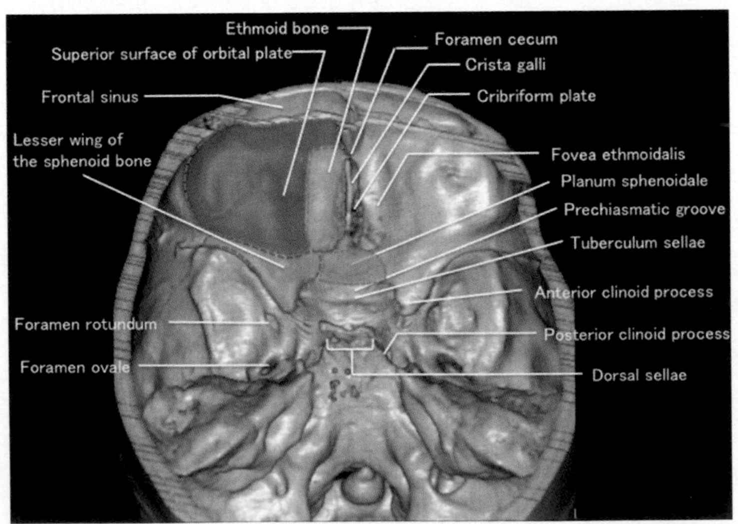

Fig. 1. Anatomy of the anterior skull base. Volume rendering CT image of the skull base demonstrates an overview of the anterior cranial fossa.

to the superior sagittal sinus but often presents as a vestigial fibrous tract.

The cribriform plate and the lateral lamella form the olfactory fossa where olfactory bulb is located. The fovea ethmoidalis, which forms the roof of the ethmoid cells connects the lateral lamella with the orbital plate of the frontal bone (**Fig. 2**). These ethmoidal components are thin and prone to injury, which may result in cerebrospinal fluid (CSF) leak. Increased depth of the olfactory fossa is associated with increased risk of injury during surgery. Keros classification is used to classify the depth of olfactory fossa and the height of the lateral lamella for the preoperative evaluation as follow: 1 to 3 mm, type I; 4 to 7 mm, type II; and 8 to 16 mm, type III.[1] The Keros type III has the higher risk of bone erosion or CSF leak.

NORMAL AND VARIANT ANATOMY OF THE SINONASAL CAVITY

Because the nasal cavity is the primary corridor to the skull base, it is pertinent to evaluate the anatomy of nasal cavity for the endoscopic approach. The nasal septum and the 3 (inferior, middle, and superior) turbinates separate the nasal cavity into 8 air chambers (the inferior, middle, and superior meatus ethmoidal, and the sphenoethmoidal recesses in each side). The vertical and basal lamellae of the middle turbinate insert into the cribriform plate and lamina papyracea, respectively, which are at risk of injury during surgery (see **Fig. 2**). The uncinate process arises from the inferior turbinate and variably inserts into the lamina papyracea or the cribriform plate. Nasal septum deviation and concha bullosa, pneumatization of the middle turbinate occasionally limit the access to the posterior nasal cavity or determine the side of access.

Sphenoid sinus is adjacent to many vital structures, including the optic nerves, the internal carotid arteries, the cavernous sinuses, and the pituitary gland. The sphenoid ostium opens to the sphenoethmoid recess at the superior part of the anterior sphenoid sinus wall (**Fig. 3**). The pneumatized nasal septum can limit access to the ostium (see **Fig. 3**).

The sphenoid sinus pneumatization is significantly variable in individuals and classified into 4 types (conchal, presellar, incomplete sellar, and complete sellar) based on the anteroposterior dimension (**Fig. 4**).[2] The complete sellar type is the most frequent and favorable for the transsphenoidal approach, whereas conchal and presellar types need drilling of bone to access to the floor of the sella.[2]

The sphenoid pneumatization can reach superiorly to the clinoid processes, laterally to the greater wing (forming the lateral recess of the sphenoid sinus), and inferolaterally to the

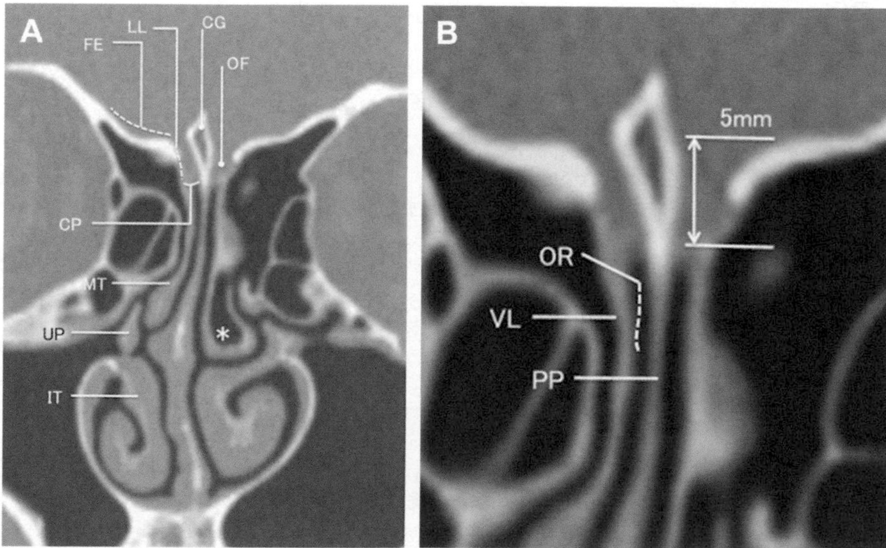

Fig. 2. Anatomy of the median anterior skull base. (*A*) Coronal CT. (*B*) Magnification of A. (*A*) The olfactory fossa (OF) is formed by the cribriform plate (CP) and lateral lamella (LL). The fovea ethmoidalis (FE) is the ethmoid roof. CG, crista galli; IT, inferior turbinate; MT, middle turbinate; UP, uncinate process. (*B*) The vertical lamella (VL) of the middle turbinate inserts to the cribriform plate forming the olfactory recess (OR) with the perpendicular plate (PP) of the ethmoid bone (*B*). The depth of the olfactory recess has a close relation with the risk of the injury to the cribriform plate. Left concha bullosa (pneumatized middle turbinate) is present (*).

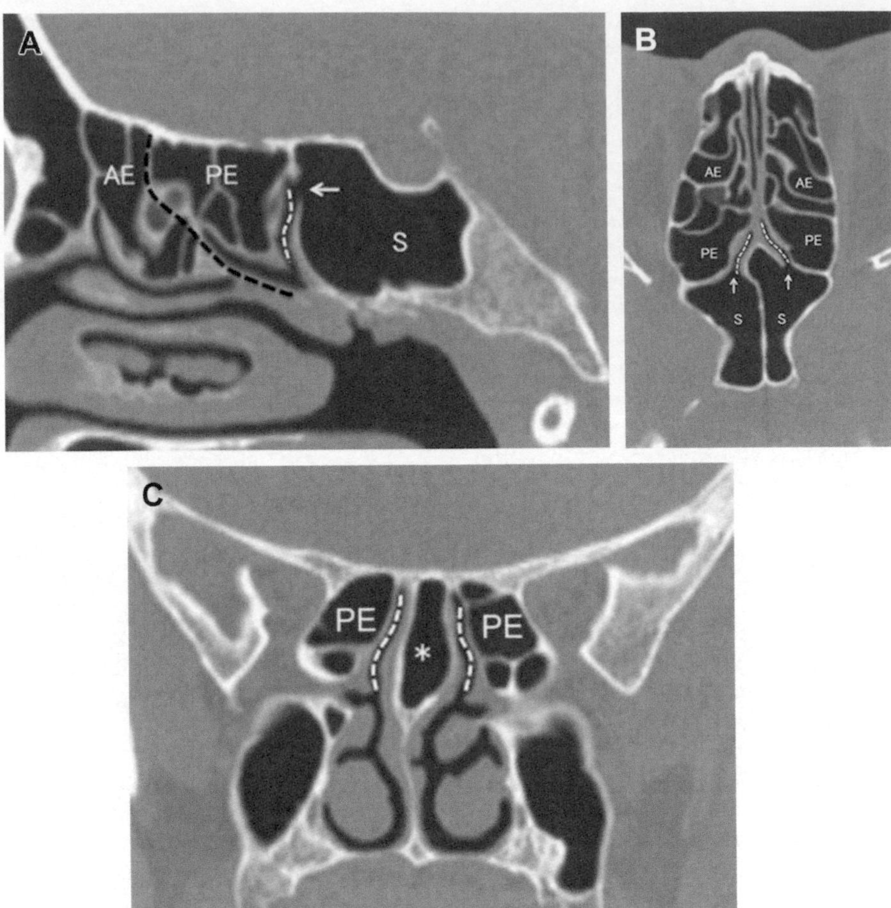

Fig. 3. CT anatomy of the ethmoid and sphenoid sinuses. (*A*) Sagittal CT. (*B*) Axial CT. (*C*) Coronal CT. Sphenoid ostia (*arrows*) locate at the superomedial part of the anterior walls of the sphenoid sinuses leading to sphenoethmoidal recesses (*white dashed lines*). The sphenovomerine bulla (*asterisk* in *C*) is present. The basal lamella of middle turbinate (*black dashed line* in *A*) divides ethmoid sinus into anterior and posterior ethmoid cells. AE, anterior ethmoid; PE posterior ethmoid; S(Sphenoid), sinuses.

pterygoid process (**Fig. 5**). Excessive pneumatization provides natural corridors for off-midline skull base lesions, although it can also increase the risk of neurovascular injury, secondary to protrusion and dehiscence of neurovascular canals (optic canal, carotid canal, pterygoid canal, and foramen rotundum).[2] Also, the intersphenoid and accessory septa potentially increase surgical risk if they insert to vital structures such as the carotid canal (see **Fig. 5**).[2,3]

The ethmoid sinus is divided into the anterior and posterior ethmoidal cells by the basal lamella of the middle turbinate (see **Fig. 3**). The agger nasi cell (the most anterior ethmoid air cell) and the ethmoid bulla (the largest anterior ethmoid air cell) are reliable anatomic landmarks for endoscopic surgery.

The anterior ethmoid canal, which houses the anterior ethmoid artery, is also an important surgical landmark. It is usually embedded in the ethmoidal roof but occasionally traverses the ethmoid air cells in a mesentery below the roof, which increases the risk of injury (**Fig. 6**).[4]

The supraorbital ethmoid air cell is an anterior ethmoid air cell located posterolateral to the frontal sinus and may be mistaken for the frontal cell (**Fig. 7**). A bony septum between the frontal and anterior ethmoid sinuses on axial and sagittal CT suggests the presence of a supraorbital ethmoid air cell. It can impose a risk of orbital and ASB injury during endoscopic surgery. Violating the supraorbital air cell during anterior cranial fossa approach to orbit increases the risk of surgical site infection.[5]

The Onodi cell, also known as the sphenoethmoidal cell, is a variant of the posterior ethmoidal cell that extends superior and/or lateral to the sphenoid sinus (**Fig. 8**). It often extends into the

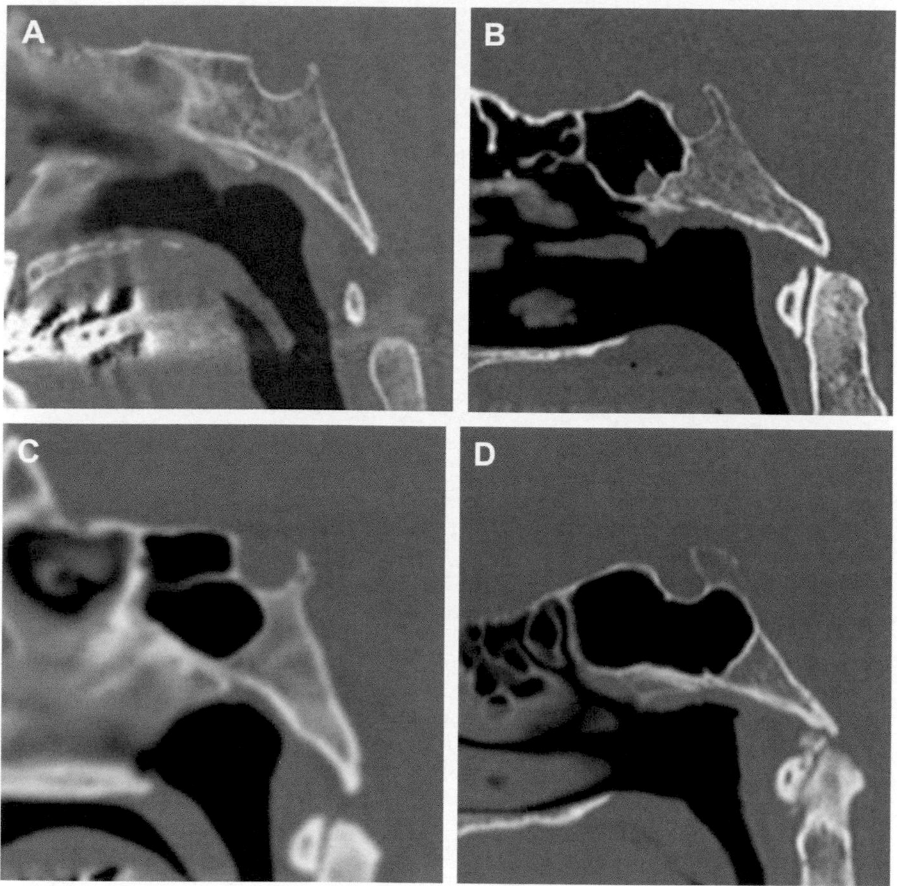

Fig. 4. Classification of sphenoid pneumatization on sagittal CT images. (*A*) Conchal type. (*B*) Presellar type. (*C*) Incomplete seller type. (*D*) Complete seller type.

anterior clinoid process, increasing risk of injury to the optic nerve and the internal carotid artery as well as CSF leakage.[6] Coronal CT images can directly demonstrate a horizontal septum between the Onodi cell and sphenoid sinus, whereas the sphenoid sinus septa only run in a vertical orientation.[2,3,7]

A dehiscence of the lamina papyracea increases the risk of orbital injury.[3] The anteroposterior diameter of the frontal sinus is related to maneuverability of the endoscopic instruments inside the sinus.[8]

ANTERIOR SKULL BASE PATHOLOGIC CONDITIONS

Sinonasal Lesions Involving the Anterior Skull Base

Both malignant and benign sinonasal diseases may involve the ASB. Extensive permeative bone destruction is associated with aggressive malignant neoplasms, whereas expansile osseous remodeling suggests slow-growing lesions, such as low-grade malignancies, benign tumors, and mucoceles.

Malignant sinonasal neoplasms

Squamous cell carcinoma is the most common malignant neoplasm of the sinonasal cavity.[9,10] Other relatively common malignancies are adenocarcinoma, melanoma, and a variety of epithelial neoplasms with differing degrees of differentiation.[10]

Malignant epithelial tumors (sinonasal carcinoma) According to the World Health Organization histologic classification, sinonasal carcinomas are classified into 6 major types: squamous cell carcinoma, adenocarcinoma, salivary gland-type carcinoma, undifferentiated carcinoma, lymphoepithelial carcinoma, and neuroendocrine tumors.[9]

Squamous cell carcinoma frequently arises from maxillary sinus, whereas adenocarcinoma often

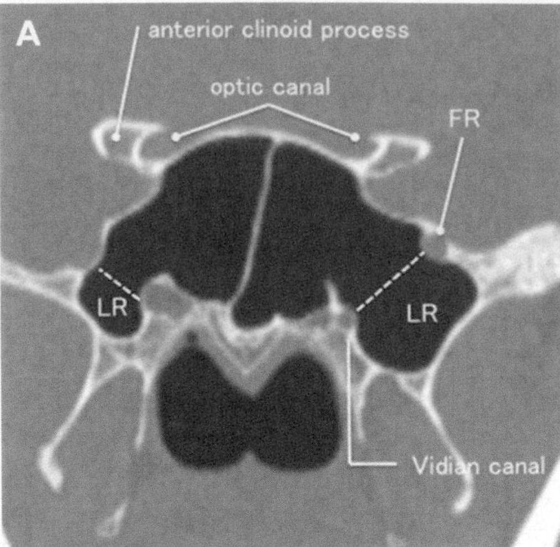

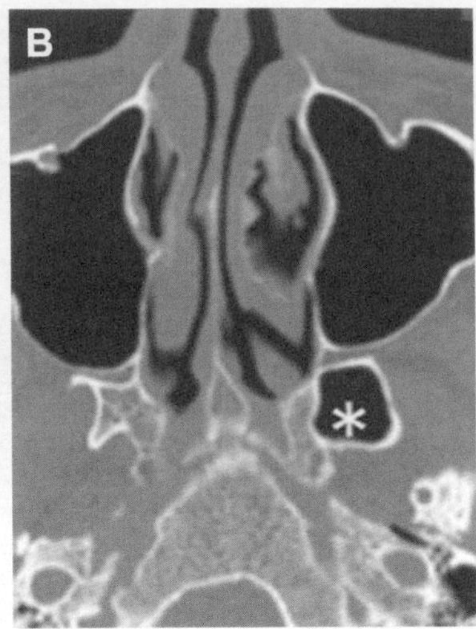

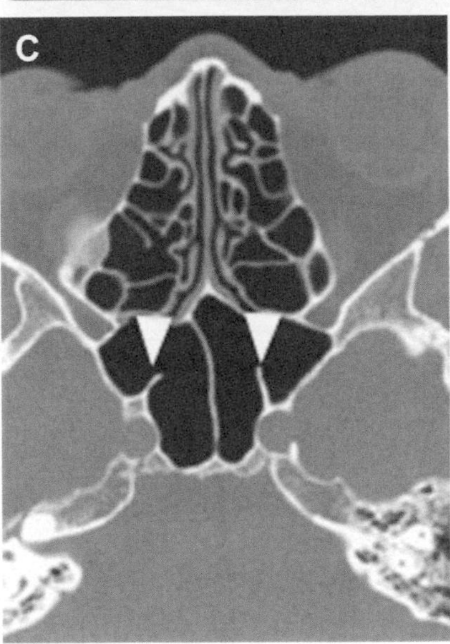

Fig. 5. Hyperpneumatized sphenoid sinus. (*A*) Coronal CT. (*B, C*) Axial CT. Coronal CT shows sphenoid pneumatization extending bilaterally over the line between vidian canal and the foramen rotundum (*dashed lines* in *A*), forming the lateral recess (LR). Left foramen rotundum (FR) protrudes into the sphenoid sinus. The pneumatization also extends to left pterygoid process (*asterisk* in *B*). Accessory septa insert into the carotid canals bilaterally (*arrowheads* in *C*).

originates from ethmoid sinus.[9] Sinonasal undifferentiated carcinoma originates from the nasal cavity and ethmoid sinus, and is associated with aggressive features with a rapidly progressive course.[11] Lymphoepithelial carcinoma, a rare tumor, is the counterpart of undifferentiated nasopharyngeal carcinoma, often arising from the nasal cavity in Southeast Asian populations, and favorably responds to radiotherapy and radiochemotherapy.[9]

The tumor-nodes-metastasis (TNM) classification and staging system, based on the 7th edition of *AJCC Staging Manual* from the American Joint Committee on Cancer (AJCC),

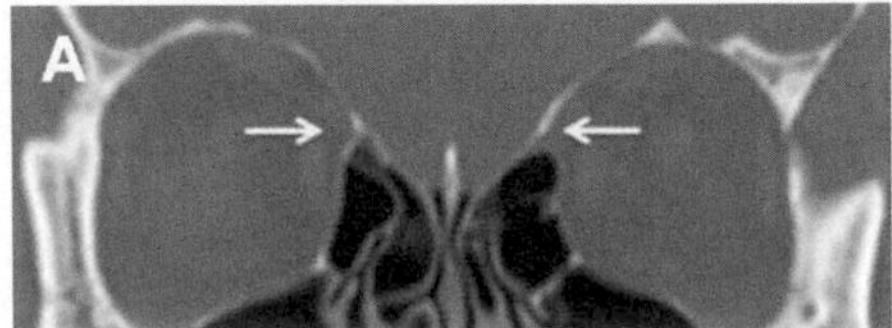

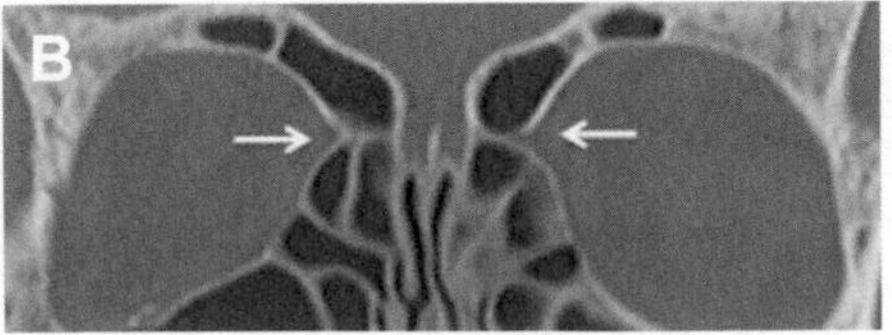

Fig. 6. Anterior ethmoid canal. The anterior ethmoid canal (*arrow*) courses in the ethmoidal roof to the lateral lamella (*A*). It occasionally traverses the ethmoid air cells in a mesentery below the roof, which increases the risk of injury to the anterior ethmoid artery (*B*).

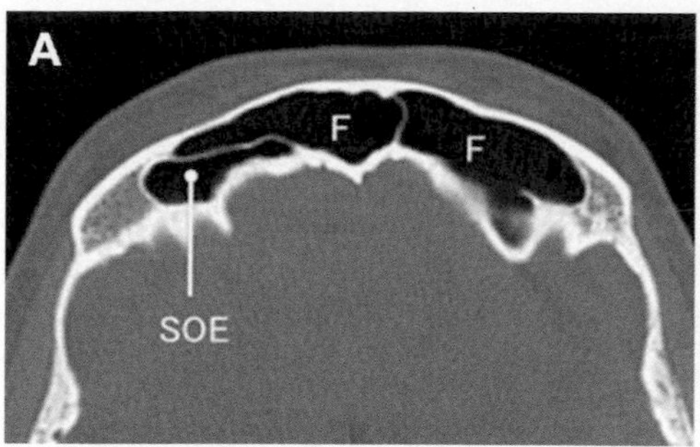

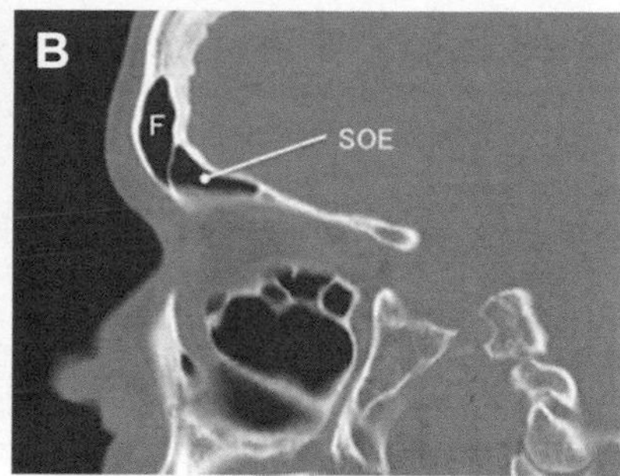

Fig. 7. Supraorbital ethmoid air cell (SOE). (*A*) Axial CT. (*B*) Sagittal CT. The supraorbital ethmoid air cell can cause disorientation during endoscopic surgery resulting in inadvertent skull base injury. F, frontal sinus.

is available for carcinomas of the maxillary sinus, nasal cavity, and ethmoid sinus but not for those in the frontal and sphenoid sinuses due to their rarity.

Sinonasal tumor invasion to the skull base, dura, brain parenchyma, and orbit affects the tumor staging for both maxillary and nasoethmoid sinus cancer and is classified into tumor stage (T)-3, T4a, or T4b (**Table 1**), which translate to stage III, IVA, or IVB disease, respectively.[12]

CT provides detailed information about bone destruction. MR imaging is superior in distinguishing tumor from inflammatory changes and fluid retention (**Figs. 9–11**). Delineation of tumor margins is best accomplished by contrast-enhanced MR imaging sequences. Aggressive sinonasal carcinomas usually present a T2WI-intermediate signal with moderate enhancement, whereas sinonasal mucosa shows T2WI hyperintense signal with avid contrast enhancement. Secretion within obstructive sinus demonstrates variable signal intensities on both T1WI and T2WI sequences, depending on the protein content but lacks contrast enhancement. Low-grade adenocarcinoma and salivary gland-type carcinomas can exhibit T2WI hyperintense signal due to abundant mucinous matrix and mimic benign tumors.[13]

Even with apparent bony erosion of the skull base or orbital wall, smooth bowing of a tumor interface suggests that the tumor is still limited by the periosteal layer of dura mater, orbital periosteum, or periorbital fascia.[9,13,14] MR imaging can demonstrate these structures as a hypointense hairline (see **Fig. 9**). In contrast, irregular or ill-defined margin is highly suggestive of tumor infiltration (see **Figs. 10** and **11**).[13,15] Nodular dural thickening and pial enhancement are highly suggestive of dural invasion (see **Fig. 10**).[13–16] Brain parenchymal or pial involvement causes vasogenic edema and parenchymal enhancement (see **Figs. 10** and **11**).[13–15]

Esthesioneuroblastoma Esthesioneuroblastoma, an uncommon tumor, arises from the olfactory epithelium in the upper third of the nasal cavity and frequently extends intracranially (**Fig. 12**).[9,17] Although not specific, marginal cysts adjacent to the intracranial tumor are characteristic imaging findings (**Fig. 13**).[18,19]

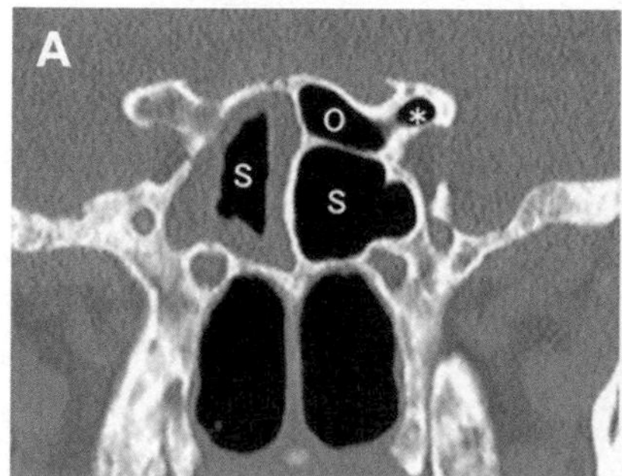

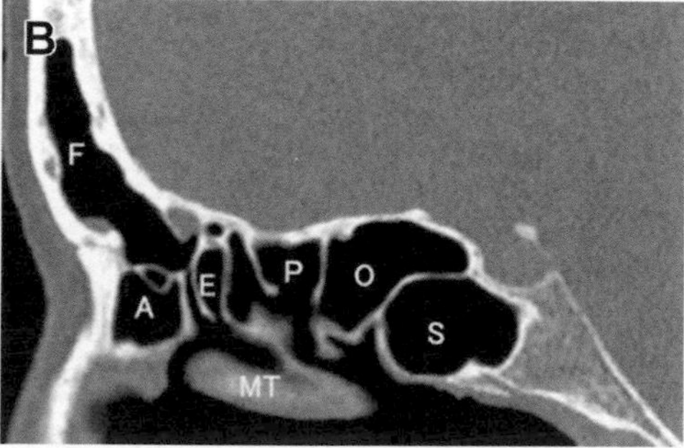

Fig. 8. Onodi cell (sphenoethmoidal cell) and pneumatized anterior clinoid process. (*A*) Coronal CT. (*B*) Sagittal CT. Coronal and sagittal CT images demonstrate left Onodi cell (O) above the left sphenoid sinus (S). Left pneumatized anterior clinoid process (*asterisk* in *A*) is also seen on coronal CT. Mucosal thickening presents in the right sphenoid sinus. A, agger nasi cell; E, ethmoid bulla; F, frontal sinus; MT, middle turbinate; P, posterior ethmoid cell.

Table 1
Tumor staging of sinonasal carcinoma relating to skull base and orbital invasion

	Maxillary Carcinoma	Nasoethmoid Carcinoma
Skull base invasion		
Cribriform plate	T4a	T3
Minimal extension to anterior cranial fossa	—	T4a
Dura, brain, middle cranial fossa, clivus cranial nerve except CNV2	T4b	T4b
Orbital invasion		
Medial wall/ inferior wall	T3	T3
Anterior orbital contents	T4a	T4a
Orbital apex	T4b	T4b

The presence of intratumoral cysts, necrosis, and hemorrhage can affect the signal intensity and homogeneity of contrast enhancement.[19,20]

Similar to sinonasal carcinomas, presence of intracranial and orbital extension leads to worse outcome.[21,22] Kadish or modified Kadish classification is used for staging of esthesioneuroblastoma (**Box 1**).[23–27] In these staging systems, Kadish stage C, modified Kadish stage C-D (orbital and intracranial extension or metastases), is related to unfavorable prognosis.[24,28–32] The occurrence of cervical lymph node metastasis is 5% at the initial presentation, whereas the cumulative rate of late lymph node metastasis is 23.4%.[24,33,34]

Surgical resection with or without irradiation is generally an optimal treatment strategy. Chemotherapy is a valid option for patients presenting with high-grade pathologic condition, residual tumor, metastases, or recurrence.[32] Long-term follow-up is necessary because late recurrences are reported.[22,33]

Lymphoma Sinonasal lymphomas are mostly non-Hodgkin lymphomas and diffuse large B-cell

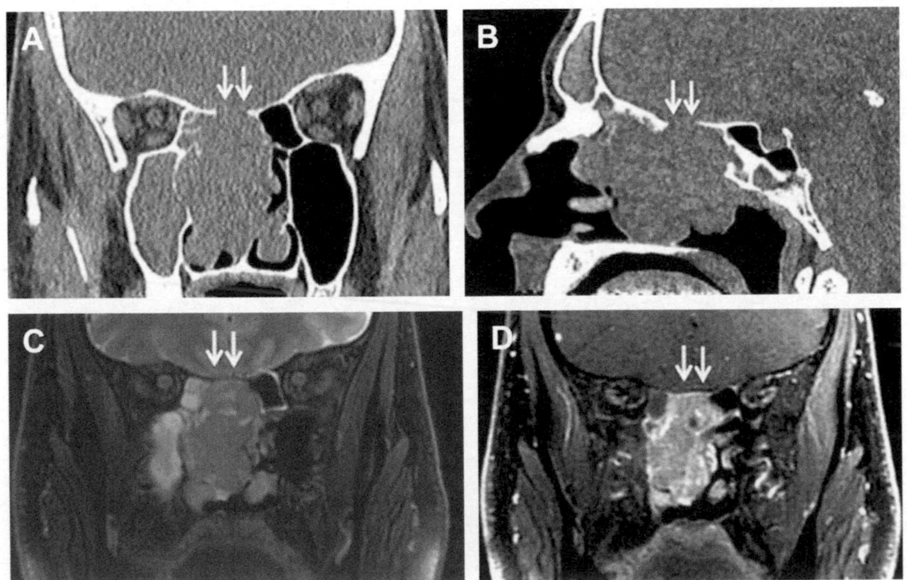

Fig. 9. Lymphoepithelial carcinoma. (*A*) Coronal CT. (*B*) Sagittal CT. (*C*) Coronal fat-saturated T2WI. (*D*) Coronal fat-saturated contrast-enhanced T1WI. Coronal and sagittal CT images show opacification in the right sinonasal cavities with bone destruction of the planum ethmoidal (*arrows* in *A, B*), nasal septum, and ethmoid cells. (*B*) MR imaging demonstrates tumor limited in the nasal cavity. A thin hypointense line between the tumor and brain parenchyma (*arrows* in *C, D*) indicates intact periosteum. T2WI hyperintense signal within the right ethmoid and maxillary cells indicates obstructive sinusitis.

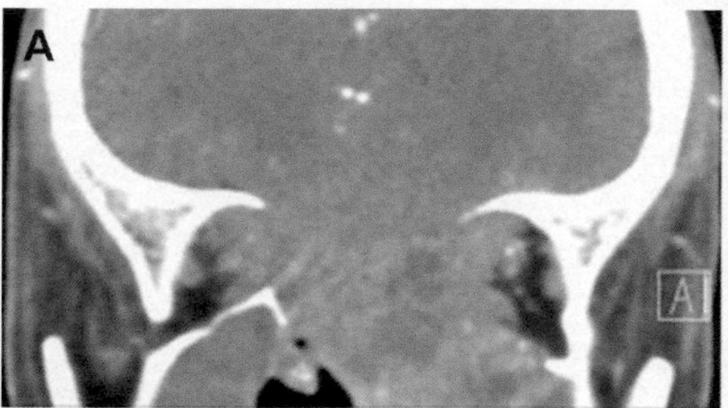

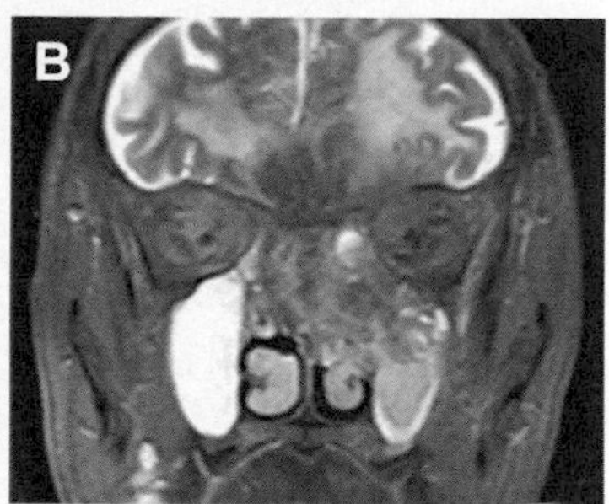

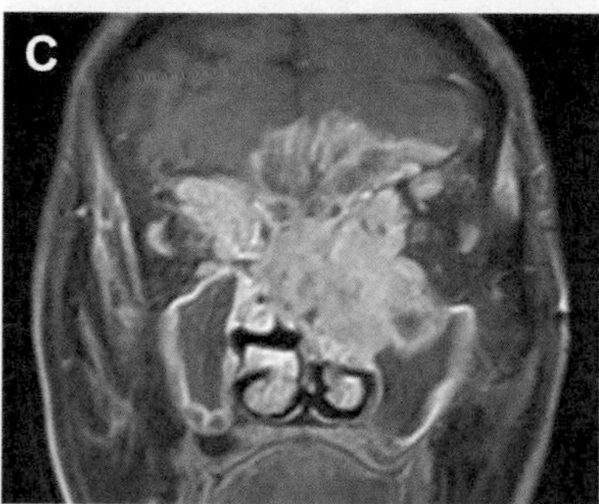

Fig. 10. Advanced sinonasal squamous cell carcinoma. (*A*) Coronal contrast-enhanced CT. (*B*) Coronal fat-saturated T2WI. (*C*) Coronal fat-saturated contrast-enhanced T1WI. (*A*) Coronal contrast-enhanced CT shows heterogeneously enhanced tumor involving bilateral orbit and anterior skull base with extensive bone destruction. (*B*) T2WI shows hypointense tumor involving bilateral frontal lobes with vasogenic cerebral edema. (*C*) Contrast-enhanced T1WI delineates the extent of the tumor. Heterogeneous enhancement within the tumor is due to presence of intratumoral necrosis.

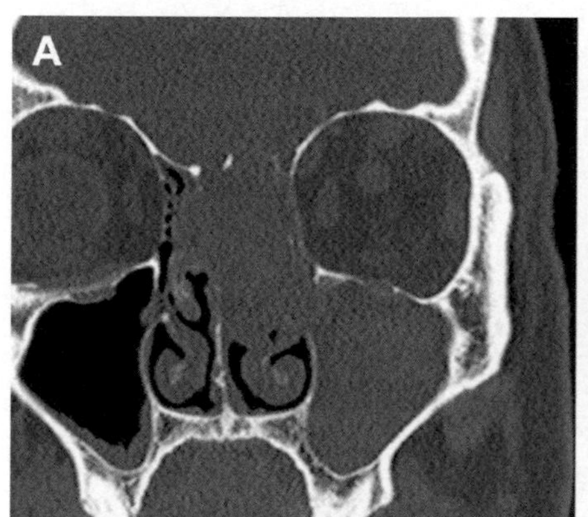

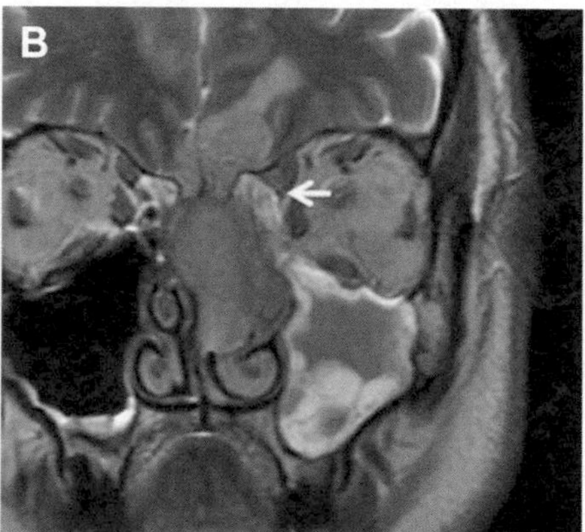

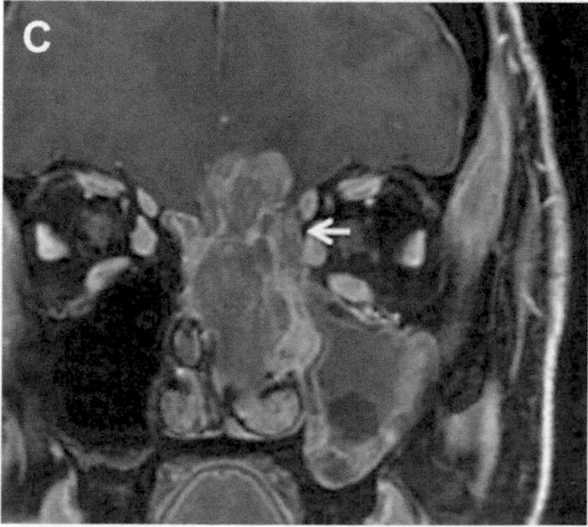

Fig. 11. Advanced sinonasal undifferentiated carcinoma. (*A*) Coronal contrast-enhanced CT. (*B*) Coronal T2WI. (*C*) Coronal fat-saturated contrast-enhanced T1WI. (*A*) Coronal CT shows opacification in the left nasal cavity and maxillary sinus with the destruction of the skull base and nasal septum. (*B*) On MR imaging, the left nasal tumor involving the anterior skull base is differentiated from the edematous mucosa and fluid in the maxillary and ethmoid sinus. T2WI hyperintense signal in the left ethmoid sinus can be confused with a tumor on contrast-enhanced T1WI alone (*arrow* in *B*, *C*).

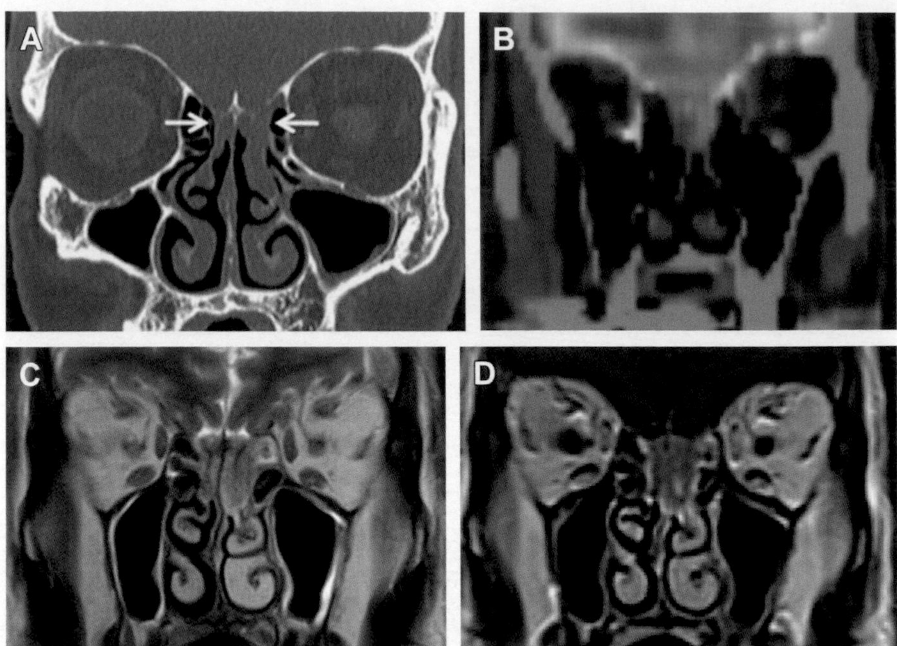

Fig. 12. Esthesioneuroblastoma. (*A*) Coronal CT. (*B*) Coronal fluorodeoxyglucose (FDG) PET/CT. (*C*) Coronal T2WI. (*D*) Coronal contrast-enhanced T1WI. Coronal CT shows subtle erosion of the cribriform plate with minimal mucosal thickening along the vertical lamella of middle turbinates (*arrows* in *A*). FDG PET/CT shows abnormal uptake corresponding to the lesion (*B*). The lesion shows intermediate T2WI signal intensity with moderate enhancement involving olfactory bulbs (*C, D*).

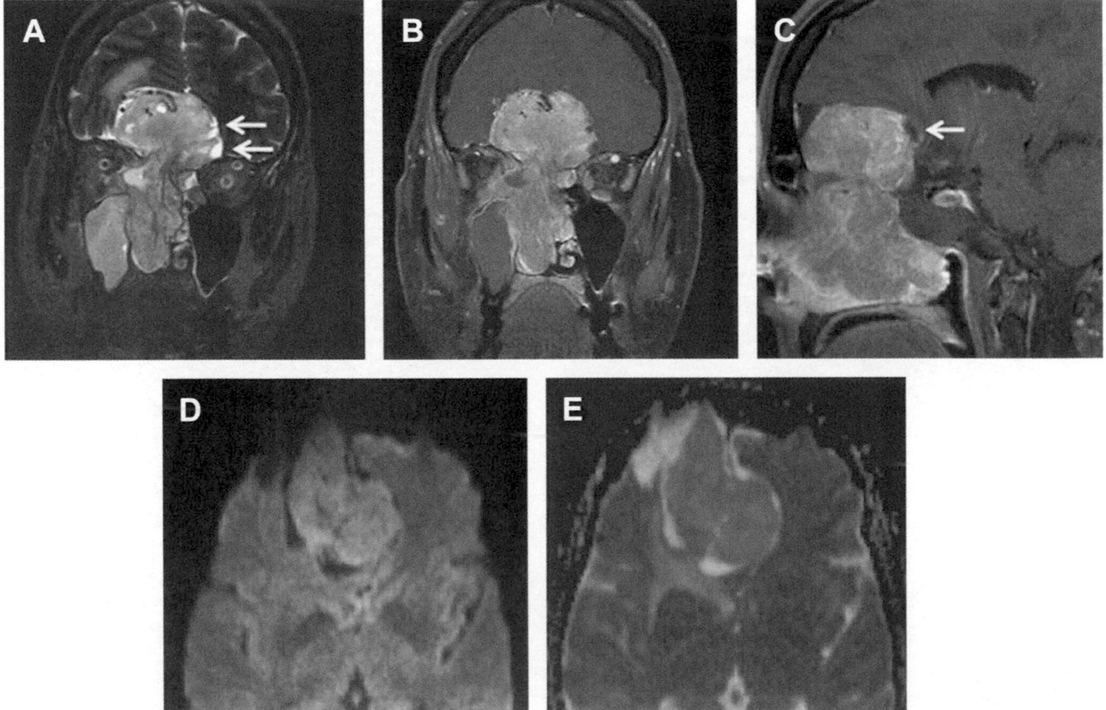

Fig. 13. Esthesioneuroblastoma with peritumoral cysts. (*A*) Coronal fat-saturated T2WI. (*B*) Coronal fat-saturated contrast-enhanced T1WI. (*C*) Sagittal fat-saturated contrast-enhanced T1WI. (*D*) Diffusion-weighted image (DWI). (*E*) Apparent diffusion coefficient (ADC) map. Esthesioneuroblastoma in the right nasal cavity shows intermediate signal intensity on T2WI with heterogeneous moderate enhancement (*A–C*). It extends to the anterior cranial fossa and right orbit. Peritumoral cysts adjacent to the intracranial component are suggestive of esthesioneuroblastoma (*arrows* in *A, C*). The tumor shows hyperintensity to the gray matter on DWI, and the mean ADC value is 1.345×10^{-3} m/s.

Box 1
Staging system for esthesioneuroblastoma

Kadish

A. Tumor confined to nasal cavity
B. Tumor involved nasal cavity and paranasal sinuses
C. Tumor spread beyond the nasal cavity and paranasal sinuses

Modified Kadish

A. Tumor confined to nasal cavity
B. Tumor involved nasal cavity and paranasal sinuses
C. Tumor extent beyond nasal cavity and paranasal sinuses, including involvement of the cribriform plate, base of skull, orbit, or intracranial cavity
D. Tumor with metastasis to cervical lymph nodes or distant sites

lymphoma (DLBCL) is the most common subtype. Lymphoma frequently occurs in the maxillary sinus as a discrete mass with homogeneous contrast enhancement, bone remodeling, and smooth erosion.[35] Due to its high cellularity, lymphoma shows high-attenuation on CT, low-to intermediate signal intensity on T2WI, and diffusion restriction on diffusion-weighted image (DWI) (**Fig. 14**).

Extranodal natural killer/T-cell lymphoma (ENKTL) is the second most common subtype having a high predilection to Asians.[10] It often affects the nasal cavity and resembles chronic sinusitis with mucosal swelling in the early stage.[14] As the lesion grows, a soft tissue mass with destructive change appears in the nasal septum, resulting in septum perforation (**Fig. 15**). Differential diagnosis of ENKTL includes squamous cell carcinoma, granulomatosis with polyangiitis, sarcoidosis, invasive fungal sinusitis, and cocaine abuse.

Better prognosis has been reported in sinonasal DLBCL with 5-year disease-specific survival rates at 72.8% compared with ENKTL at 38.4%.[10]

Melanoma Sinonasal melanoma most often arises from the nasal septum or turbinates.[14] Melanoma typically presents T1WI hyperintense signal due to intratumoral hemorrhage and paramagnetic effects of melanin, although 10% to 30% of sinonasal melanomas are amelanotic and exhibit nonspecific T1WI hypointense and T2WI hyperintense signal (**Fig. 16**). Contrast enhancement might be difficult to observe on MR imaging for melanotic melanoma due to intrinsic T1WI

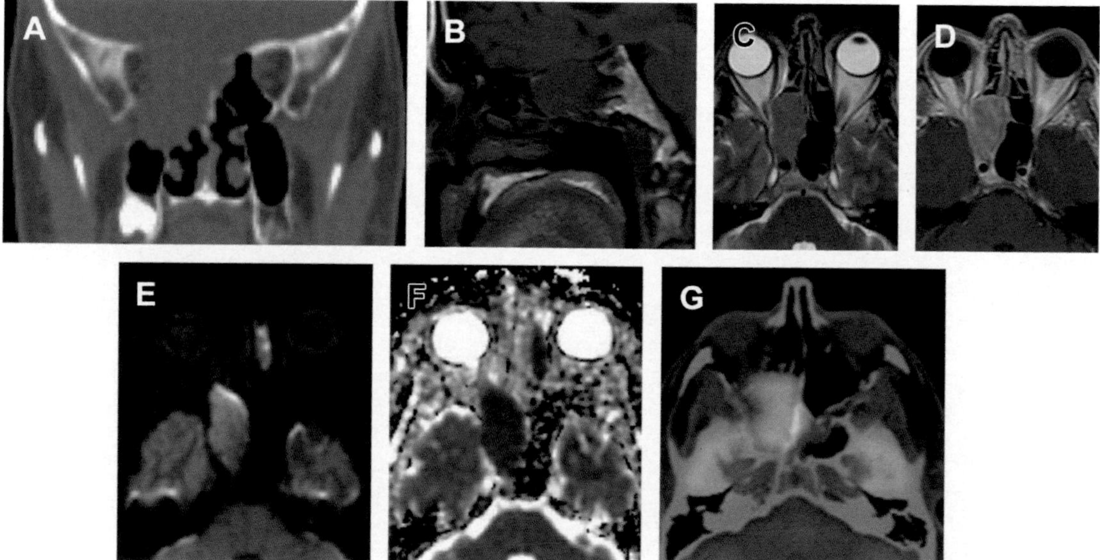

Fig. 14. DLBCL in the sphenoid sinus. (*A*) Coronal CT. (*B*) Sagittal T1WI. (*C*) Axial T2WI. (*D*) Axial contrast-enhanced T1WI. (*E*) DWI. (*F*) ADC map. (*G*) Axial FDG PET/CT. Coronal CT shows soft tissue density mass in the right sphenoid sinus involving the orbit and maxillary sinus with extensive skull base destruction (*A*). Subtle linear hypointense-signal on sagittal T1WI indicates the periosteum on the planum sphenoidale containing the tumor invasion (*B*). The tumor shows T2WI intermediate signal with moderate enhancement and marked diffusion restriction (ADC: 457×10^{-6} m/s), suggesting high cellularity (*C–F*). PET/CT demonstrates avid FDG uptake corresponded to the sphenoid lesion (*G*).

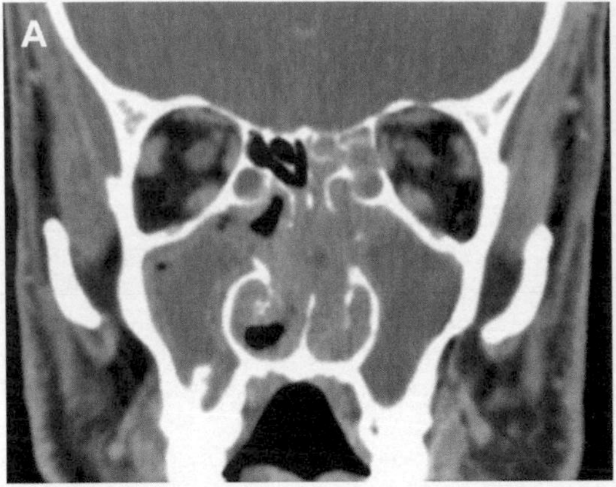

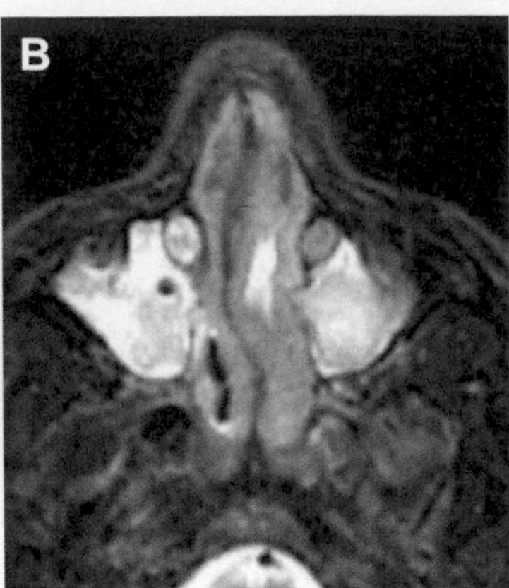

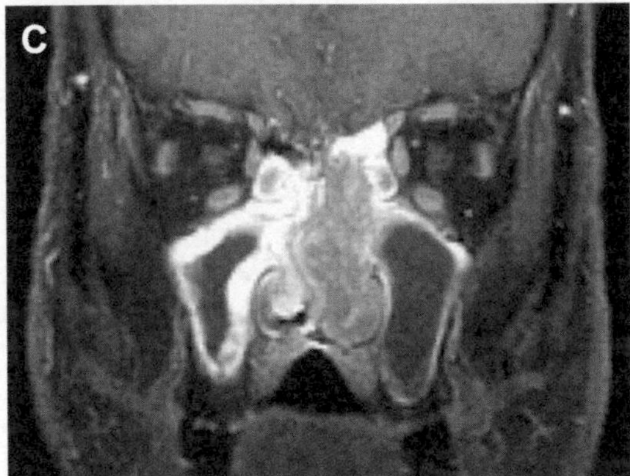

Fig. 15. ENKTL in the nasal cavity. (*A*) Coronal contrast-enhanced CT. (*B*) Axial fat-saturated T2WI. (*C*) Coronal fat-saturated contrast-enhanced T1WI. Coronal contrast-enhanced CT (*A*) shows mild enhanced soft tissue in the nasal cavity and left ethmoid sinus with nasal septum perforation. The lesion presents intermediate T2WI signal intensity with moderate enhancement (*B, C*). Avid mucosal enhancement indicates tumor contained within the nasal cavity (*C*).

hyperintensity. Lymph node metastasis is common (40%), and perineural extension and hematogenous metastasis are also reported.[3,36]

Involvement to adjacent muscle, skull base, and orbit is a negative survival predictor.[37] According to the 2010 AJCC staging system for mucosal melanoma of the head and neck, the mucosal disease is already considered as T3 regardless of the tumor size.[12] Skull base and intracranial involvement constitute a T4b disease.

Standard treatment of melanoma is surgical resection followed by radiotherapy. Chemotherapy is a treatment option for patients with metastasis or recurrence. The prognosis is poor with 5-year survival of 20% to 30%.[38]

Sinonasal or benign neoplasm

Juvenile nasopharyngeal angiofibroma Juvenile angiofibroma is a highly vascular benign tumor with a strong predilection for adolescent males. It most often arises from the sphenopalatine foramen and extends laterally to the infratemporal fossa through the pterygopalatine fissure and superiorly to the sphenoid sinus and skull base. Tumor invasion into the sphenoid bone is associated with a high risk of residual tumor after surgery and recurrence (**Fig. 17**).[39] Although intracranial extension is uncommon, the middle cranial fossa is the most frequent site through the skull base foramina and fissures (**Fig. 18**). Due to its hypervascular nature, it exhibits avid enhancement and signal voids within and along the periphery of the tumor (see **Fig. 18**).

Preoperative embolization is often performed to decrease intraoperative blood loss. The internal maxillary artery and the ascending pharyngeal artery are the common main feeders. In case of intracranial extension, blood supply comes from the branches of the internal carotid artery.[40] Transnasal endoscopic resection has become an established treatment option for relatively small juvenile angiofibroma without intracranial extension.

Sinonasal papilloma Sinonasal papilloma is histopathologically classified into 3 types: inverted (62%), exophytic (32%), and oncocytic (6%) papillomas. Malignant transformation occurs in approximately 10% of inverted papillomas and 4% to 17% of oncocytic papillomas but is exceedingly rare in exophytic papillomas.[41–43]

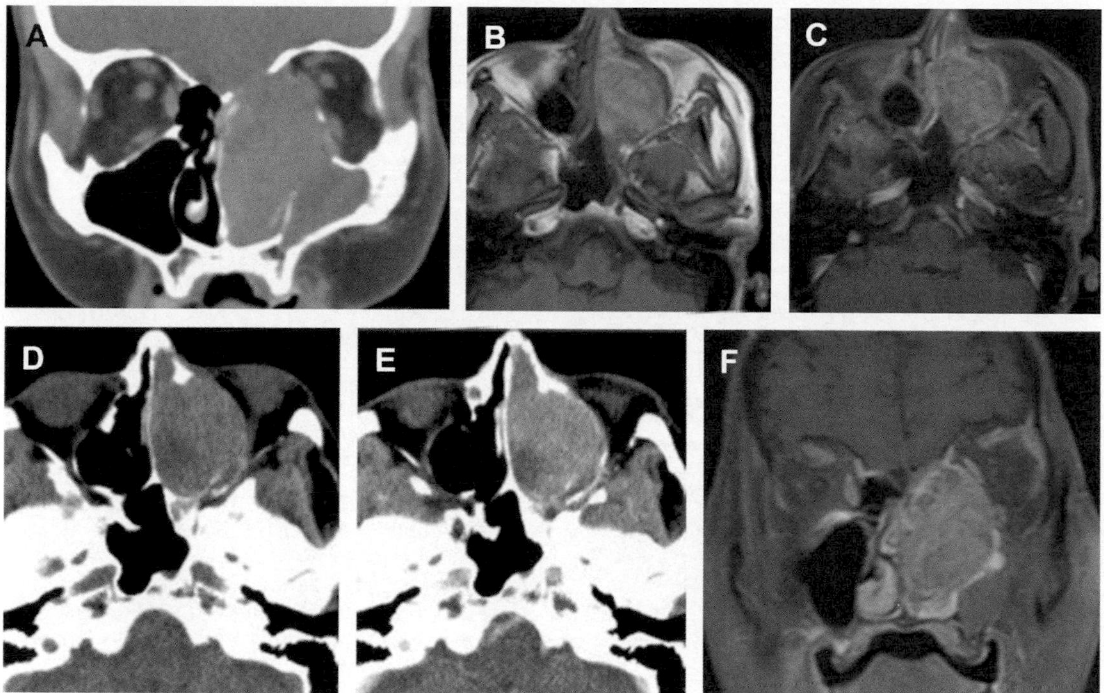

Fig. 16. Sinonasal malignant melanoma. (*A*) Coronal CT. (*B*) Axial T1WI. (*C*) Axial fat-saturated contrast-enhanced T1WI. (*D*) Axial CT. (*E*) Axial contrast-enhanced CT. (*F*) Coronal fat-saturated contrast-enhanced T1WI. Coronal CT (*A*) demonstrates a large expansile tumor in the left nasal cavity with destruction of the adjacent lamina papyracea, medial orbital floor, medial maxillary wall, and cribriform plate. T1WI-hyperintense signal in the tumor is suggestive of melanotic melanoma (*B*). Contrast enhancement in the tumor is difficult to affirm on contrast-enhanced T1WI alone because of the intrinsic T1WI hyperintensity (*C*). A combination of plain and contrast-enhanced CT is useful to confirm the enhancement (*D, E*). Smooth bowing of the interface with the orbital contents suggests the periorbital fascia still contains the tumor infiltration.

CT usually shows a localized soft tissue mass in the early stage and extensive soft tissue opacification with bone remodeling in the advanced stage.

In inverted papilloma cases, T2WI and contrast-enhanced T1WI show a convoluted cerebriform pattern that is the combination of linear or curvilinear hyperintense and hypointense

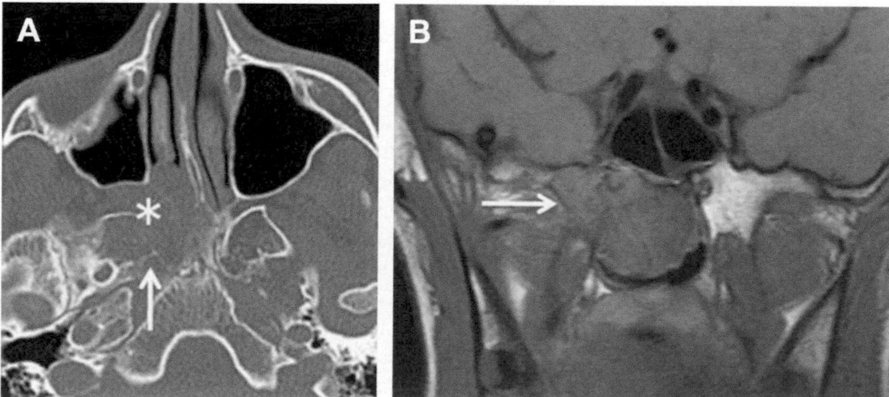

Fig. 17. Juvenile angiofibroma in a 14-year-old boy. (*A*) Axial CT. (*B*) Coronal T1WI. CT shows soft tissue density mass (*asterisk* in *A*) in right sphenopalatine foramen extending laterally to pterygopalatine fossa. The right pterygoid process demonstrates a lytic change on CT, and decreased signal intensity on T1WI, suggesting tumor infiltration (*arrows* in *A, B*).

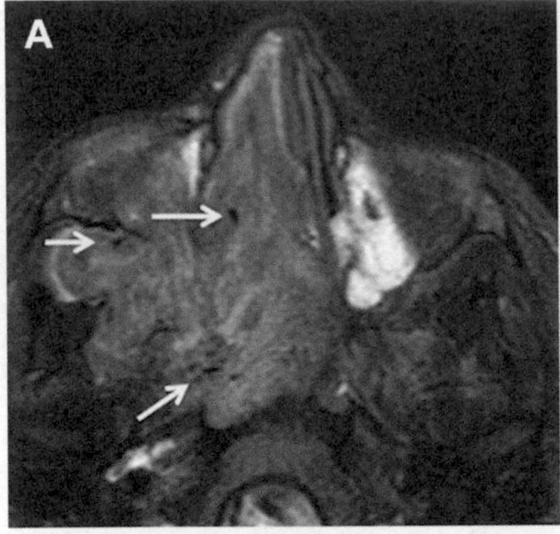

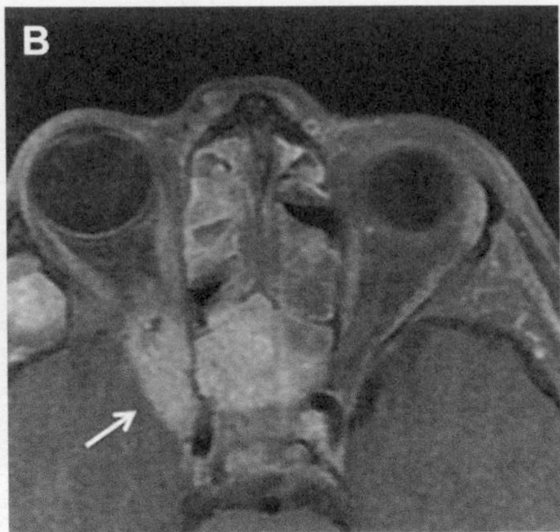

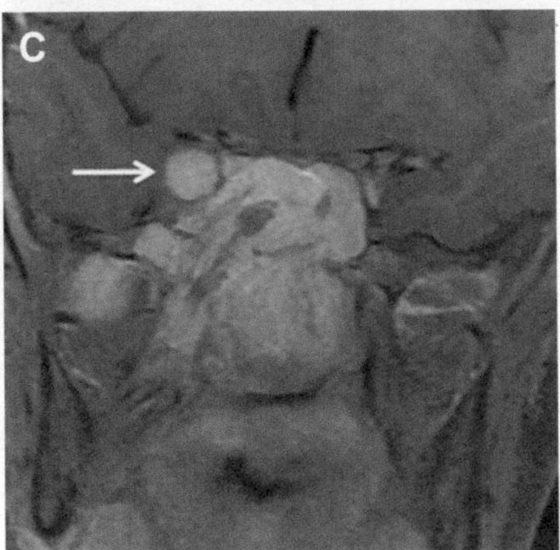

Fig. 18. Juvenile angiofibroma in a 13-year-old boy. (*A*) Axial fat-saturated T2WI. (*B*) Axial fat-saturated contrast-enhanced T1WI. (*C*) Coronal fat-saturated contrast-enhanced T1WI. T2WI hyperintense mass extends anterior to the nasal cavity, posterior to the nasopharynx, and lateral to the infratemporal fossa and maxillary sinus. Multiple flow-related signal voids in the tumor suggest hypervascularity (*arrows* in *A*). Contrast-enhanced T1WI shows intracranial tumor extension through superior orbital fissure (*arrows* in *B*, *C*).

striations in the solid components of the tumor (**Fig. 19**).[44]

Identification of the tumor origin is important for the complete resection because the inverted papilloma exhibits a centrifugal growth pattern.[45] It most often arises from the lateral nasal wall (52.6%), followed by the maxillary (25%) and anterior ethmoid sinuses (21.6%). Exophytic papillomas originate from the lower anterior nasal septum.[41,45] Focal hyperostosis of the sinonasal wall is a useful finding to identify its origin (see **Fig. 19**).[45]

Krouse classification (T1 to T4) is the most widely accepted staging system for inverted papilloma.[46] Intracranial extension is rare (1.8%) and classified as T4.[47,48]

The diagnosis of synchronous carcinoma is often difficult because it is distributed widely in the papilloma as multiple small foci.[44,49] However, presence of synchronous carcinoma is suggested when the following findings are present: extrasinonasal extension with aggressive bone destruction, T2WI hypointense signal with loss of convoluted cerebriform pattern, intratumoral necrosis, and lymph node metastasis.[44,49]

Surgical excision is the treatment of choice and local recurrence is often seen in 2 to 3 years after surgery.[41] According to a recent study, the recurrence rate of inverted papilloma is 25.3%.[43]

Infectious disease

Fungal rhinosinusitis Fungal rhinosinusitis (FRS) is classified into invasive and noninvasive FRS. Invasive sinusitis includes acute (fulminant), chronic, and granulomatous, whereas noninvasive includes mycetoma and allergic FRS.

Acute invasive fungal sinusitis (AIFRS) presents a rapidly progressive course (<4 weeks), whereas chronic and granulomatous FRS have an indolent course (>4–12 weeks). Acute and chronic invasive FRS is common in immunocompromised patients and histopathologically shows fungal hyphae in the affected tissue. In contrast, granulomatous invasive FRS predominantly occurs in immunocompetent hosts, forming noncaseating granulomas with scanty fungal hyphae.

AIFRS often involves the middle turbinate as the initial site. It can rapidly extend to the orbit, skull base, and intracranial cavities. Once the intracranial contents are involved, the mortality rate is

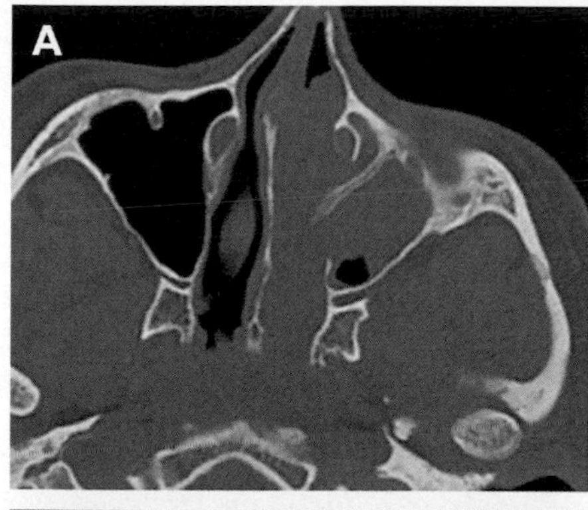

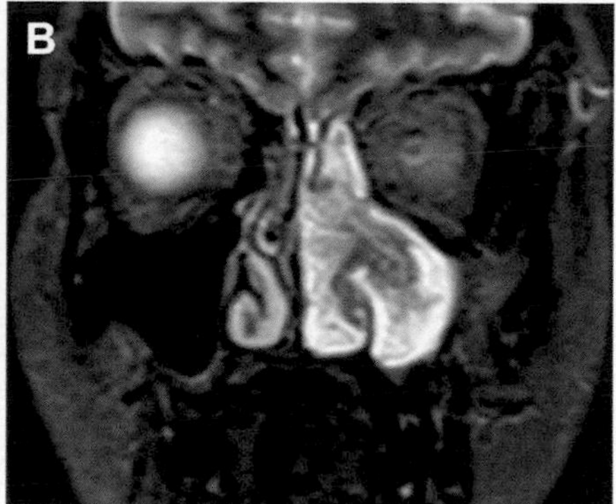

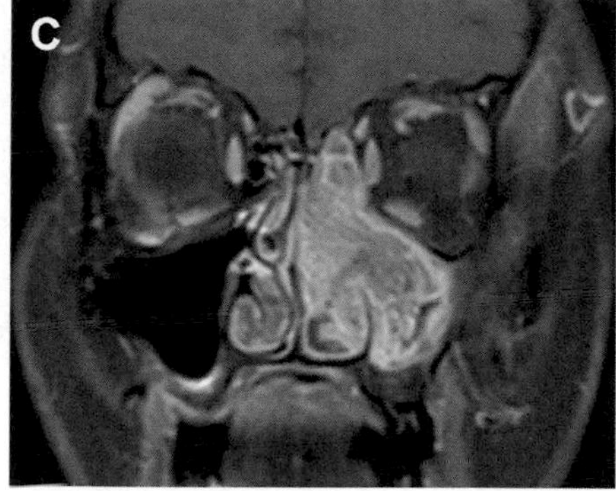

Fig. 19. Inverted papilloma. (*A*) Axial CT. (*B*) Coronal fat-saturated T2WI. (*C*) Coronal fat-saturated contrast-enhanced T1WI. Axial CT shows a soft tissue density mass filling the left maxillary sinus and nasal cavity. A thick bony stalk arising from the anterior wall of the maxillary sinus is likely the site of tumor attachment. T2WI and contrast-enhanced T1WI demonstrate convoluted cerebriform pattern in the tumor on consistent with inverted papilloma (*B*, *C*).

very high. Fungal invasion of the vasculature can cause vasculitis, thrombosis, infarction, necrosis, hemorrhage, and pseudoaneurysm. Due to profound tissue necrosis, AIFRS exhibits lack of mucosal enhancement in the affected middle turbinate (**Fig. 20**). As the disease progresses, invasive FRS shows progressive bone destruction and extension to the orbit and the intracranial compartment. Timely wide surgical debridement and intravenous administration of antifungals are critical for cure of invasive FRS.

Mucocele

Sinonasal mucoceles occur with obstruction of the sinus ostium followed by the continuous collection of mucus secretion, leading to expansile

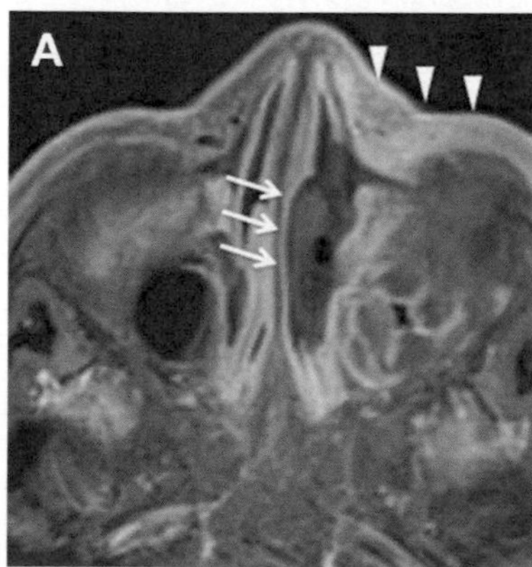

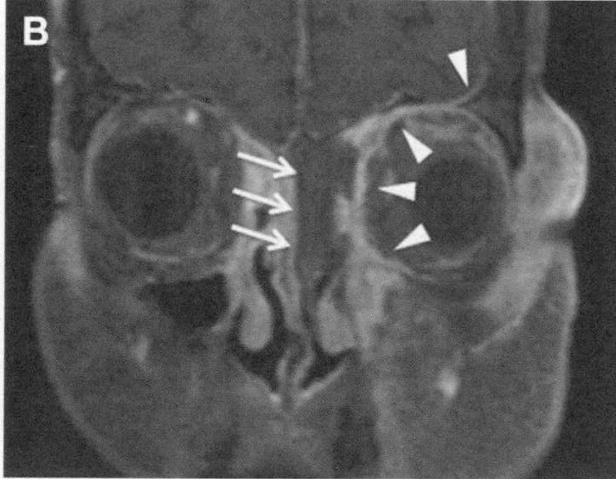

Fig. 20. Acute invasive fungal sinusitis in a patient with immunocompromised state presenting progressive orbital swelling. (*A*) Axial fat-saturated contrast-enhanced T1WI. (*B*) Coronal fat-saturated contrast-enhanced T1WI. Contrast-enhanced T1WIs show the lack of mucosal enhancement (*arrows* on *A* and *B*) of the left middle turbinate and left ethmoid sinus suggesting tissue necrosis in the setting of invasive fungal sinusitis. In contrast, left subcutaneous facial tissue shows strong enhancement with swelling, indicating inflammatory extension (*arrowheads* in *A*). Dural thickening and enhancement are also evident, as well as periorbital fascia (*arrowheads* in *B*).

remodeling of the sinus wall. The frontal sinus is the most common site for mucoceles, followed by the ethmoid, maxillary, and sphenoid sinuses in a decreasing order of frequency.[50] Mucoceles usually present with symptoms due to mass effect upon the adjacent structures. When a mucocele is infected symptoms include those of acute sinus infection.

CT is useful to evaluate the bony remodeling and mass effect to neighboring structures (**Fig. 21**).

MR imaging can reveal extrasinus complications, such as orbital cellulitis, meningitis, and intracranial abscess, all of which are rare occurrences.

CT attenuation and MR imaging signal intensity of mucoceles are variable depending on its protein concentration. A contrast-enhanced study shows a thin rim of contrast enhancement with no enhancement of the contents of the mucocele otherwise. Nodular or mass-like enhancement suggests neoplastic lesion with a secondary mucocele.

Intrinsic Anterior Skull Base Lesions

Osseous and fibro-osseous lesions in sinonasal cavity and anterior skull base

The osseous and fibro-osseous lesions involving the ASB and sinonasal cavities include fibrous dysplasia (FD), osteoma, ossifying fibroma, and osteoblastoma. These lesions are often asymptomatic and incidentally found. Common symptoms include headache, nasal obstruction, anosmia, and craniofacial deformity. Facial swelling and pain may occur due to chronic sinusitis, and proptosis and diplopia can be seen when the lesion extends to the orbit.

The osseous element presents bony or ground-glass attenuation and the fibrous elements present soft tissue density on CT. On MR imaging, fibro-osseous lesions may exhibit highly complex signal characteristics. The osseous parts show T1WI and T2WI hypointense signals, whereas fibrous elements demonstrate T1WI hypointensity, variable T2WI signal, and moderate to marked

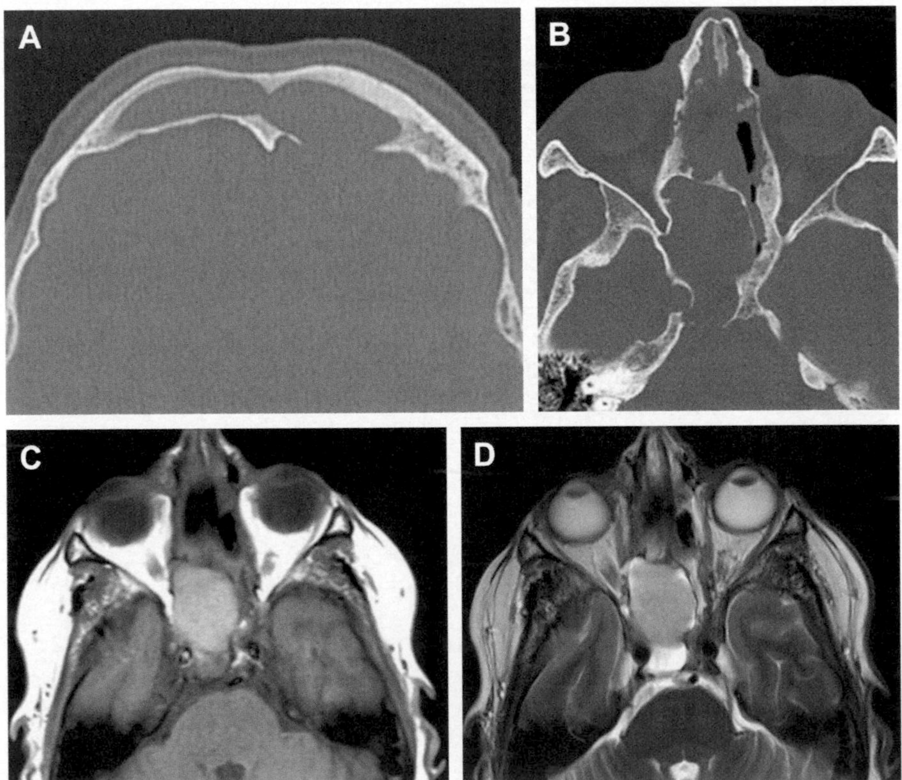

Fig. 21. (*A*) Frontal mucocele. (*B–D*) sphenoid mucocele. (*A*) Axial CT. (*B*) Axial CT. (*C*) Axial T1WI. (*D*) Axial T2WI. (*A*) Axial CT demonstrates opacification in bilateral frontal sinus with focal dehiscence at the left posterior wall. (*B–D*) Axial CT of another patient with a history of ethmoidectomy demonstrates expansile opacification in right sphenoid sinus with dehiscence at the posterior wall (*B*). Both T1WI and T2WI hyperintense signals in the sphenoid sinus suggest proteinous fluid consistent with mucocele (*C, D*).

contrast enhancement. T1WI hyperintensity may be present in the lesion, indicating fatty marrow.

Compressive cranial neuropathies due to involvement of neural foramina are a major indication for surgical intervention. Specifically, compression of the orbital apex and optic canal with acute or progressive visual deterioration requires immediate orbital decompression surgery. Fat-saturated T2WI and DWI may directly visualize the abnormal high signal intensity in the affected optic nerve (**Fig. 22**).

Fibrous dysplasia

FD is a developmental disorder affecting the medullary bone and histologically consists of varying amounts of spindle cell bundles (fibrous tissue) and immature woven trabecular bone (osseous tissue).[51,52] It presents as an expansile fibro-osseous lesion with an ill-defined border to the normal medullary bone, often involving multiple craniofacial bones diffusely.

It demonstrates combinations of 3 CT attenuation patterns (ground-glass, sclerotic, and cystic), depending on the ratio of fibrous to osseous tissue (see **Fig. 22**). Ground-glass pattern is the typical finding, reflecting histologic findings of mixture of the fibrous and osseous tissues.[51,53,54]

Variable MR imaging signal patterns of FD may be mistaken for malignant neoplasms. Radiologists must consider FD in the differential diagnosis for skull base lesions and recommend additional CT examination before biopsy, especially when the abnormal findings are incidentally found on MR imaging examinations.

Ossifying fibroma

Ossifying fibroma is a benign fibro-osseous tumor consisting of fibrous tissue containing variable amounts of mineralized material resembling bone and cementum.[55] It most frequently presents in the mandible in the second decade of life with a female predominance.[11,56]

Sinonasal ossifying fibroma is presumed to originate from ectopic periodontal membrane and frequently occurs in the ethmoid and maxillary sinuses.[57] Typically, it forms an oval or spherical expansile mass with a well-defined border. The osseous elements surround the fibrous tissue (**Fig. 23**). Multicystic appearance with fluid-fluid levels suggests secondary aneurysmal bone cysts.[11,58] Tumor vascularity should be evaluated preoperatively because severe bleeding can occur during surgery.[57]

Endoscopic surgery is safe and effective in managing ossifying fibromas but an external approach may be necessary for tumors located in the frontal sinus or larger tumors with intracranial extension.[57]

Osteoma

Osteoma is a benign lesion composed of mature bone with a predominantly lamellar structure. It

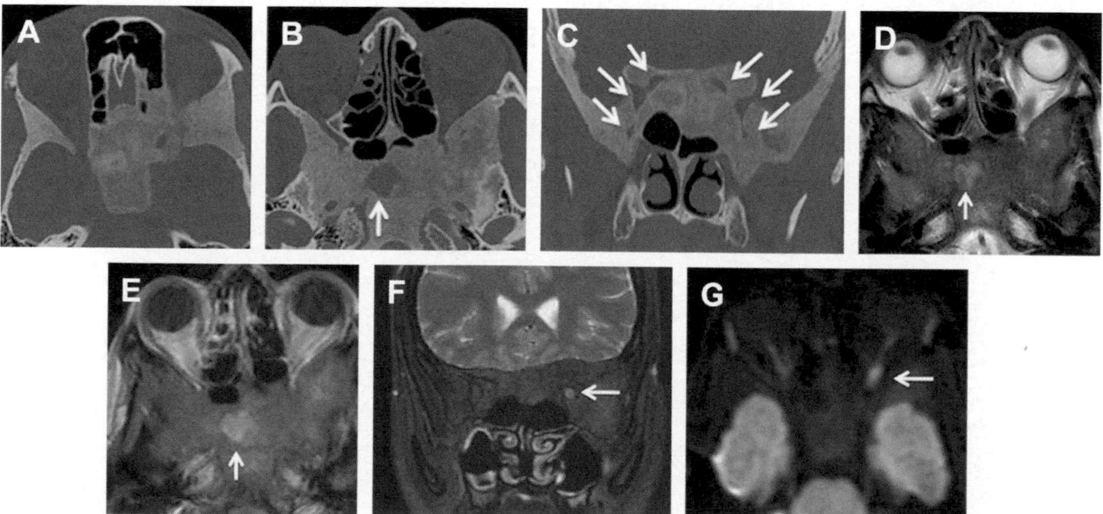

Fig. 22. A patient with FD (Fibrous Dysplasia) complaining of left visual disturbance. (*A*) Axial CT. (*B*) Axial. (*C*) Coronal CT. (*D*) Axial fat-saturated T2WI. (*E*) Axial fat-saturated contrast-enhanced T1WI. (*F*) Coronal fat-saturated T2WI. (*G*) Axial DWI. Axial and coronal CT (*A–C*) shows ground glass attenuated expansile lesion diffusely involving the sphenoid bones. There is severe stenosis in the optic canals, superior orbital fissures, and foramen rotundum bilaterally (*arrows* in *C*). Cystic attenuation area in the sphenoid body (*arrow* in *B*) presents T2WI hyperintensity with moderate contrast enhancement (*arrow* in *D*, *E*), indicating fibrous tissue. Left optic nerve (*arrow* in *F* and *G*) shows hyperintensity at the orbital apex on coronal T2WI and DWI, suggesting compressive neuropathy (*F*, *G*).

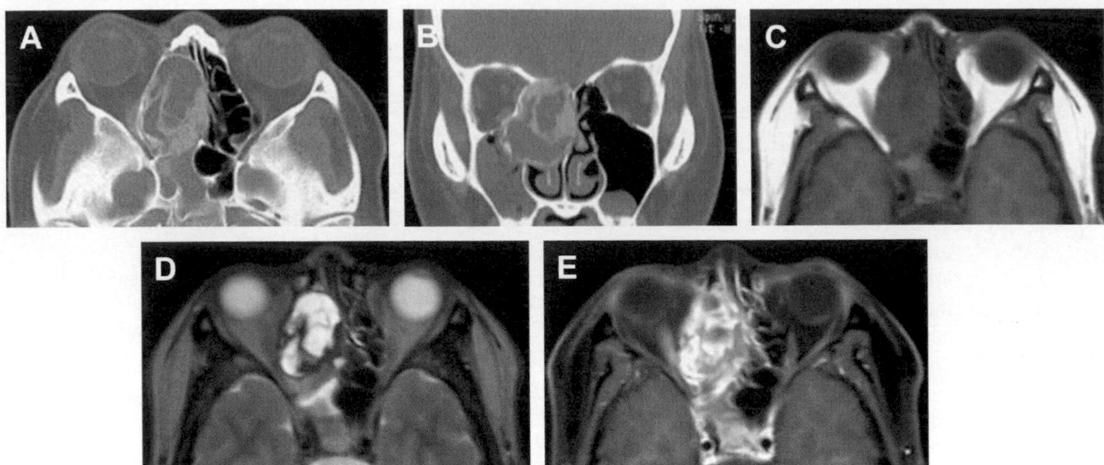

Fig. 23. Ossifying fibroma. (*A*) Axial CT. (*B*) Coronal CT. (*C*) Axial T1WI. (*D*) Axial T2WI. (*E*) Axial fat-saturated contrast-enhanced T1WI. Axial and coronal CT images demonstrate well-demarcated expansile mass involving the anterior skull base and medial orbital wall (*A*, *B*). The ossified area shows T2WI hypointensity and mild enhancement, whereas the central cystic attenuated areas show T1WI isointensity and T2WI hyperintensity and heterogeneous enhancement, indicating fibrous tissue (*C–E*).

occurs most commonly in the frontal and ethmoid sinuses and appears as a well-circumscribed, dense bony mass. It is generally asymptomatic though it occasionally obstructs sinus drainage pathway resulting in sinusitis or mucocele (**Fig. 24**). If that happens, endoscopic surgery is suitable for many cases. Combined external and endoscopic approach is necessary for lesions extending lateral to a sagittal plane passing through the lamina papyracea.[8,59,60]

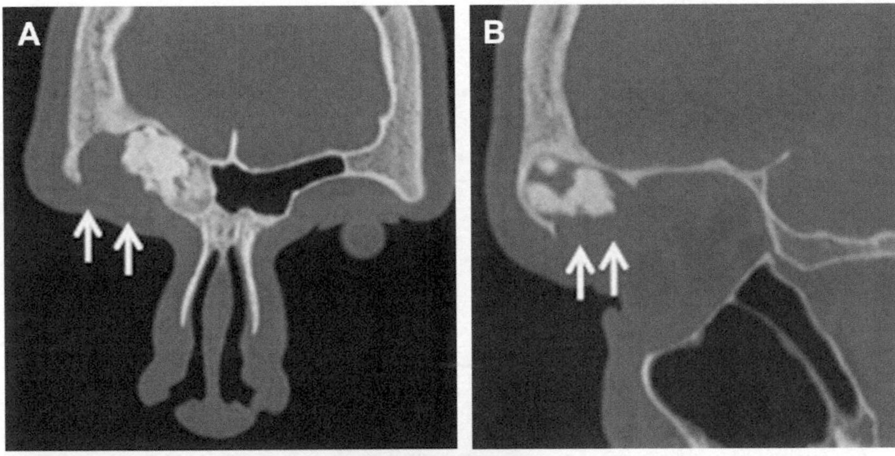

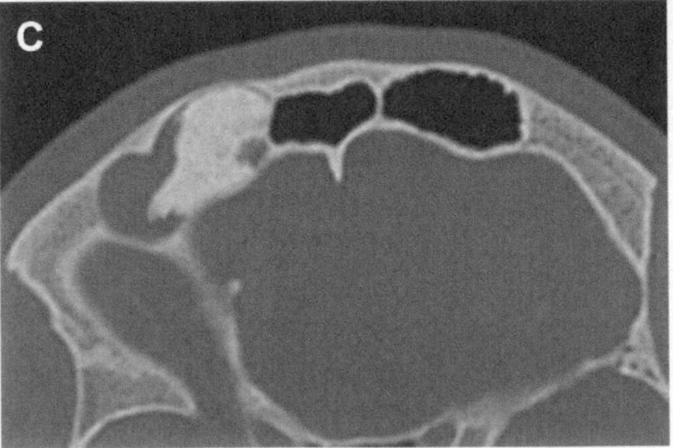

Fig. 24. Frontal osteoma with mucocele. A lobulated osteoma obstructs the right frontal ostium, resulting in mucocele with dehiscence of the inferior wall (*arrows* in *A*, *B*). Notice a well-defined bone expansion of right frontal sinus (*C*).

Intracranial Lesions Involving the Anterior Skull Base

Meningioma

ASB meningiomas are classified into olfactory groove meningioma, planum sphenoidale meningioma, or tuberculum sellae meningioma based on the site of the dural attachment (**Fig. 25**).[61] They appear as well-circumscribed, smooth, or lobulated lesions. Dural thickening, known as the dural tail sign, is suggestive of meningioma, although it may be present in other neoplastic and nonneoplastic lesions.[62] Hyperostosis is often present in the adjacent bone. CT demonstrates isoattenuating to hyperattenuating mass. Intratumoral calcifications may be present. On MR imaging, the tumor shows isointense signal to the cortex on T1WI and T2WI. Peritumoral edema can present in variable degrees. Imaging plays a significant role in evaluating the extent of the ASB meningioma and in determining the optimal surgical approach and reconstruction procedure. Complete resection may be difficult if the tumor involves vital structures, such as the cavernous sinuses and optic nerves, or encases the anterior cerebral arteries or internal carotid arteries.[63]

Nasal cephalocele

Cephalocele is a congenital or acquired herniation of intracranial contents through a skull defect and divided into encephalocele and meningocele. Whereas encephalocele contains brain tissue, meninges, and CSF, meningocele contains meninges and CSF only without brain tissue in its content. The frontoethmoidal (sincipital) and basal cephaloceles are associated with ASB and sinonasal cavity.

CT can demonstrate the extent of skull base defect (**Fig. 26**). MR imaging is suitable for determination of herniated content. Because the skull base ossification is not yet complete in infants, CT may overestimate the size of the bone defect.[14] Most of the ASB is completely ossified by 24 months.[64] Encephalocele contains (see **Fig. 26**) a herniated brain tissue, which is isointense to brain parenchyma. MR imaging allows a close inspection of the herniated contents in preoperative evaluation. Particularly, basal encephaloceles can contain critical structures, such as pituitary gland and hypothalamus, olfactory nerve, optic pathways, and branches of the anterior cerebral artery.

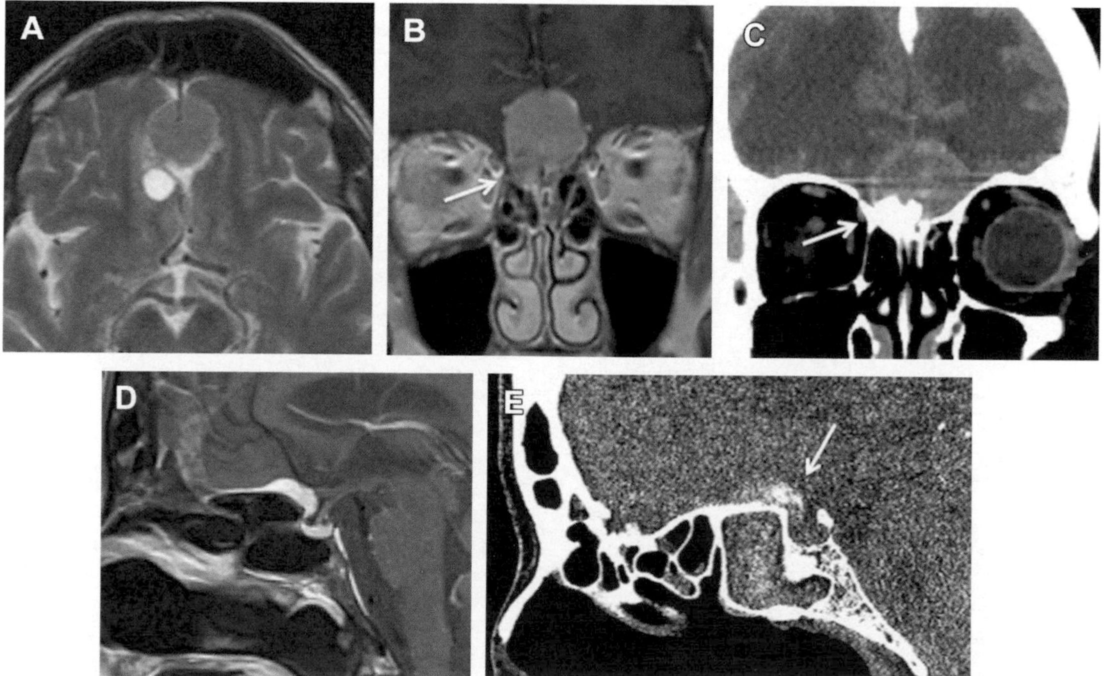

Fig. 25. (*A–C*) Olfactory groove meningioma. (*D, E*) Tuberculum sellae meningioma. (*A*) Axial T2WI. (*B*) Coronal contrast-enhanced T1WI. (*C*) Coronal CT. (*D*) Sagittal contrast-enhanced T1WI. (*E*) Sagittal CT. (*A–C*) Axial T2WI shows a lesion in the olfactory groove with a peritumoral cyst. Homogeneous enhancing tumor involves the right upper nasal vault through the cribriform plate with hyperostosis (*arrows* in *B, C*). (*D, E*) Sagittal contrast-enhanced T1WI shows a small tuberculum sellae meningioma with adjacent dura thickening (*D*). Sagittal CT image shows calcification (*arrow* in *E*) in the lesion (*E*).

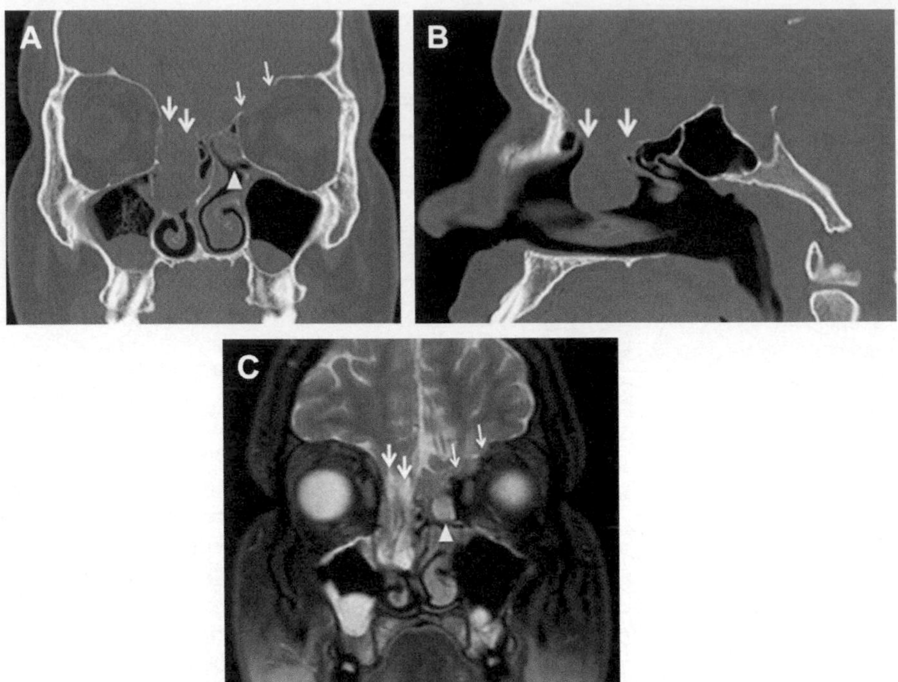

Fig. 26. Transethmoid encephalocele. (*A*) Coronal CT. (*B*) Sagittal CT. (*C*) Coronal fat-saturated T2WI. Coronal and sagittal CT images show the bone defect in the right ethmoid roof (*large arrows* in *A* and *C*) and the left orbital plate (*small arrows* in *A*). Soft tissue density masses fill the right ethmoid sinus and upper nasal cavity. Coronal T2WI demonstrates a mixed intensity mass with a direct connection to intracranial space, confirming the right transethmoidal encephalocele. Left frontal parenchyma slightly protrudes into left orbit through the dehiscence of the left orbital plate. A cystic lesion (*arrowheads* in *A*, *C*) in the left ethmoid cell is another transethmoidal encephalocele (the connection with an intracranial cavity is not demonstrated in the figures).

SUMMARY

The ASB has a close relation to the sinonasal cavity. In addition to the intrinsic ASB lesions, sinonasal and intracranial diseases extend inferiorly to involve the ASB. CT and MR imaging play a complementary role in evaluating the ASB pathologic conditions. Radiologists should be familiar with the detailed anatomy, identify dangerous anatomic variations, provide appropriate differential diagnosis, and assess the extent of the lesion for optimal treatment planning.

REFERENCES

1. Keros P. Über die praktische Bedeutung der Niveauunterschiede der Lamina cribrosa des Ethmoids. Z Laryngol Rhinol Otol 1962;41:808–13.
2. García-Garrigós E, Arenas-Jiménez JJ, Monjas-Cánovas I, et al. Transsphenoidal approach in endoscopic endonasal surgery for skull base lesions: what radiologists and surgeons need to know. Radiographics 2015;35(4):1170–85.
3. Mossa-Basha M, Blitz AM. Imaging of the paranasal sinuses. Semin Roentgenol 2013;48(1):14–34.
4. Hoang JK, Eastwood JD, Tebbit CL, et al. Multiplanar sinus CT: a systematic approach to imaging before functional endoscopic sinus surgery. AJR Am J Roentgenol 2010;194(6):W527–36.
5. Nouraei SA, Elisay AR, Dimarco A, et al. Variations in paranasal sinus anatomy: implications for the pathophysiology of chronic rhinosinusitis and safety of endoscopic sinus surgery. J Otolaryngol Head Neck Surg 2009;38(1):32–7.
6. Shpilberg KA, Daniel SC, Doshi AH, et al. CT of anatomic variants of the paranasal sinuses and nasal cavity: poor correlation with radiologically significant rhinosinusitis but importance in surgical planning. AJR Am J Roentgenol 2015;204(6):1255–60.
7. Beale TJ, Madani G, Morley SJ. Imaging of the paranasal sinuses and nasal cavity: normal anatomy and clinically relevant anatomical variants. Semin Ultrasound CT MR 2009;30(1):2–16.
8. Turri-Zanoni M, Dallan I, Terranova P, et al. Frontoethmoidal and intraorbital osteomas: exploring the limits of the endoscopic approach. Arch Otolaryngol Head Neck Surg 2012;138(5):498–504.

9. Barnes L, Eveson JW, Reichart P, et al. World Health Organization classification of tumours. Pathology and genetics of head and neck tumours. Lyon (France): IARC; 2005. p. 210–81.
10. Dubal PM, Dutta R, Vazquez A, et al. A comparative population-based analysis of sinonasal diffuse large B-cell and extranodal NK/T-cell lymphomas. Laryngoscope 2015;125(5):1077–83.
11. Kendi AT, Kara S, Altinok D, et al. Sinonasal ossifying fibroma with fluid-fluid levels on MR images. AJNR Am J Neuroradiol 2003;24(8):1639–41.
12. Edge S, Byrd D, Compton C, et al. AJCC Cancer Staging Manual. 7th edition. New York: Springer-Verlag; 2010.
13. Connor SEJ. The skull base in the evaluation of sinonasal disease: role of computed tomography and MR imaging. Neuroimaging Clin N Am 2015;25(4): 619–51.
14. Parmar H, Gujar S, Shah G, et al. Imaging of the anterior skull base. Neuroimaging Clin N Am 2009; 19(3):427–39.
15. Maroldi R, Ravanelli M, Borghesi A, et al. Paranasal sinus imaging. Eur J Radiol 2008;66(3):372–86.
16. Eisen MD, Yousem DM, Montone KT, et al. Use of preoperative MR to predict dural, perineural, and venous sinus invasion of skull base tumors. AJNR Am J Neuroradiol 1996;17(10):1937–45.
17. Gallagher KK, Spector ME, Pepper JP, et al. Esthesioneuroblastoma: updating histologic grading as it relates to prognosis. Ann Otol Rhinol Laryngol 2014;123(5):353–8.
18. Som PM, Lidov M, Brandwein M, et al. Sinonasal esthesioneuroblastoma with intracranial extension: marginal tumor cysts as a diagnostic MR finding. AJNR Am J Neuroradiol 1994;15(7):1259–62.
19. Yu T, Xu YK, Li L, et al. Esthesioneuroblastoma methods of intracranial extension: CT and MR imaging findings. Neuroradiology 2009;51(12): 841–50.
20. Pickuth D, Heywang-Kobrunner SH, Spielmann RP. Computed tomography and magnetic resonance imaging features of olfactory neuroblastoma: an analysis of 22 cases. Clin Otolaryngol Allied Sci 1999;24(5):457–61.
21. Tajudeen BA, Arshi A, Suh JD, et al. Esthesioneuroblastoma: an update on the UCLA experience, 2002-2013. J Neurol Surg B Skull Base 2015; 76(1):43–9.
22. Patel SG, Singh B, Stambuk HE, et al. Craniofacial surgery for esthesioneuroblastoma: report of an international collaborative study. J Neurol Surg B Skull Base 2012;73(3):208–20.
23. Dulguerov P, Calcaterra T. Esthesioneuroblastoma: the UCLA experience 1970-1990. Laryngoscope 1992;102(8):843–9.
24. Petruzzelli GJ, Howell JB, Pederson A, et al. Multidisciplinary treatment of olfactory neuroblastoma: patterns of failure and management of recurrence. Am J Otolaryngol 2015;36(4):547–53.
25. Snyderman CH, Carrau RL, Kassam AB, et al. Endoscopic skull base surgery: principles of endonasal oncological surgery. J Surg Oncol 2008;97(8):658–64.
26. Kadish S, Goodman M, Wang CC. Olfactory neuroblastoma. A clinical analysis of 17 cases. Cancer 1976;37(3):1571–6.
27. Morita A, Ebersold MJ, Olsen KD, et al. Esthesioneuroblastoma: prognosis and management. Neurosurgery 1993;32(5):706–14 [discussion: 714–5].
28. Feng L, Fang J, Zhang L, et al. Endoscopic endonasal resection of esthesioneuroblastoma: a single center experience of 24 patients. Clin Neurol Neurosurg 2015;138:94–8.
29. Van Gompel JJ, Giannini C, Olsen KD, et al. Long-term outcome of esthesioneuroblastoma: hyams grade predicts patient survival. J Neurol Surg B Skull Base 2012;73(5):331–6.
30. Song CM, Won TB, Lee CH, et al. Treatment modalities and outcomes of olfactory neuroblastoma. Laryngoscope 2012;122(11):2389–95.
31. Ozsahin M, Gruber G, Olszyk O, et al. Outcome and prognostic factors in olfactory neuroblastoma: a rare cancer network study. Int J Radiat Oncol Biol Phys 2010;78(4):992–7.
32. Kane AJ, Sughrue ME, Rutkowski MJ, et al. Post-treatment prognosis of patients with esthesioneuroblastoma. J Neurosurg 2010;113(2):340–51.
33. Dulguerov P, Allal AS, Calcaterra TC. Esthesioneuroblastoma: a meta-analysis and review. Lancet Oncol 2001;2(11):683–90.
34. Rinaldo A, Ferlito A, Shaha AR, et al. Esthesioneuroblastoma and cervical lymph node metastases: clinical and therapeutic implications. Acta Otolaryngol 2002;122(2):215–21.
35. Peng KA, Kita AE, Suh JD, et al. Sinonasal lymphoma: case series and review of the literature. Int Forum Allergy Rhinol 2014;4(8):670–4.
36. Chang PC, Fischbein NJ, McCalmont TH, et al. Perineural spread of malignant melanoma of the head and neck: clinical and imaging features. AJNR Am J Neuroradiol 2004;25(1):5–11.
37. Roth TN, Gengler C, Huber GF, et al. Outcome of sinonasal melanoma: clinical experience and review of the literature. Head Neck 2010;32(10):1385–92.
38. Khan MN, Kanumuri VV, Raikundalia MD, et al. Sinonasal melanoma: survival and prognostic implications based on site of involvement. Int Forum Allergy Rhinol 2014;4(2):151–5.
39. Boghani Z, Husain Q, Kanumuri VV, et al. Juvenile nasopharyngeal angiofibroma: a systematic review and comparison of endoscopic, endoscopic-assisted, and open resection in 1047 cases. Laryngoscope 2013;123(4):859–69.
40. Ballah D, Rabinowitz D, Vossough A, et al. Preoperative angiography and external carotid artery

embolization of juvenile nasopharyngeal angiofibromas in a tertiary referral paediatric centre. Clin Radiol 2013;68(11):1097–106.

41. Barnes L, Tse LLY, Hunt JL, et al. Tumours of the nasal cavity and paranasal sinuses. Pathology and Genetics of Head and Neck Tumors. Proceeding of IARC (International Agency for Research on Cancer) Press Lyon, France, July 13–16, 2003.
42. von Buchwald C, Bradley PJ. Risks of malignancy in inverted papilloma of the nose and paranasal sinuses. Curr Opin Otolaryngol Head Neck Surg 2007;15(2):95–8.
43. Nygren A, Kiss K, Von Buchwald C, et al. Rate of recurrence and malignant transformation in 88 cases with inverted papilloma between 1998-2008. Acta Otolaryngol 2016;136(3):333–6.
44. Jeon TY, Kim HJ, Chung SK, et al. Sinonasal inverted papilloma: value of convoluted cerebriform pattern on MR imaging. AJNR Am J Neuroradiol 2008;29(8):1556–60.
45. Lee DK, Chung SK, Dhong HJ, et al. Focal hyperostosis on CT of sinonasal inverted papilloma as a predictor of tumor origin. AJNR Am J Neuroradiol 2007; 28(4):618–21.
46. Krouse JH. Development of a staging system for inverted papilloma. Laryngoscope 2000;110(6): 965–8.
47. Lawson W, Ho BT, Shaari CM, et al. Inverted papilloma: a report of 112 cases. Laryngoscope 1995; 105(3):282–8.
48. Mohan S, Nair S, Sharma M, et al. Inverted papilloma of frontal sinus with intracranial extension. Med J Armed Forces India 2015;71:S152–5.
49. Ojiri H, Ujita M, Tada S, et al. Potentially distinctive features of sinonasal inverted papilloma on MR imaging. AJR Am J Roentgenol 2000;175(2):465–8.
50. Capra GG, Carbone PN, Mullin DP. Paranasal sinus mucocele. Head Neck Pathol 2012;6(3):369–72.
51. Brown EW, Megerian CA, McKenna MJ, et al. Fibrous dysplasia of the temporal bone: Imaging findings. AJR Am J Roentgenol 1995;164(3):679–82.
52. Kransdorf MJ, Moser RP Jr, Gilkey FW. Fibrous dysplasia. Radiographics 1990;10(3):519–37.
53. Fries JW. The roentgen features of fibrous dysplasia of the skull and facial bones; a critical analysis of thirty-nine pathologically proved cases. Am J Roentgenol Radium Ther Nucl Med 1957; 77(1):71–88.
54. Chong VFH, Khoo JBK, Fan YF. Fibrous dysplasia involving the base of the skull. AJR Am J Roentgenol 2002;178(3):717–20.
55. Urs AB, Kumar P, Arora S, et al. Clinicopathologic and radiologic correlation of ossifying fibroma and juvenile ossifying fibroma - An institutional study of 22 cases. Ann Diagn Pathol 2013;17(2): 198–203.
56. Manes RP, Ryan MW, Batra PS, et al. Ossifying fibroma of the nose and paranasal sinuses. Int Forum Allergy Rhinol 2013;3(2):161–8.
57. Wang H, Sun X, Liu Q, et al. Endoscopic resection of sinonasal ossifying fibroma: 31 cases report at an institution. Eur Arch Otorhinolaryngol 2014;271(11): 2975–82.
58. Yang BT, Wang YZ, Wang XY, et al. Imaging study of ossifying fibroma with associated aneurysmal bone cyst in the paranasal sinus. Eur J Radiol 2012; 81(11):3450–5.
59. Schick B, Steigerwald C, El Tahan AER, et al. The role of endonasal surgery in the management of frontoethmoidal osteomas. Rhinology 2001;39(2): 66–70.
60. Karligkiotis A, Pistochini A, Turri-Zanoni M, et al. Endoscopic endonasal orbital transposition to expand the frontal sinus approaches. Am J Rhinol Allergy 2015;29(6):449–56.
61. Refaat MI, Eissa EM, Ali MH. Surgical management of midline anterior skull base meningiomas: experience of 30 cases. Turk Neurosurg 2015; 25(3):432–7.
62. Wallace EW. The dural tail sign. Radiology 2004; 233(1):56–7.
63. Shin M, Kondo K, Saito N. Current status of endoscopic endonasal surgery for skull base meningiomas: review of the literature. Neurol Med Chir (Tokyo) 2015;55(9):735–43.
64. Belden CJ, Mancuso AA, Kotzur IM. The developing anterior skull base: CT appearance from birth to 2 years of age. AJNR Am J Neuroradiol 1997;18(5): 811–8.

Imaging of the Central Skull Base

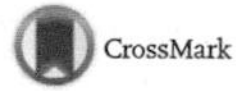

Lindsey M. Conley, MD*, C. Douglas Phillips, MD

KEYWORDS

• Central skull base • Skull base anatomy • Skull base pathology

KEY POINTS

- The skull base is divided in to anterior, middle, and posterior.
- Multiple entities from notochord remnants, to neoplasm, to infection, and other interesting cases occur in the central skull base.
- Understanding embryology and anatomy aids in recognition of the characteristic location and imaging features of this diverse group of developmental variants and pathologic entities.

INTRODUCTION

The skull base is a complex bony and soft tissue interface that is divided anatomically into compartments. It provides a separation between intracranial and extracranial anatomy. This article will focus specifically on the central skull base, which has complex embryologic development and anatomy. Other articles will deal with other segments of the skull base. Multiple entities from notochord remnants, neoplasm, infection, and other abnormalities may occur in the central skull base. As this is not a structure that can be evaluated on physical examination, imaging is critical for depicting skull base pathology and its intimate relationship with the surrounding structures, such as nerves and arteries.

ANATOMY

The central skull base is limited anteriorly by the lesser wing of the sphenoid bone and posteriorly by the dorsum sella. It contains multiple foramina and fissures that are important pathways into and out of the skull (**Box 1**; **Figs. 1** and **2**). Numerous cranial nerves traverse this region:

- CNII through the optic canal; CNIII, CNIV, and CNVI via the superior orbital fissure
- The infraorbital orbital nerve through the inferior orbital fissure
- The maxillary division of CNV through foramen rotundum
- The mandibular division of CNV through foramen ovale
- The meningeal branch of CNV3 through the foramen spinosum
- The vidian nerve (a branch of CN VII) via the vidian canal

There is also an intimate relationship with the internal carotid artery (ICA) through carotid canal and foramen lacerum, ophthalmic artery and vein via the optic canal and superior orbital fissure, respectively, and the inferior orbital artery and vidian artery (**Fig. 3**).

The skull base is formed mostly through endochondral ossification from posterior to anterior and begins at about 12 and one-half weeks. Over 100 ossification sites have been identified in the fetal calvarium. During the fourth week of gestation, the mesoderm and neural crest cells begin to form the cartilaginous and bony portions of the skull base. By the eighth week, it is almost completely chondrocranium. From 12 to 17 weeks, ossification begins from the occipital bone to the sphenoid bone. The important ossification centers

Disclosure Statement: The authors have nothing to disclose.

Department of Radiology, Weill Cornell Medical College, NewYork-Presbyterian Hospital, 525 East 68th Street, New York, NY 10065, USA
* Corresponding author.
E-mail address: Conley.lindsey@gmail.com

Radiol Clin N Am 55 (2017) 53–67
http://dx.doi.org/10.1016/j.rcl.2016.08.007
0033-8389/17/Published by Elsevier Inc.

Box 1
Central skull base foramina and fissures

Foramen ovale
Foramen spinosum
Foramen rotundum
Foramen lacerum
Superior orbital fissure
Inferior orbital fissure
Optic canal
Carotid canal
Vidian canal

are orbitosphenoid and alisphenoid, which form the lesser wing and greater wing of the sphenoid, respectively, the pre- and postsphenoid, and the basiocciput. The postsphenoid and basiocciput form the clivus (**Fig. 4**).[1]

There is also an intimate relationship of the central skull base and the notochord. The notochord develops along a tract from the primitive node to the buccopharyngeal membrane. The most craniad portion is a hook-like extension into the region of the future dorsum sella. The notochord crosses the clivus multiple times in the fifth week of life. The medial basal canal is considered the cephalad exit tract of the notochord, as it moves from its intraclival location ventrally into the midline

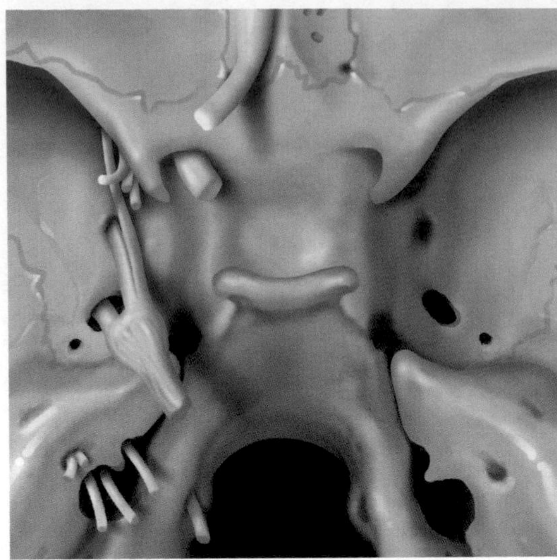

Fig. 2. Central skull base and the nerves traversing though the foramina. (*From* Harnsberger HR, Osborn AG, Macdonald AJ, et al. Diagnostic and surgical imaging anatomy: brain, head and neck, spine. Salt Lake City: Amirsys, 2006; with permission.)

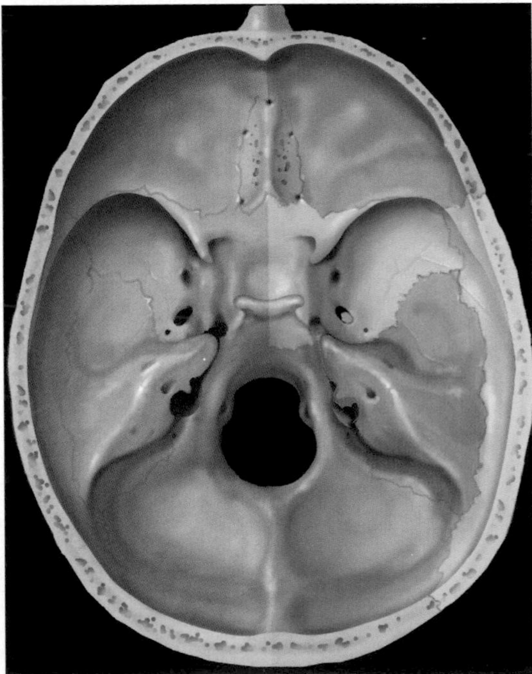

Fig. 1. Skull base and foramina. (*From* Harnsberger HR, Osborn AG, Macdonald AJ, et al. Diagnostic and surgical imaging anatomy: brain, head and neck, spine. Salt Lake City: Amirsys, 2006; with permission.)

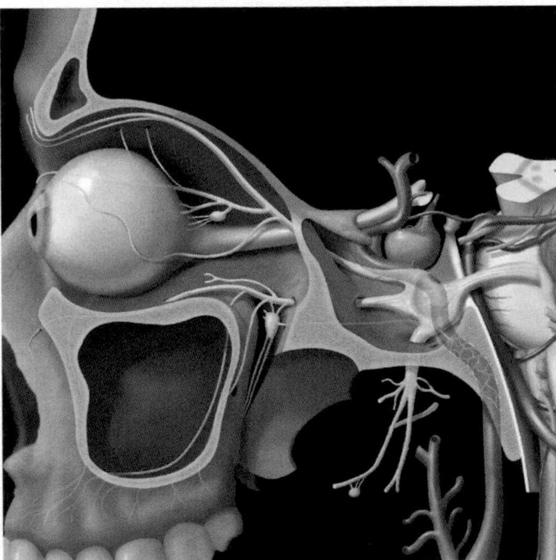

Fig. 3. Sagittal view of the central skull base. (*From* Harnsberger HR, Osborn AG, Macdonald AJ, et al. Diagnostic and surgical imaging anatomy: brain, head and neck, spine. Salt Lake City: Amirsys, 2006; with permission.)

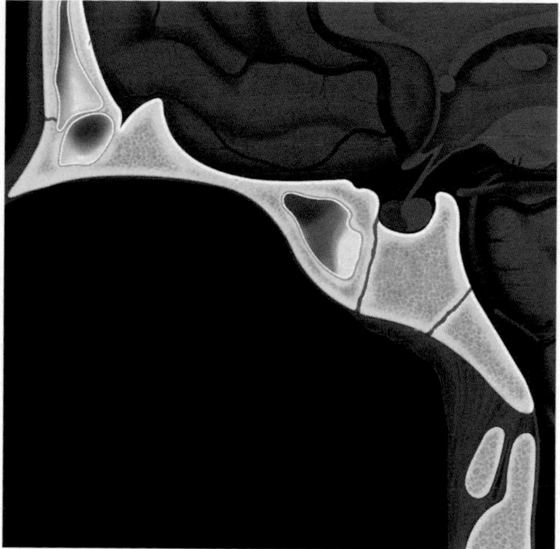

Fig. 4. Central skull base major ossification centers. (*From* Harnsberger HR, Osborn AG, Macdonald AJ, et al. Diagnostic and surgical imaging anatomy: brain, head and neck, spine. Salt Lake City: Amirsys, 2006; with permission.)

nasopharyngeal soft tissues. At each stage of notochordal development, remnants may be left behind, creating a spectrum of normal variants and pathology. Understanding of the relevant embryology aids in recognition of the characteristic location and imaging features of this diverse group (**Fig. 5**).[2–4]

IMAGING TECHNIQUE

Imaging of the central skull base can be performed with the complementary techniques of computed tomography (CT) and MR imaging. CT is useful for the bony landmarks and foramen and also to see ossification or chondroid matrix, while MR imaging can highlight perineural tumor spread and subtle soft tissue anatomic details.

PATHOLOGY

There are multiple benign etiologies involving the central skull base, from congenital to neoplastic, infection, and other diverse entities, such as toxin effects. This article will concentrate on several lesions that are primary to the central skull base, and also discuss lesions that arise superior to the skull base and lesions that arise below the skull base.

Benign etiologies are shown in **Box 2**.

NOTOCHORD REMNANTS

Although the notochord typically regresses by postnatal life, various remnants can be found along its embryologic path. This section will review remnants occurring at the cranial end, which range from the mundane Tornwaldt cyst to the esoteric, ecchordosis physaliphora.

Ecchordosis Physalipohora

Ecchordosis physalipohora (EP) is an intra- and extradural focus of gelatinous tissue that is widely accepted to represent a notochordal remnant. The presentation of EP is usually as an incidental finding in an asymptomatic patient. This entity is found in the prepontine cistern and attached to the dorsal wall of the clivus. The lesion classically extends through the dura into the prepontine cistern. CT imaging demonstrates a low-density structure related to a well-defined midline clival defect; this may project through the defect into the adjacent sphenoid sinus. On MR imaging, this lesion is classically T1 hypointense and T2 hyperintense, and the extension into the

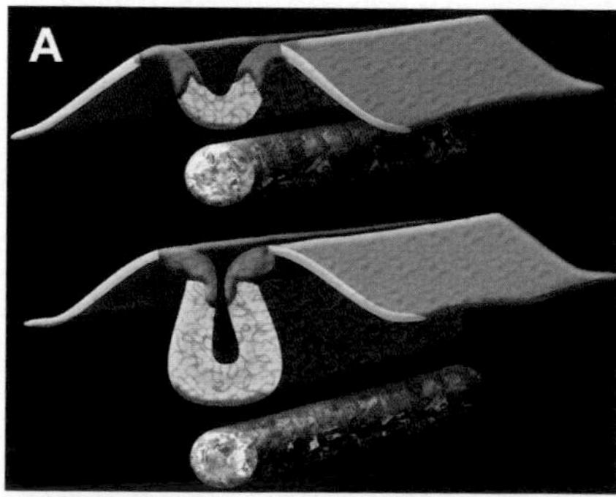

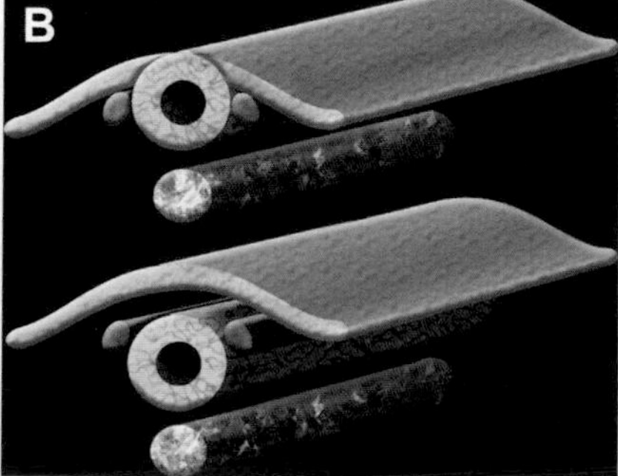

Fig. 5. (*A, B*) Neural tube closure starts at 4 weeks and the center will become the central canal of the spinal cord and the ventricular system of the brain. (*From* Woodward PJ, Kennedy A, Sohaey S. Diagnostic imaging: obstetrics. Salt Lake City: Amirsys, 2016; with permission.)

Box 2
Benign central skull base pathology

Notochord remnants
Arachnoid granulations
Langerhans histiocytosis
Fibrous dysplasia
Paget disease
Cephalocele

prepontine cistern can be better appreciated. Postgadolinium sequences typically demonstrate no enhancement. The absence of enhancement is an important imaging characteristic that distinguishes EP from a chordoma. There are subtypes of EP based on the appearance on high-resolution MR imaging. There is classical, which is further divided into type A, a hyperdense excrescence on the dorsal surface of the clivus, and type B, which is the excrescence on the clivus along with a hyperdense lesion within the clivus. All lesions that do not fit into this category are considered incomplete, which is a T2 hypointense protrusion of the clivus or variant, which is only the hyperintense lesion within the clivus alone.[5] EP requires no intervention, although MR imaging follow-up may be performed to assure stability (**Fig. 6**).

Fossa Navicularis Magna

The cranium begins as a cartilaginous structure, which will be replaced with bone through fetal development. Specifically, the clivus develops by enchondral formation in the second month. There are parachordal cartilages along each side of the cephalic notochord, which grow and eventually fuse; this, with the notochord, forms the basal plate. The attachment of the notochord then forms the pharyngeal bursa. Persistence of the notochord prevents complete ossification of the basiocciput, resulting in a defect along its anterior inferior margin. Fossa navicularis magna (FNM) is uncommon and usually an incidental finding on head and neck imaging. CT scans demonstrate a well-circumscribed osseous defect, which may be air- or soft tissue-filled. The defect may be filled with lymphoid tissue, a finding that may be demonstrated on MR imaging when signal within the FNM is identical to contiguous adenoidal tissue. This lesion also requires no intervention (**Fig. 7**).

Persistent Canalis Basilaris Medianus

Persistent canalis basilaris medianus (PCBM) is a remnant of the notochord in the caudal basiocciput, which may be incomplete or traverse entirely through the basioccipital bone. There are 6 variants of PCBM, which are classified based on the extension through the basiocciput, and can be divided into complete and incomplete forms. The complete form can then be further subdivided into superior, inferior and bifurcates. The incomplete form has 3 subtypes; 1 subtype is a channel that begins in the basiocciput and continues to the post basisphenoid. The other 2 subtypes are superior or inferior recesses in the basiocciput[6] (**Figs. 8** and **9**). On CT imaging, there is a well-defined canal originating on the intracranial surface of the basiocciput near the foramen magnum. It is important to be able to distinguish PCBM from FNM. FNM is a notch-like defect in the basiocciput, whereas PCBM is an actual canal. This is often best seen on sagittal imaging[7,8] (**Fig. 10**).

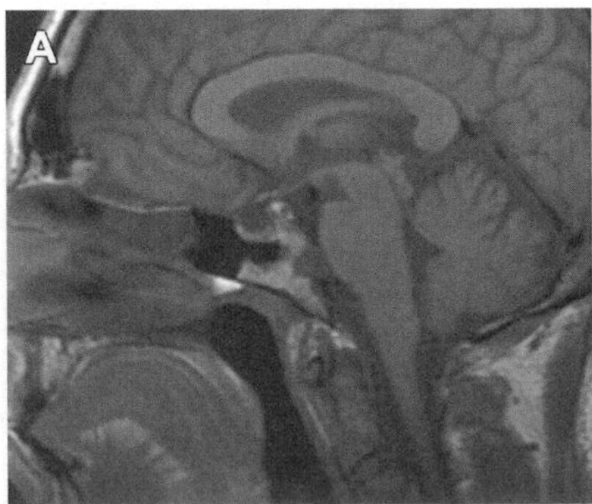

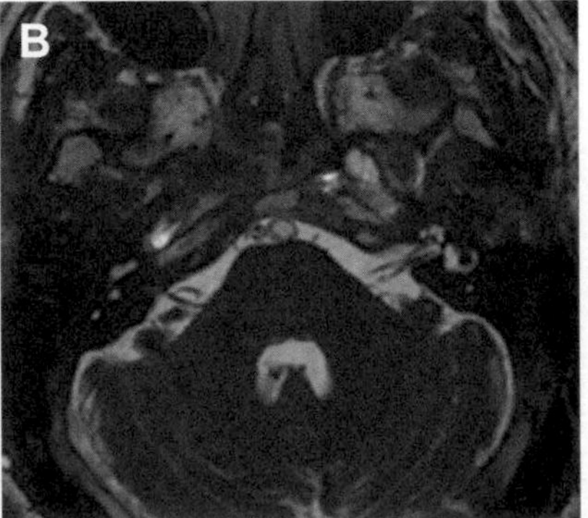

Fig. 6. (*A, B*) Sagittal TIWI and axial heavily T2 weighted MR imaging demonstrates a T1 hypointense and T2 hyperintense lesion with extension into the prepontine cistern.

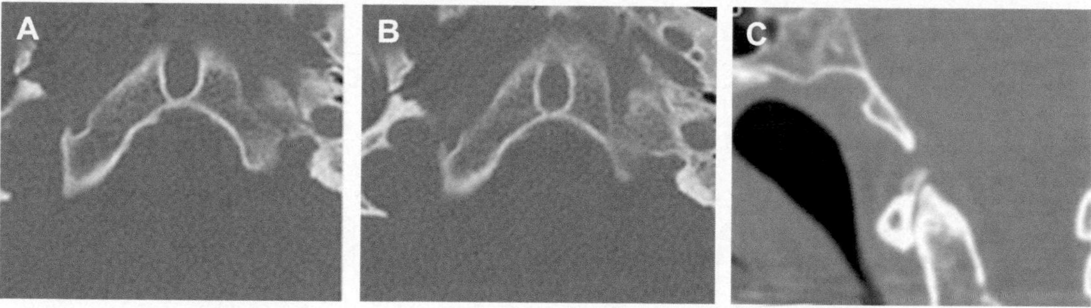

Fig. 7. (*A–C*) Consecutive axial and sagittal CT demonstrates a well circumscribed osseous defect.

Persistent Craniopharyngeal Canal

Persistent craniopharyngeal canal is a bony defect extending from the floor of the sella to the nasopharyngeal roof.[9] Although this is not a notochord remnant, it is relevant in the differential diagnosis of PCBM. The relationship of these 2 entities to the sphenooccipital synchondrosis can help differentiate them.[10] The craniopharyngeal canal is anterior to the synchondrosis, while the PCBM is posterior. There are 3 subtypes; the first is an incidental canal without anatomic contents. The second subtype contains ectopic adenohypophysis, and the third includes benign and malignant tumors such as pituitary adenomas or gliomas. Based on the subtype, treatment and surgical approach differ.[9]

Tornwaldt Cyst

Tornwaldt cyst is a cystic lesion in the roof of the nasopharynx. It is usually an asymptomatic incidental entity. Rarely, this lesion has been associated with chronic halitosis. When large, it may also cause otitis media secondary to eustachian tube obstruction. CT imaging demonstrates a well-circumscribed, low-density midline cyst. On MR imaging, the signal may vary on T1WI due to variable protein content, although T2 hyperintensity is a more consistent finding. These lesions do not typically demonstrate enhancement, although some rim enhancement is possible if the cyst becomes infected. If the patient is asymptomatic, no intervention is necessary.

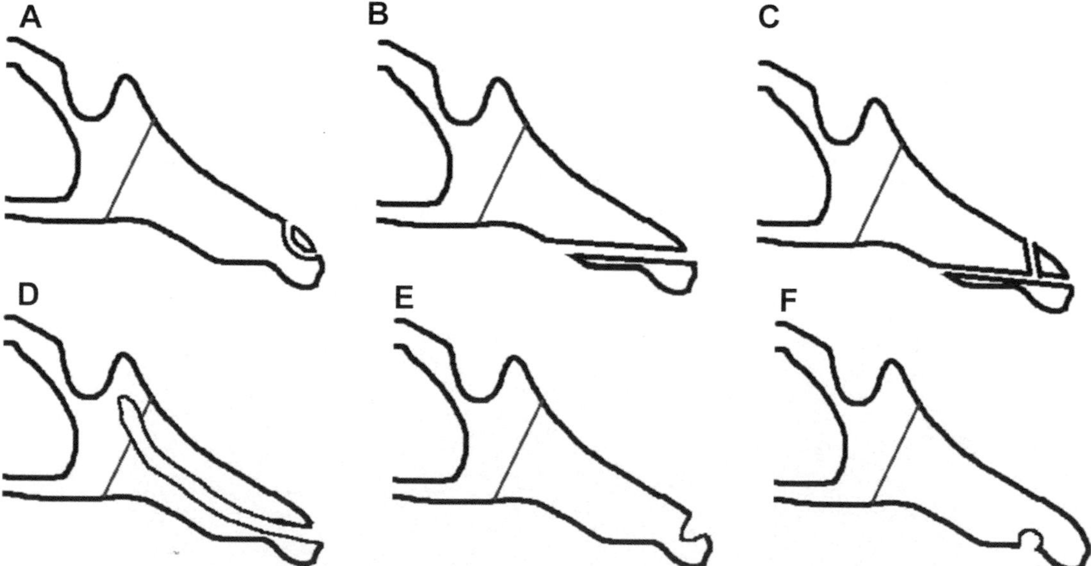

Fig. 8. (*A–F*) Illustration adapted from *Canalis Basilaris Medianus and Related Defects of the Basiocciput* showing the variants of PCBM. Complete forms: (*A*) CBM superior, (*B*) CBM inferior, (*C*) CBM bifurcates. Incomplete forms: (*D*) long channel in basiocciput and postbasisphenoid, (*E*) superior recess in basiocciput, (*F*) inferior recess in basiocciput. (*Data from* Currarino G. Canalis basilaris medianus and related defects of the basiocciput. AJNR Am J Neuroradiol 1988;9:208–11.)

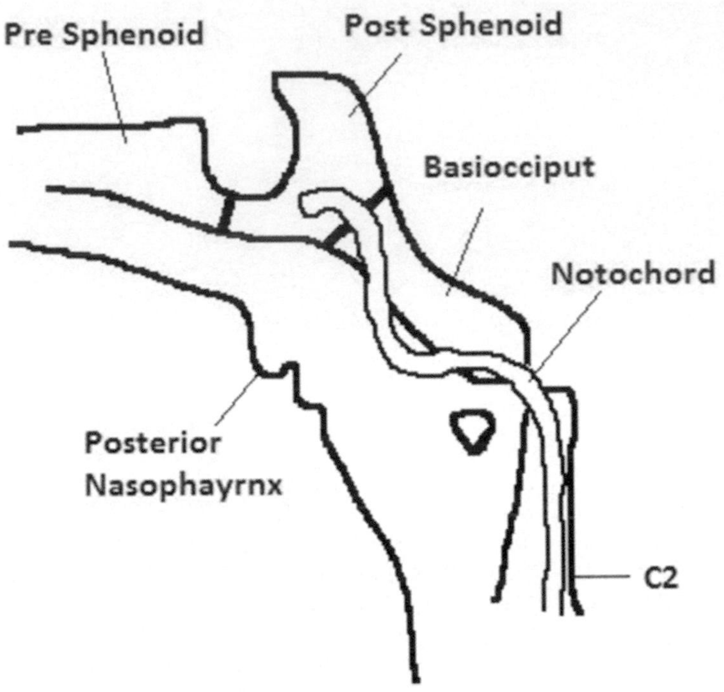

Fig. 9. Illustration adapted from *Canalis Basilaris Medianus and Related Defects of the Basiocciput* showing the development of the notochord through the basiocciput and posterior sphenoid. (*Data from* Currarino G. Canalis Basilaris Medianus and Related Defects of the Basiocciput. AJNR Am J Neuroradiol 1988;9:208–11.)

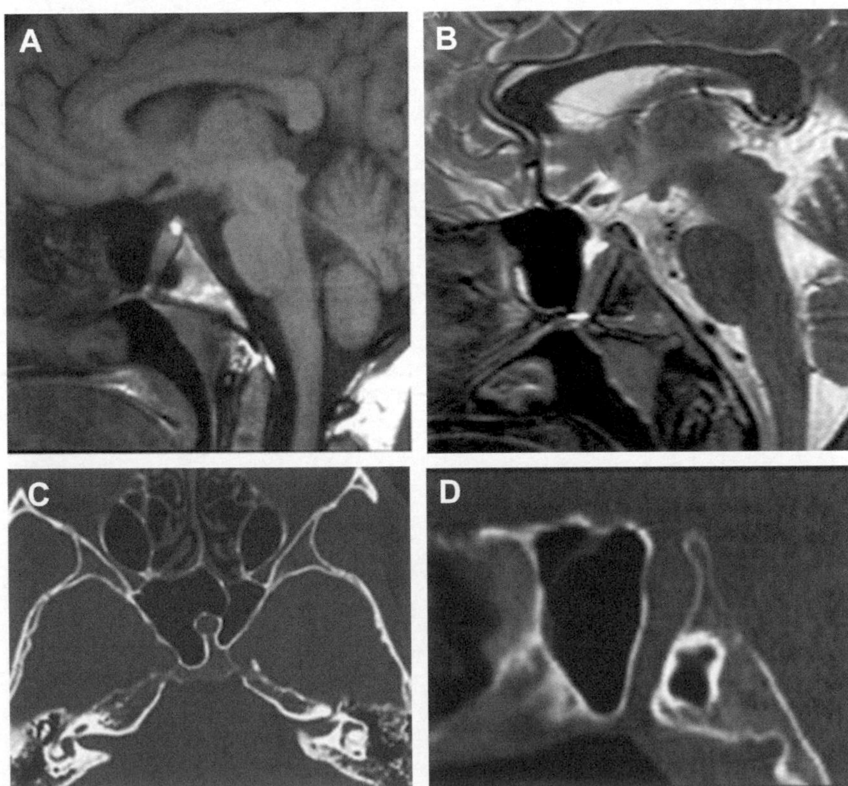

Fig. 10. (*A, B*) Sagittal T1WI and T2WI MR imaging and (*C, D*) axial and sagittal CT demonstrate a well-defined canal through the basiocciput.

ARACHNOID GRANULATIONS

Arachnoid granulations (AGs) are appendages of the arachnoid membrane into dural sinuses and venous spaces. They are usually found along the dural sinuses or skull surface. Aberrant AGs penetrate the dura but do not reach the sinus and are typically in the sphenoid bone. AGs are well defined nonenhancing lesions that may erode through the inner table of the calvarium; alternatively, they may appear as focal pits. It has been suggested that AGs are related to intracranial hypertension. AGs may be one of the causes of intracranial hypertension (ICH) by obstructing the sinus venous flow.[11] However, it has also been proposed that AGs may be the sequelae of ICH. These lesions tend appear in areas where there is dural weakness and possibly secondary to cerebral spinal fluid (CSF) pulsation at elevated intracranial pressures.[12] ICH may be suggested as a possible etiology of multiple arachnoid granulations in some patients. On CT, these lesions appear lytic. On MR imaging, they follow CSF signal. Venograms show the filling defect and the communication with the arachnoid membrane. No treatment is needed for AGs (**Fig. 11**).

LANGERHANS HISTIOCYTOSIS

Langerhans histiocytosis is a rare disease most common in young males. It caused by the proliferation of Langerhans cells and has recently been recategorized. It is commonly seen in the calvarium and may involve the central skull base. It varies from 1 small lesion to more diffuse involvement of the entire skull base. CT demonstrates a punched-out lytic lesion with an associated soft tissue mass. The soft tissue extent is better evaluated on MR imaging. The T1 and T2 signal varies; however, avid enhancement is common. This entity usually responds to chemotherapy and has a high cure rate, averaging up to 90% (**Fig. 12**).

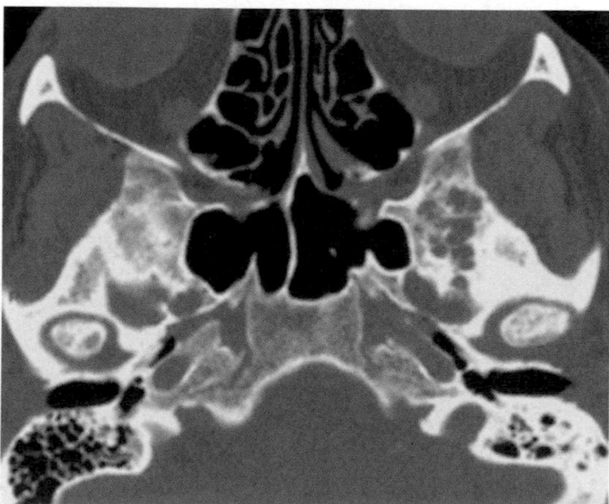

Fig. 11. Axial CT demonstrates lytic lesions along the left skull base.

FIBROUS DYSPLASIA

Fibrous dysplasia (FD) is a rare disorder where bone is replaced by fibroosseous tissue.[13] Although the cause of FD is not completely clear, there is clear evidence supporting mosaic genetics with a mutation of the GNAS gene.[14,15] Genetic testing can aid in the diagnosis of these cases. Interestingly, there has also been suggestion of the normalization of FD in the adult population secondary to apoptosis of the GNAS gene.[16] FD is usually seen in younger women and is described in 2 forms, monostotic or polyostotic based on single or multiple sites of involvement. There are 3 types that are best defined by CT imaging features: sclerotic, which has the classic ground glass appearance, a pagetoid variant that is mixed sclerotic and lytic, and a cystic form that appears lucent with a thin sclerotic border. On MR imaging, markedly hypointense T2 signal is an important point to differentiate FD from other lesions. Surgery is typically reserved for decompression of neural foramen or other compressive symptoms. Otherwise, conservative management and monitoring of disease status with imaging and clinical evaluation are utilized. Bisphosphonate therapy has been utilized to treat FD-related bone pain, but does nothing to arrest the disease progression or improve bone quality[17] (**Fig. 13**).

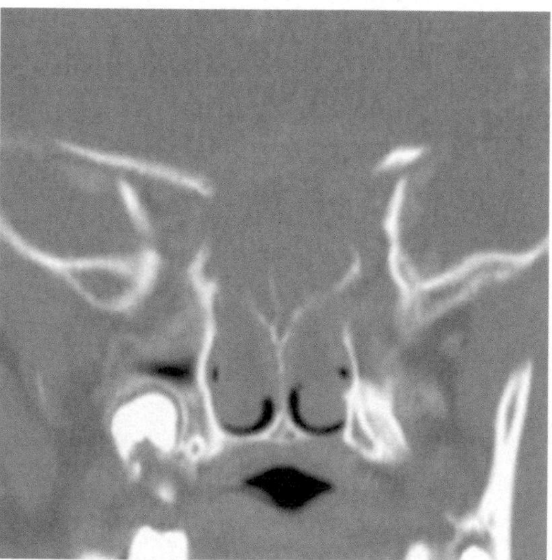

Fig. 12. Coronal CT demonstrates a punched-out lytic lesion with soft tissue mass. (*Courtesy of* R Wiggins, MD, Salt Lake City, UT.)

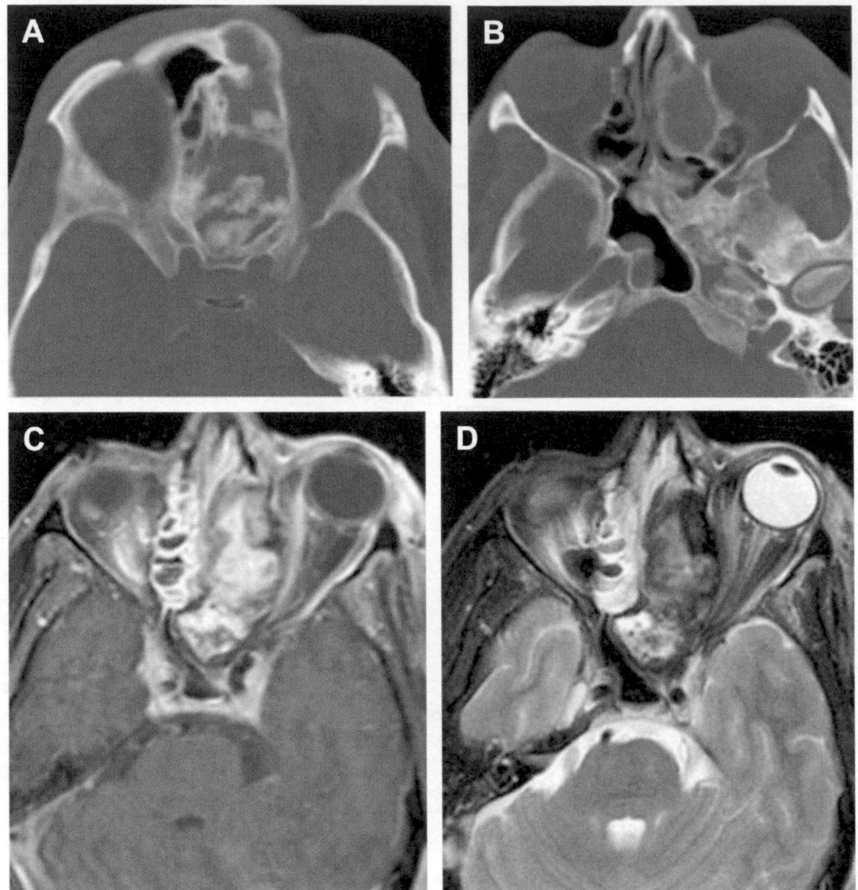

Fig. 13. (*A, B*) Axial CT demonstrates classic sclerotic ground glass appearance. (*C, D*) Axial post gadolinium TIWI and T2WI MR imaging demonstrates enhancement and T2 hypointensity.

PAGET DISEASE

Paget disease is abnormal growth and destruction of bone and is more common in older males. Although there is not a clear etiology of Paget disease, genetic and environmental factors contribute, so family history may be useful. A large environmental factor has been the measles virus. Notably, since the measles vaccination was developed and became a standard of care, the

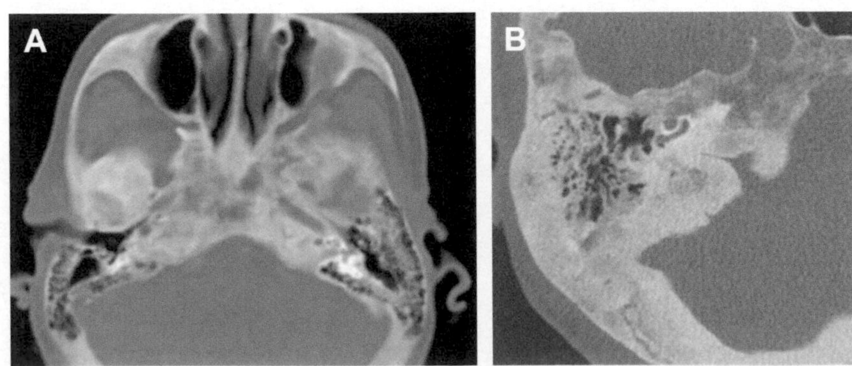

Fig. 14. (*A, B*) Axial CT and coned down view demonstrates classic cotton wool appearance.

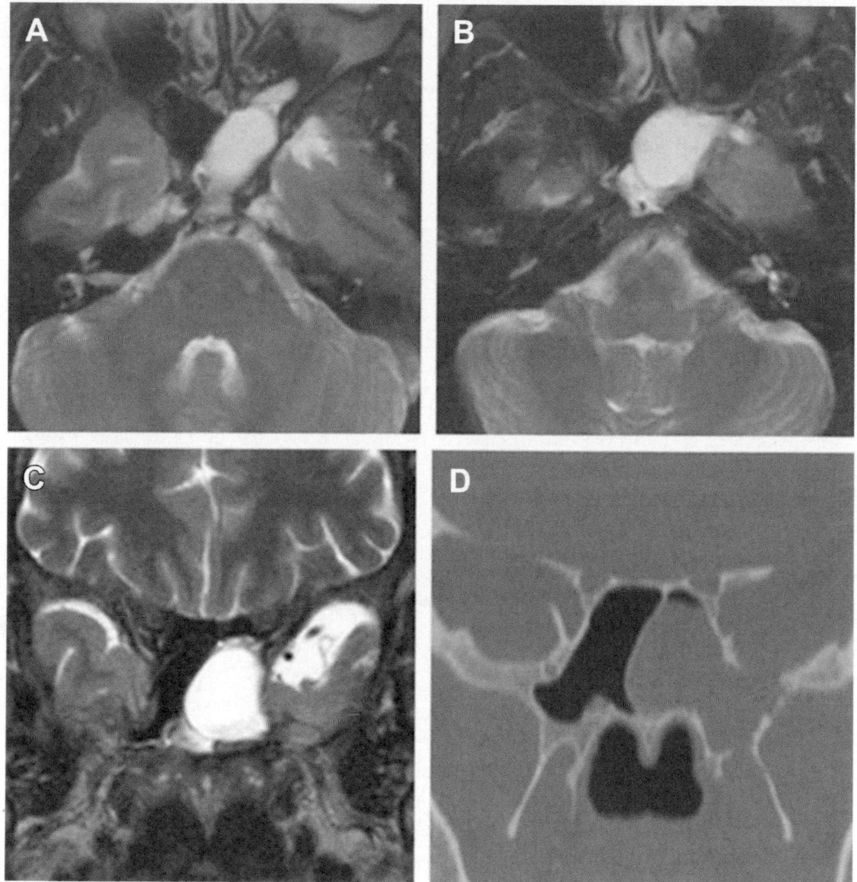

Fig. 15. (*A–C*) Consecutive axial and coronal MR imaging demonstrates a T2 uniformly hyperintense lesion protruding through bony defect. (*D*) Coronal CT demonstrates bony defect.

incidence of Paget disease has decreased considerably.[18,19] CT demonstrates sclerosis and lytic areas with a classic cotton wool appearance. On MR imaging, Paget is T1 hypointense with heterogenous signal on T2WI, with heterogeneous

Box 3
Neoplasm

Benign
- Meningioma
- Juvenile angiofibroma with invasion

Malignant
- Chordoma
- Chondrosarcoma
- Clival invasion from nasopharynx ca
- Rhabdomyosarcoma
- Metastasis

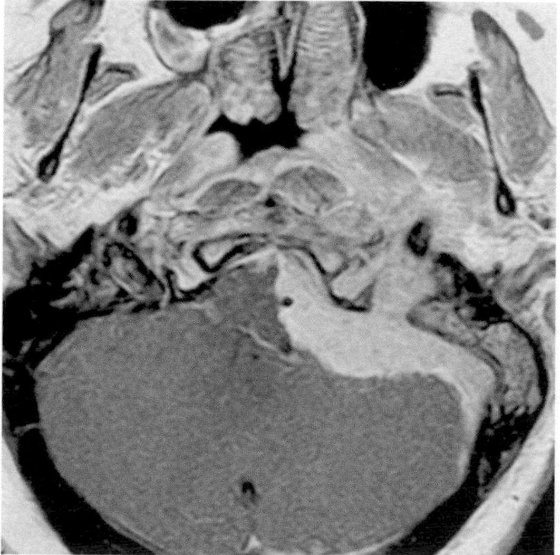

Fig. 16. Axial postgadolinium TIWI MR imaging demonstrates enhancing extra-axial dural-based mass.

enhancement. Medical treatment is standard for this disease (**Fig. 14**).

CEPHALOCELE

Basal cephaloceles are herniation of meninges and/or brain through a defect in the sphenoid, ethmoid, or basiocciput. These are usually congenital but may be post-traumatic. Basal cephaloceles are variously classified according to the location: sphenoorbital, sphenomaxillary, and nasopharyngeal, which includes transethmoid, sphenoethmoid, sphenonasopharyngeal, and basioccipital–nasopharyngeal. It was thought that 1 common congenital cause of a lateral sphenoid cephalocele was the presence of Sternberg canal, which is an incomplete bony fusion of the posterior sphenoid sinus that creates a lateral craniopharyngeal canal.[20] However, is has been shown that only a few patients have this persisting to adulthood, and when it is present it is just inferior to the cavernous sinus.[21,22] A lateral sphenoid cephalocele most commonly occurs lateral to the foramen rotundum, suggesting that most cases are not secondary to a persistent Sternberg canal.[22] It is important for surgical planning to detect central nervous system (CNS) tissue within a defect. Therefore CT and MR imaging are frequently used in conjunction to demonstrate the bony defect and the presence of brain tissue, respectively. They are well circumscribed lesions and are widely variable in size. Treatment is surgical (**Fig. 15**).

Neoplastic etiologies are shown in **Box 3**.

BENIGN MENINGIOMA

Meningiomas are a benign extra-axial tumor of arachnoid cap cells, usually seen in older women. They can occur anywhere in the skull base; petroclival and paracavernous meningiomas are described in the central skull base, although the lesions may appear anywhere along a dural surface. CT classically demonstrates a hyperdense dural-based mass, occasionally with intratumoral calcification. There may be associated hyperostosis, a relatively specific sign of meningioma. On MR imaging, the lesions are hypointense on T2WI and T1WI with avid enhancement. They may extend in a transosseous fashion, but may also extend via neural or vascular foramen. When contiguous with vascular structures,

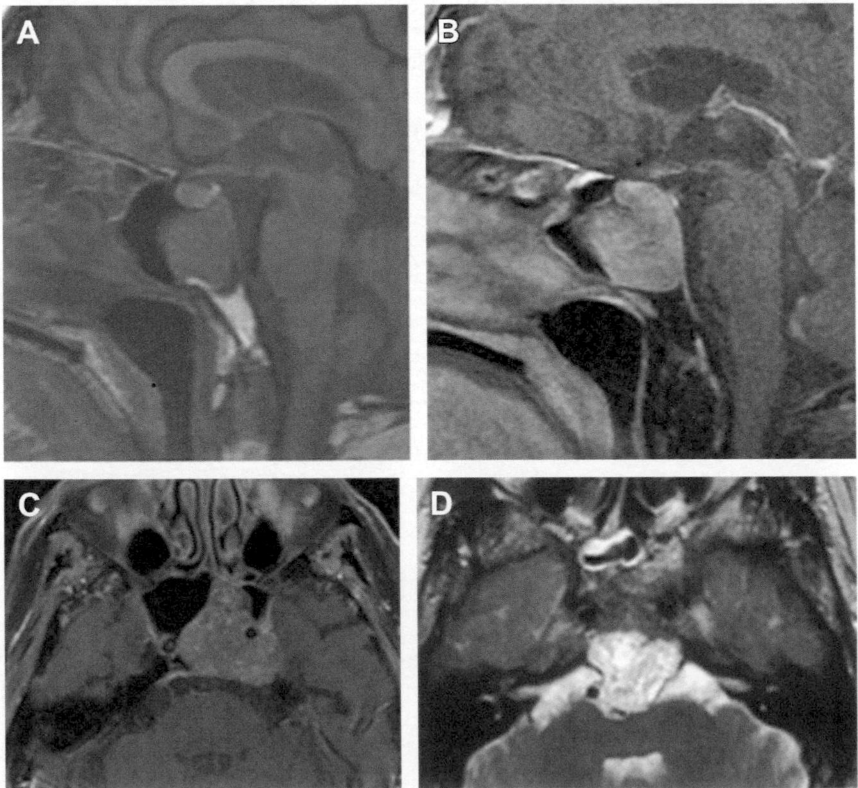

Fig. 17. (*A–C*) Sagittal pre- and sagittal and axial postgadolinium T1WI MR imaging demonstrates enhancing clival mass. (*D*) Axial T2WI MR imaging demonstrates marked hyperintensity.

meningiomas may result in narrowing of the vessel, such as the ICA in paracavernous meningiomas (**Fig. 16**).

JUVENILE ANGIOFIBROMA

Juvenile angiofibroma is a benign vascular mass that arises from in proximity to the sphenopalatine foramen in a younger male. This is discussed in greater detail (See Jindal and colleagues article, "Imaging Evaluation and Treatment of Vascular Lesions at the Skull Base," in this issue).

MALIGNANT CHORDOMA

Chordoma is felt to represent the malignant counterpart of ecchordosis physaliphora. It is a slow-growing neoplasm that may present with a variety of intracranial or extracranial components, but typically arises broadly from the clivus and results in compression of the pons. Symptoms are typically caused by the mass effect on the brainstem or cranial nerves, notably CN VI. CT imaging demonstrates a well-circumscribed, low attenuation midline or paramedian mass with lytic bone destruction, with modest contrast enhancement. On MR imaging, this lesion appears intermediate to profoundly hypointense signal on T1WI and is markedly hyperintense on T2WI. Postgadolinium T1WI demonstrates heterogeneous enhancement with a described characteristic honeycomb appearance,[23] although in some cases enhancement is minimal. Treatment Is radiation therapy in combination with surgical excision; chemotherapy has been occasionally used (**Fig. 17**).

CHONDROSARCOMA

Chondrosarcoma is chondroid neoplasm that usually arises off midline centered on the petro-occipital fissure. The location helps to distinguish this entity from a chordoma, which is more commonly midline. It often has characteristic ring and arc calcifications that are seen best on CT.

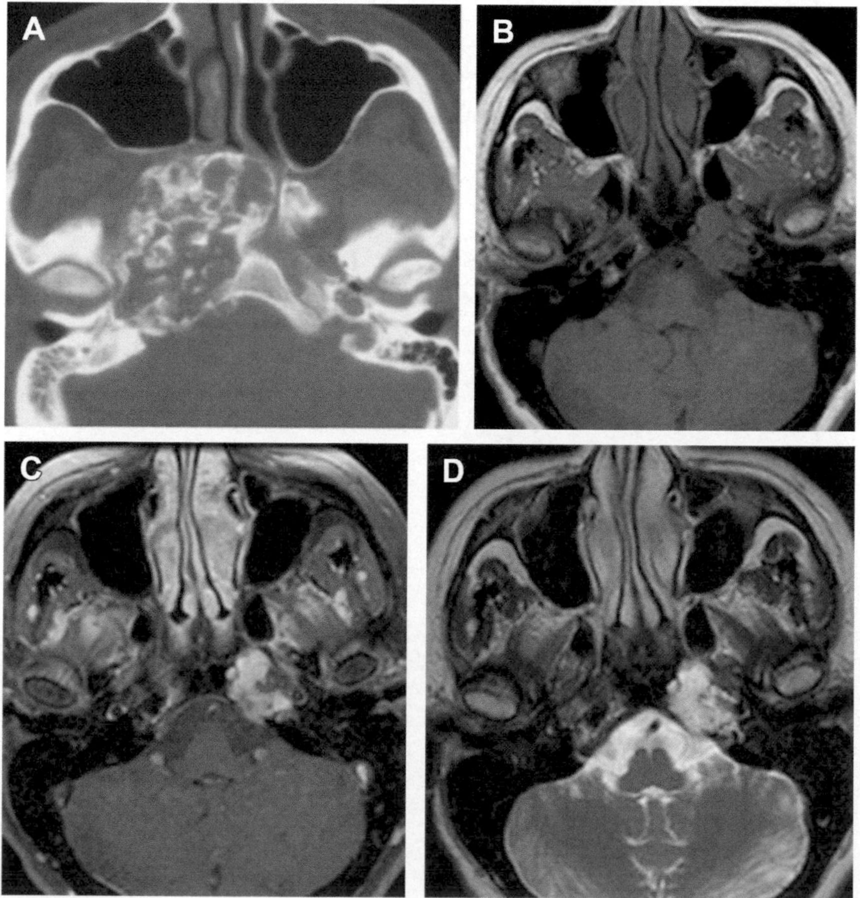

Fig. 18. (*A*) Axial CT demonstrates ring and arc calcifications. (*B–D*) Axial pre- and postgadolinium T1WI and T2WI MR imaging demonstrates heterogenous enhancement and marked T2 hyperintensity.

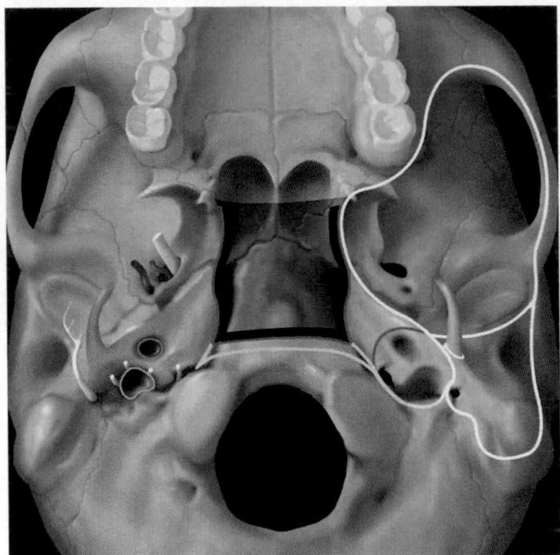

Fig. 19. The blue outlines the nasopharynx abutting the central skull base. (*From* Harnsberger HR, Osborn AG, Macdonald AJ, et al. Diagnostic and surgical imaging anatomy: brain, head and neck, spine. Salt Lake City: Amirsys, 2006; with permission.)

Chondrosarcoma, like many other chondroid lesions, has considerable hyperintensity on T2WI and demonstrates heterogenous enhancement. Surgery is the treatment of choice, but these lesions may be difficult to resect in entirety; radiation therapy may follow debulking (**Fig. 18**).

CLIVAL INVASION FROM NASOPHARYNX NEOPLASM

There is an intimate relationship of the nasopharynx with the clivus (**Fig. 19**). Nasopharyngeal neoplasia often invades the clivus in a direct fashion. Frank cortical bone destruction may be seen, but marrow space involvement (best depicted on MR imaging) may also occur (**Fig. 20**).

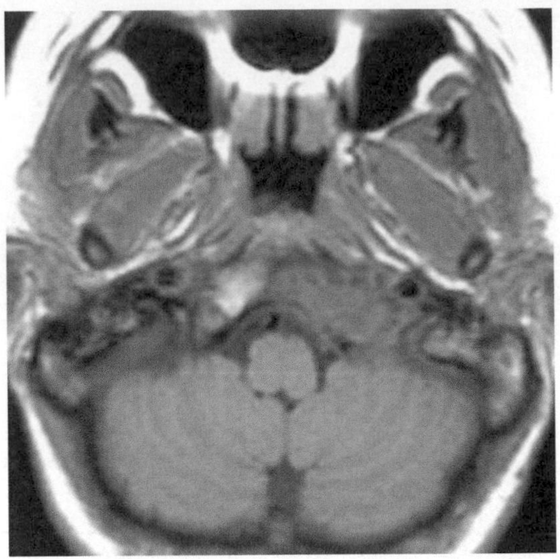

Fig. 21. Axial T1WI MR imaging demonstrates infiltrative hypointense clival lesion.

RHABDOMYOSARCOMA

Rhabdomyosarcoma is the most common childhood soft tissue sarcoma. There is common involvement of the head and neck, with slightly under one-half of cases occurring in this region. Involvement of the central skull base can be seen in tumors involving the midface or nasopharynx. The appearance may be nonspecific with an invasive soft tissue mass. Patient age is a critical concern. Most lesions occur in the first decade of life.[24] The lesions may result in considerable bone destruction and also may spread via a perineural route.[24] CT is useful for cortical bone involvement. MR imaging is most useful to depict the entire extent of disease. MR imaging is crucial to depict perineural tumor spread.[24] Treatment may involve surgery with adjuvant chemotherapy and radiation.

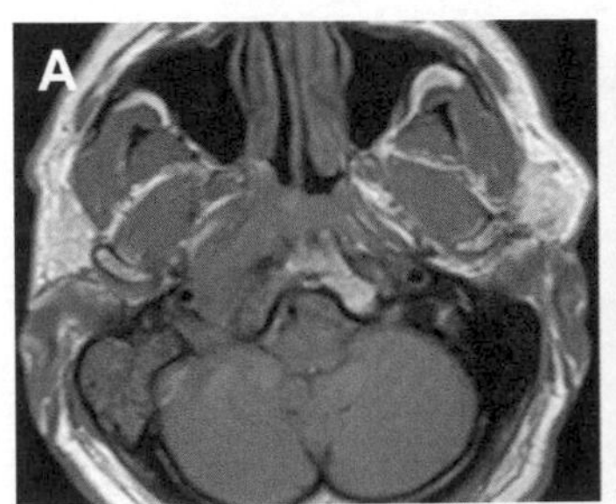

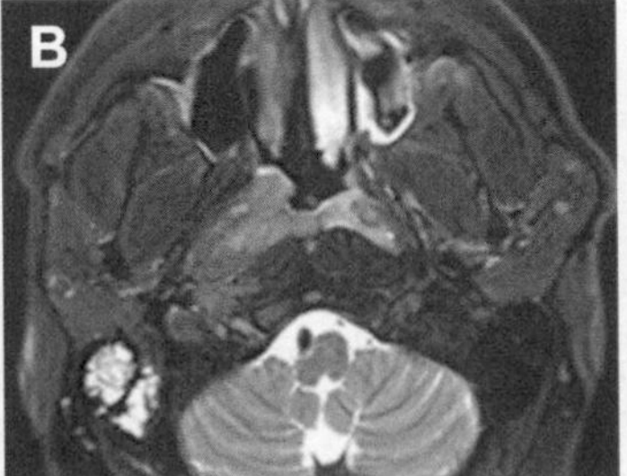

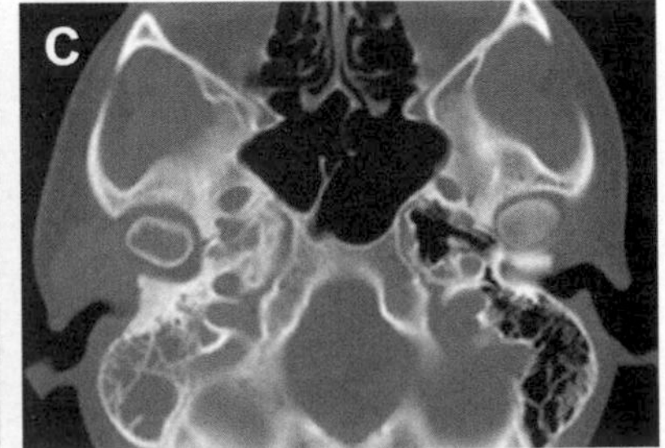

Fig. 20. (*A, B*) Axial T1WI and T2WI MR imaging demonstrate mass extending from right nasopharynx into the clivus. (*C*) Axial CT demonstrates how relatively insensitive CT is to bone marrow invasion.

Box 4 Infection
Osteomyelitis
Gradenigo syndrome

METASTASIS

Any malignant neoplasm may metastasize to the skull base; however, breast and prostate are the most common. An aggressive central skull base lesion may always represent a metastasis; knowledge of an existing primary malignancy is an important consideration in generating a differential diagnosis (**Fig. 21**).

Infectious etiologies are shown in **Box 4**.

OSTEOMYELITIS

Osteomyelitis is an infection of the bone of the skull base that is usually bacterial and may be acute or chronic. *Staphylococcus aureus* is by far the most common organism. CT may demonstrate a permeative lytic lesion. On MR imaging, osteomyelitis may appear T1 hypointense with high T2 signal because of the edema. Sequestra may result in fluid within the bone, which may peripherally enhance and restrict diffusion.

GRADENIGO SYNDROME

Gradenigo syndrome is an uncommon complication of otitis media from infection extending to and involving the petrous apex. There is involvement of the petrous temporal bone that causes a classic triad, periorbital pain (unilateral), diplopia, and otorrhea (**Fig. 22**).

Other etiologies are shown in **Box 5**.

Box 5 Other interesting pathology
Cocaine use
Pseudotumor
Invasive pituitary macroadenoma

COCAINE

The constant use of cocaine and other illicit pharmaceutical compounds can cause significant necrosis in the nasal cavity and contiguous soft tissues due to vasoconstriction. Chronic nasal inhalation of toxic materials may result in loss of soft tissue and bone (in extreme cases) and may involve the central skull base (**Fig. 23**).

PSEUDOTUMOR

Pseudotumor is a benign inflammatory process with a mixed inflammatory cell (predominantly lymphoid) infiltration that results in fibrous reaction. Fibrosis is typically hypointense on T2WI, an important point to remember in consideration of this diagnosis. Pseudotumor also usually

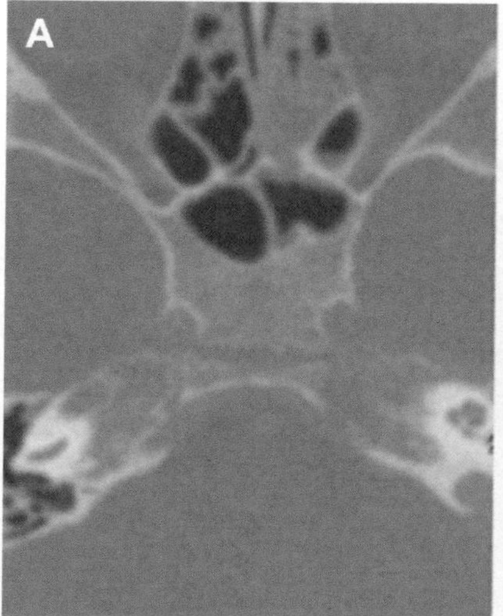

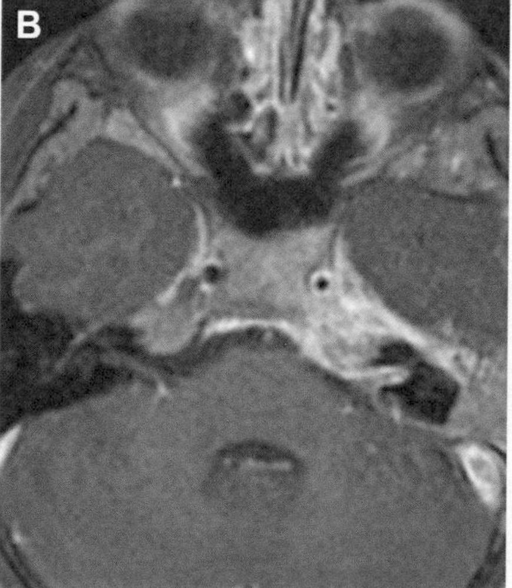

Fig. 22. (*A*) Axial CT demonstrates osseous destruction involving the petrous apex. (*B*) Axial postgadolinium T1WI MR imaging demonstrates avid enhancement.

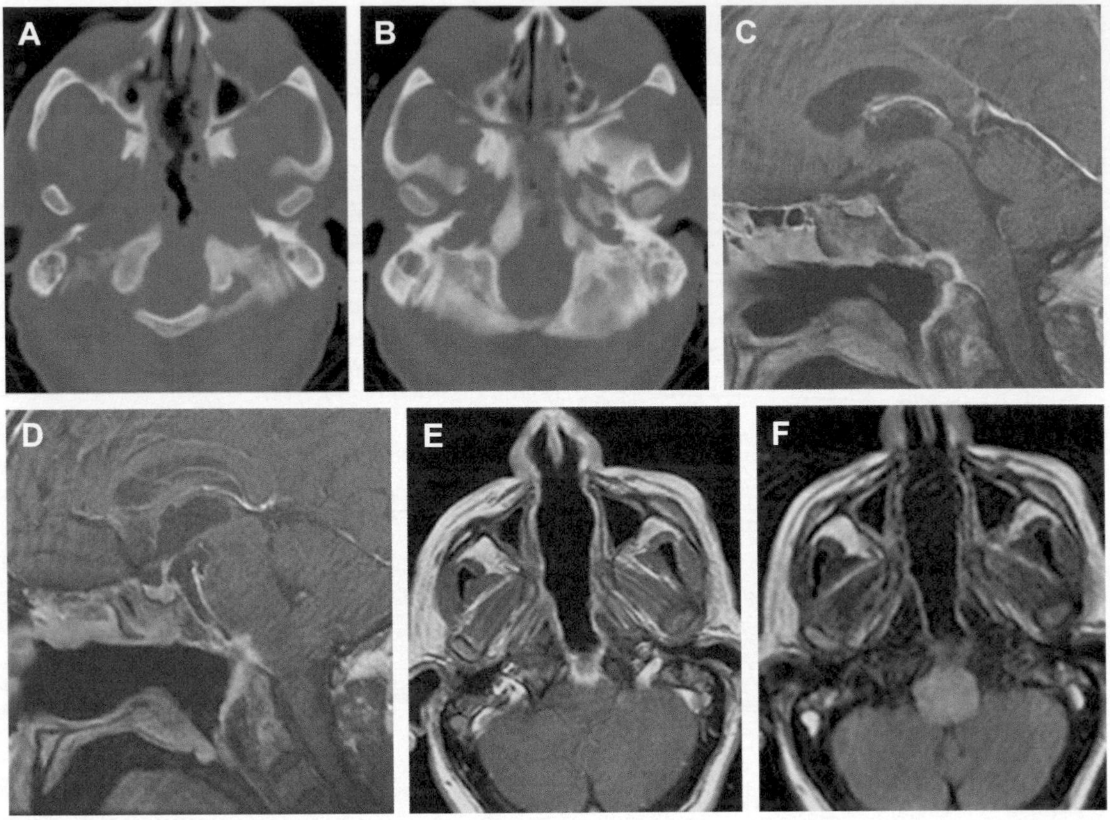

Fig. 23. (*A, B*) Axial CT demonstrates soft tissue necrosis and bone destruction extending from posterior nasopharynx to central skull base. (*C–F*) Sagittal and axial postgadolinium T1WI MR imaging demonstrates extension to and enhancement of the brainstem.

demonstrates avid enhancement. This is usually a diagnosis of exclusion and requires biopsy for pathology. The etiology of pseudotumors is unclear; there are some indications that this may represent another manifestation of IgG4 disease (**Fig. 24**).[25,26]

PITUITARY MACROADENOMA

A large pituitary adenoma may invade the central skull base (See John L. Go and Anandh G. Rajamohans' article, "Imaging of the Sella and Parasellar Region," in this issue.)

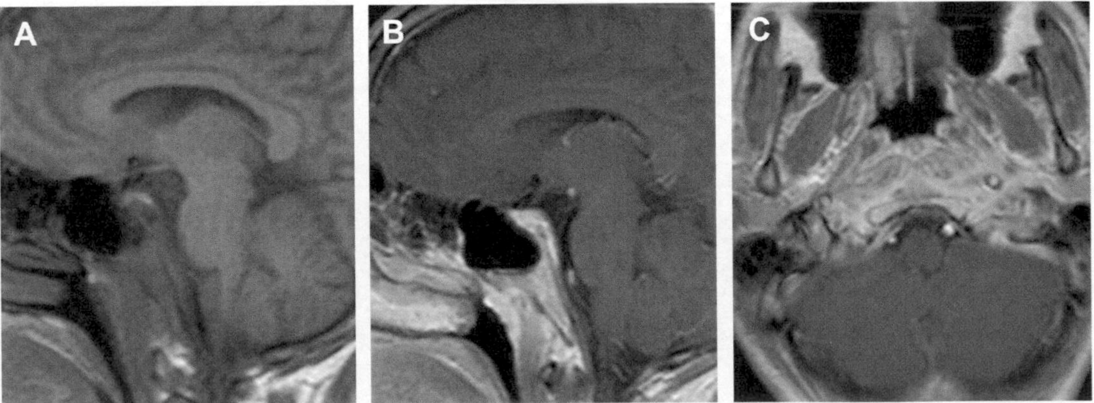

Fig. 24. (*A–C*) Sagittal pre- and sagittal and axial postgadolinium T1WI MR imaging diffuse infiltration with avid enhancement.

SUMMARY

The central skull base is complex separation between the intracranial and extracranial contents, with obvious anatomic continuity between the 2 compartments because of the traversing vascular and neural structures. Multiple pathologies can be primary to the central skull base, many of which have unique and interesting imaging characteristics. Understanding of the relevant embryology and anatomy aids in recognition of the characteristic location and imaging features of this diverse group of developmental variants and pathologic entities.

REFERENCES

1. Nemzek W. MR, CT and plain film imaging of the developing skull base in fetal specimens. AJNR Am J Neuroradiol 2000;21:1699–706.
2. Laine F. CT and MR imaging of the central skull base. Radiographics 1990;10:591–602.
3. Christopherson L. Persistence of the notochordal canal: MR and plain film appearance. AJNR Am J Neuroradiol 1999;20:33–6.
4. Lohman BD. Not the typical Tornwaldt's cyst this time? A nasopharyngeal cyst associated with canalis basilaris medianus. Br J Radiol 2011; 84(1005):e169–71.
5. Chihara C. Ecchordosis physalipohora and its variants: proposed new classification based on high-resolution fast MR imaging employing steady-state acquisition. Eur Radiol 2013;10:2854–60.
6. Currarino G. Canalis basilaris medianus and related defects of the basiocciput. AJNR Am J Neuroradiol 1988;9:208–11.
7. Beltramello A. Fossa Navicularis Magna. AJNR Am J Neuroradiol 1998;19:1796–8.
8. Mehnert F. Retroclival ecchordosis physaliphora: MR imaging and review of the literature. AJNR Am J Neuroradiol 2004;25:1851–5.
9. Abele T. Craniopharyngeal canal and its spectrum of pathology. AJNR Am J Neuroradiol 2013;35(4):772–7.
10. Nguyen RP. Extraosseous Chordoma of the Nasopharynx. AJNR Am J Neuroradiol 2009;30:803–7.
11. Arjona A. Intracranial Hypertension Secondary to Giant Arachnoid Granulations. J Neurol Neurosurg Psychiatry 2003;74:418.
12. Amlashi SFA. Intracranial hypertension and giant arachnoid granulations. J Neurol Neurosurg Psychiatry 2004;75:172.
13. Kransdorf MJ. Fibrous Dysplasia. Radiographics 1990;10(3):519–37.
14. Bianco P. Mutation of the GNAS1 gene, stromal cell dysfunction, and osteomalacic changes in non-mccune-albright fibrous dysplasia of bone. J Bone Miner Res 2000;1:120–8.
15. Shi RR. GNAS mutational analysis in differentiating fibrous dysplasia and ossifying fibroma of the jaw. Mod Pathol 2013;8:1023–31.
16. Kuznetsov S. Age-dependent demise of GNAS-mutated skeletal stem cells and "normalization" of fibrous dysplasia of bone. J Bone Miner Res 2008; 11:1731–40.
17. Chapurlat RD. Medical therapy in adults with fibrous dysplasia of bone. J Bone Miner Res 2006;2:114–9.
18. Singer F. Paget's disease of bone—genetic and environmental factors. Nat Rev Endocrinol 2015;11: 662–71.
19. Gudino LC. Epidemiology of Paget's disease of bone: a systematic review and meta-analysis of secular changes. Bone 2013;55:347–51.
20. Aladioglu K. MRI and CT imagining of an intrasphenoidal encephalocele: a case report. Pol J Radiol 2014;79:360–2.
21. Sternberg M. Ein bisher Nicht beschriebener Kanal im Keilbein des Menschen. Anat Anz 1888; 23:784–6.
22. Settecase F. Spontaneous lateral sphenois cephaloceles: anatomic factors contributing to pathogenesis and proposed classification. AJNR Am J Neuroradiol 2014. http://dx.doi.org/10.3174/ajnr.A3744.
23. Erdem E. Comprehensive review of Intracranial Chordoma. Radiographics 2003;23(4):995–1009.
24. Freling N. Imaging findings in craniofacial childhood rhabdomyosarcoma. Pediatr Radiol 2010;40(11): 1723–38.
25. Toyoda K. MR Imaging of IgG4-Related Disease in the Head and Neck and Brain. AJNR Am J Neuroradiol 2012. http://dx.doi.org/10.3174/ajnr.A3147.
26. Chen A. Clival invasion on multi-detector CT in 390 pituitary macroadenomas: correlation with sex, subtype and rates of operative complication and Recurrance. AJNR Am J Neuroradiol 2011;32: 785–9.

Diplopia: What to Double Check in Radiographic Imaging of Double Vision

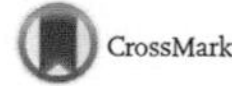

Claudia F.E. Kirsch, MD[a,*], Karen Black, MD[b]

KEYWORDS

• Diplopia • MR imaging • Computed axial tomography

KEY POINTS

- Binocular diplopia may be caused by life-threatening causes requiring careful neuroimaging in patients who have new onset, progressive symptoms, more than one symptom, or history of neoplasm.
- In patients with a new onset ptosis and binocular diplopia, a careful assessment of the vasculature adjacent to cranial nerves III, IV, and VI is needed to exclude an aneurysm.
- An awareness of the radiographic anatomy of cranial nerves III, IV, and VI from their respective nuclei, cisternal and cavernous segments, terminal innervation, and connective pathways is helpful in assessing imaging for binocular diplopia.

Diplopia or "double vision" comes from the Greek terms "diplous" meaning double and "ops" for eye. Diplopia is distressing for patients and may occur from an extensive list of causes. Because certain causes may be life threatening, patients with diplopia require an accurate clinical physical assessment, and in certain cases, a careful radiographic review. Patients with diplopia are often first evaluated by a neurologist or ophthalmologist, who determines whether the diplopia is "monocular" or "binocular." If the patient has "monocular" diplopia, this means they see double with only one eye open. In monocular diplopia, doctors and patients can usually breathe a sigh of relief because causes are often related to eye issues from refractive difficulties, poor glasses, dry eyes, uveitis, or cornea warping, and radiographic imaging may not be required.[1–3]

However, in "binocular" diplopia, the patients see double with both eyes open. Binocular diplopia requires physicians and radiologists assessing these patients to be on high alert and double check everything, including history and images, because these life-threatening causes need to be excluded in the myriad of possible causes. So, when should radiographic studies be obtained in patients with binocular diplopia? Previous general guidelines for imaging patients with binocular diplopia included new onset diplopia in a patient less than 50 years old, presence of more than one neurologic symptom, or a progressive course or history of cancer[1,2]; an easy way to remember it is the rhyme, "In diplopia, if the patient is young, and symptoms are progressing more than one, then neuroimaging should be done!"

Disclosures: Consultant Primal Pictures 3D Anatomy; Grant Funding: Idiopathic Intracranial Hypertension Foundation, RTOG: Radiation Therapy Oncology Group 3504 (C.F.E. Kirsch). K. Black has nothing to disclosure.
[a] Neuroradiology, Department of Radiology, North Shore University Hospital, Long Island Jewish Medical Center, Northwell Health, Hofstra Northwell School of Medicine, 300 Community Drive, Manhasset, NY 11030, USA; [b] Department of Radiology, North Shore University Hospital, Northwell Health, 300 Community Drive, Manhasset, NY 11030, USA
* Corresponding author.
E-mail addresses: ckirsch@northwell.edu; cfekirsch@gmail.com

Radiol Clin N Am 55 (2017) 69–81
http://dx.doi.org/10.1016/j.rcl.2016.08.008
0033-8389/17/© 2016 Elsevier Inc. All rights reserved.

radiologic.theclinics.com

Recent studies, however, have shown that the guidelines for not imaging a patient regardless of age, elderly or not, with a monocular palsy of cranial nerve (CN) III, IV, or VI, are less clear and controversial. These publications advocate that imaging, including a contrast-enhanced MR imaging, may be necessary for all patients presenting with an oculomotor neuropathy resulting in a diplopia.[3] Therefore, a better rhyme to remember is, "If a patient is binocular seeing more than one, than accurate neuroimaging should be done!" Before imaging, a thorough physical examination is essential, especially if patients complain of tiredness at rest and have diplopia. In these cases, myasthenia gravis needs to be excluded, and a good second rule of thumb is, "If the diplopia occurs at rest, also do a tensilon test."

Because an accurate imaging assessment is imperative in certain life-threatening causes of diplopia, understanding the pertinent anatomic pathways of CN III, IV, and VI, including the paramedian pontine reticular formation (PPRF) and medical longitudinal fasiculus (MLF) for lateral gaze, is invaluable.[4] This article presents a few key examples of critical anatomy, abnormality, and radiographic findings affecting these nerves from the cranial nuclei to their distal innervation. A complete list of causes and radiographic findings for binocular diplopia is extensive and beyond the scope of this article.

This article's main focus (pardon the pun) is to present the pertinent anatomy and critical abnormality radiologists should double check on imaging using the acronym, VISION - including the *V*essels, *I*nfection or Inflammation, *S*kull base, *S*uperior orbital fissure, and not forgetting the *S*calp for giant cell temporal arteritis, *I*ncreased *I*ntracranial pressure, *O*nset of new or worst headaches of life, or *O*nset new psychosis, and *N*eoplastic, all of which may cause binocular diplopia and need to be excluded to reduce morbidity and mortality.

ORBITAL ANATOMY

Double checking the course of the nerves involved in orbital imaging requires an awareness of the radiographic course of the cranial nerves, CN III, CN IV, and CN VI, from the brainstem, subarachnoid space, cavernous sinus, superior orbital fissure, and orbit. In addition, a lack of coordinated eye movements may cause diplopia if there is abnormality affecting thePPRF coordinating CN III and CN VI via ascending fibers of the MLF for lateral gaze.[4] Therefore, disruptions of the medial longitudinal fasciculus by upper motor neurons or any other cause can cause diplopia.[1–4] Remembering the orbital cranial nerve muscle innervation is easy with the chemical formula $LR_6\ SO_4$ and all the rest are 3, meaning the lateral rectus muscle is innervated by CN VI the abducens nerve, the superior oblique by CN IV, the trochlear nerve, and remaining orbital musculature by CN III the oculomotor nerve.[5,6] **Fig. 1** is a sagittal T1 MR image, delineating the location of CN III, IV, and IV in the brainstem.

The oculomotor nerve or CN III is a somatic motor nerve with efferent fibers supplying the levator palpebrae superioris, superior, inferior, medial, and lateral rectus and inferior oblique muscles, and a visceral motor efferent with parasympathetic supply constricting the pupil and ciliary muscles, via the ciliary ganglion.[3,5,6] The combined somatic motor fibers and parasympathetic fibers form the CN III oculomotor nerve as it leaves the brainstem.

As demonstrated in **Fig. 2**A, the CN III nucleus somatic motor component is "V" shaped and is located in the midbrain at the level of the superior colliculus, just anterior to the cerebral aqueduct, with the medial longitudinal fasciculus as its neighbor laterally and inferiorly. In the brainstem, the oculomotor complex is composed of lateral subnuclei with the posterior component supplying the *ipsilateral* inferior rectus, the intermediate nucleus supplying the inferior oblique, and the anterior ventral nuclei supplying the medial rectus muscles. The medial subnucleus gives supply to the *contralateral* superior rectus, and the central

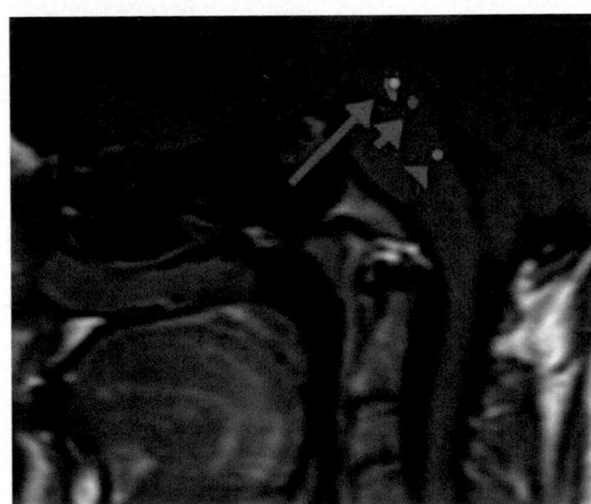

Fig. 1. Sagittal T1-weighted MR imaging with the large arrow showing the location of the nucleus for the oculomotor nerve CN III, including both the visceral motor Edinger-Westphal nucleus posteriorly in blue that innervates the parasympathetics for the pupil constrictor muscles and ciliary muscles, and the anterior pink somatic nucleus. The short arrow demarcates the trochlear CN IV nucleus located below the CN III nucleus, and the arrowhead demarcates the lateral abducens CN IV nucleus.

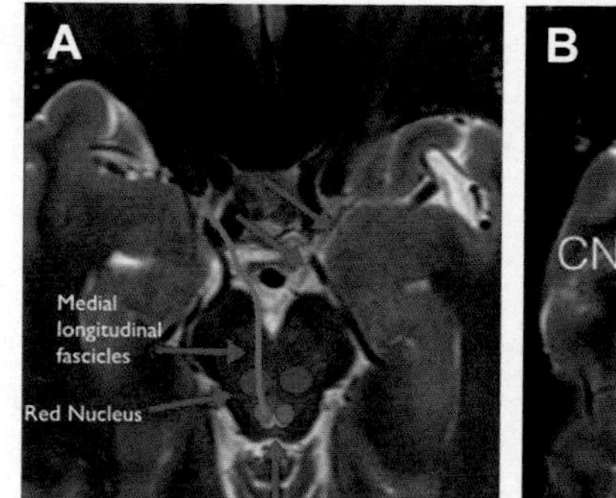

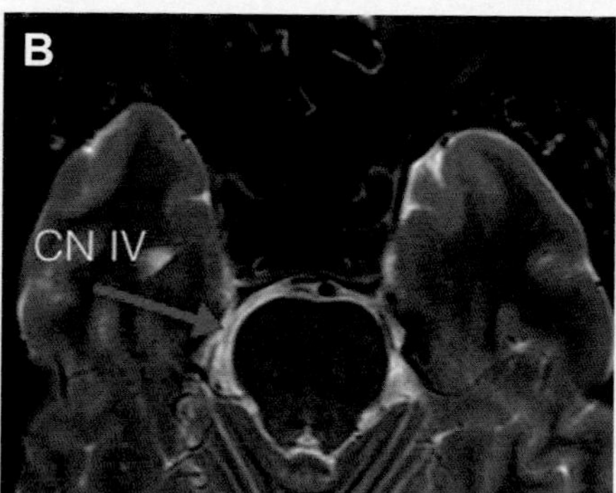

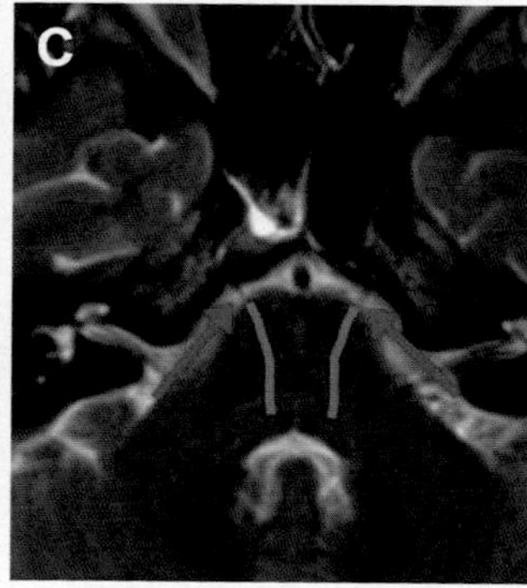

Fig. 2. The course of the cranial nerves. (*A*) Axial T2 MR imaging at the level of the CN III oculomotor nucleus demonstrates the course of CN III from its nucleus, through the medial longitudinal fasciculus, and into the interpeduncular cistern as it extends underneath the posterior communicating artery. Red arrows are the cisternal segment of CN III, pink line is the intracranial course of CN III, red circles are the red nuclei, pink circles are the CN III nuclei, the tiny blue dot is the CN III Edinger-Westphal nucleus. (*B*) Axial T2 MR imaging taken a slice below (*A*), demonstrating the trochlear nerve CN IV, whose nucleus is located at the midbrain tegmentum near the midline anterior to the cerebral aqueduct. CN IV decussates exiting dorsally, going around the cerebral peduncles marked by the red arrow and with CN III going between the PCA and SCA, underneath the posterior communicating artery and then piercing the tentorial free and attached border to enter the cavernous sinus located below CN III. (*C*) Axial T2 MR image of pons at the level of the fourth ventricle. The expected course of CN VI (*pink lines*) is shown with the red arrows pointing to the CN VI cisternal segments in the prepontine cistern, where it then pierces the dura and extends superiorly.

subnucleus gives supply to the bilateral levator palpebrae superiorus muscles, with the Edinger-Westphal (visceral motor) nucleus located posteriorly, giving rise to the parasympathetic fibers.

The CN III axons for the lower motor neurons extend anteriorly through midbrain tegmentum, through the red nucleus, emerging in the medial interpeduncular cistern where the pons and midbrain merge. CN III runs between the superior cerebellar artery (SCA) and posterior cerebral artery (PCA), just below the posterior communicating artery. CN III enters the dura into the cavernous sinus, running along the superior lateral wall above the trochlear nerve. The CN III nerve exits via the superior orbital fissure into the tendinous ring, and entering the orbit, divides into superior and inferior components. The superior nerve of CN III goes upward and lateral to the optic nerve supplying the superior rectus and levator palpebrae. The inferior CN III separates into 3 parts, supplying the inferior rectus, and medial rectus muscles along the medial ocular margin and the inferior oblique muscle along its posterior aspect.[3,5]

The Edinger-Westphal visceral motor neurons course along with the somatic motor axons, from the middle cranial fossa, cavernous sinus, and superior orbital fissure. The nerves separate from the neural components supplying the inferior oblique muscle and terminate in the ciliary ganglion at the apex of the orbital cone. Exiting from the ciliary ganglion are short ciliary nerves that join with sympathetic fibers from the internal carotid artery (ICA), that enter into the globe at the posterior margin near the optic nerve. These nerves control the constrictor pupillae muscles and ciliary muscles and run in between the sclera and choroid of the eye ending up in the ciliary body and iris of the globe where the fibers control pupil size and lens shape.[6]

As noted in **Fig. 2**B, CN IV, the trochlear nerve, is smallest cranial nerve, with the longest intracranial course. CN IV is a somatic motor nerve only innervating the superior oblique muscle, with the nucleus located in the midbrain tegmentum below CN III, in the inferior colliculus.[5,6] Most motor neurons are located medially as is the nucleus, located just ventral to the cerebral aqueduct. CN IV is unique because it is the only nerve exiting from the back (dorsal) brainstem and crossing to the opposite side. Because CN IV decussates or crosses from the brainstem, each superior oblique muscle is innervated by the trochlear nucleus located in the contralateral brainstem. CN IV runs with CN III between the PCA and SCA arteries, along the margin of the free and attached margin of the tentorium cerebelli. CN IV runs below CN III in the cavernous sinus, and through the superior orbital fissure crossing diagonally across the levator palpebrae and superior rectus muscle to the superior oblique muscle.[6] When CN IV is not functioning, the CN III and CN VI take over the globe, and the globe is rotated outwardly by abduction from CN VI and inferiorly from unopposed action of the muscles innervated by CN III.[3,5] Therefore, this is sometimes referred to as the "bum's muscle" because a lack of a functioning CN IV has you looking down and out.

As shown in **Fig. 2**C, the abducens nerve CN VI is a somatic efferent nerve to the lateral rectus muscle. The CN VI nucleus is in the pontine tegmentum, and like additional somatic motor nuclei, is located closer to the midline anterior to the fourth ventricle. As the seventh cranial nerve (CN VII) circles over the sixth nerve nuclei, it creates a little bump or hill, "colliculus" along the fourth ventricular anterior margin. The CN VI emerges where the pons and medullary pyramid meet, extends through the prepontine cistern entering the dura lateral to the dorsum sella, and then travels through the petroclival confluence (Dorello canal) under the petrosphenoidal "Gruber ligament."[7] It is important to be aware of the actual course of CN VI and the true definition of the "Dorello canal." The course of CN VI is well outlined by Umansky and colleagues,[8] who note 3 curves. The first curve of CN VI is at the dural foramen where CN VI curves upward to lateral to the petrous apex; the second curve of CN VI is over the petrous apex where CN VI must angle inferiorly and laterally to reach the posterior aspect of the cavernous ICA, and the third curve as CN VI extends around the posterior ICA and then runs next to the vessel in the medial cavernous sinus (**Fig. 3**).[7–9] In Dorello's original 1905 paper, he defined the canal as the "Triangular space bordered by Gruber's superior petrosphenoidal ligament (PSL) superolaterally, superior clivus inferiorly, petrous apex inferolaterally. The space at the 2nd bend of the CN VI, with CN VI always below Gruber's ligament and containing the ostium of the inferior petrosal sinus (IPS) within the canal."[7,8] However, this definition has many problems, as modern microneurosurgery and imaging demonstrate. First, there are no bony margins like the optic canal! Second, since 1991, studies demonstrated that CN VI can go above Gruber ligament.[7] On thin-section MR imaging, follow this nerve closely and you may notice this finding as well! Third, in microneurosurgery, it is noted that the ostium of the IPS is outside of this space; therefore, more recently, clinicians have referred to this space as the "petroclivus venous confluence."[7–9]

The extension of the CN VI through the petrovenous confluence (Dorello canal) over the petrous ridge is where CN VI is at highest risk for injury. The risk of injury is greater partly because CN VI is tethered inferiorly entering the dura and superiorly as it enters the cavernous sinus. Therefore, the curved segment of the nerve extending over the petrous apex of the temporal bone is the site most at risk to trauma, infection, or increased intracranial pressure.[7–9] After CN VI extends over the petrous apex, CN VI, into the cavernous sinus, it is the most medial of the cranial nerves, next to the ICA, as shown in **Fig. 4**. The CN VI then extends into the superior orbital fissure. In patients with a lower motor neuronal lesion, the lateral rectus muscle is denervated, and the patient cannot abduct the globe laterally; the globe is pulled medially due to the unopposed action of CN III on the medial rectus muscle.

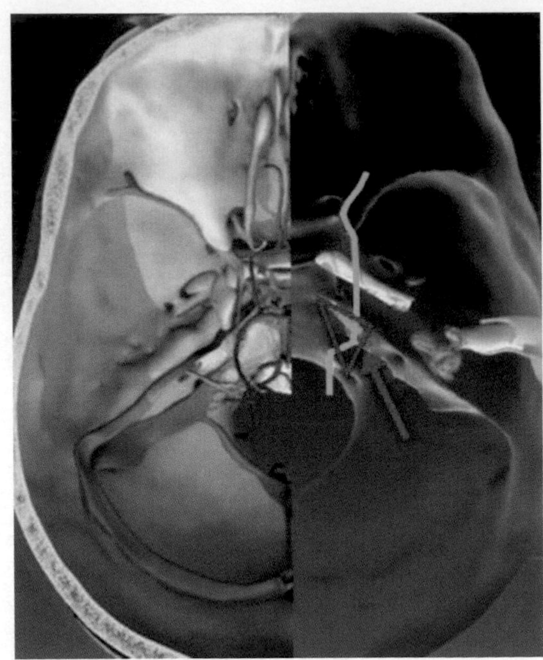

Fig. 3. The course of CN VI (*green line*) through the petroclival confluence or "Dorello canal" marked by the triangle in red. The arrow is pointing to the location of Dorello's canal. (*From* Berkovitz B, Kirsch C, Moxham B, et al. 3D head & neck anatomy with special senses and basic neuroanatomy [DVD]. Primal Pictures; 2007; with permission.)

What to Double Check Using the Acronym VISION

In assessing patients with binocular diplopia, it is helpful to have a checklist to rule out the most critical causes. Using the acronym VISION is a good way to double check for abnormality causing double vision: *V*asculature, *I*nfectious or *I*nflammatory, remembering to check the *S*calp for a giant cell arteritis, *S*kull base and *S*uperior orbital fissure in trauma, *I*ncreased *I*ntracranial pressure, *O*nset of new or worst headaches, or *O*nset new psychosis,

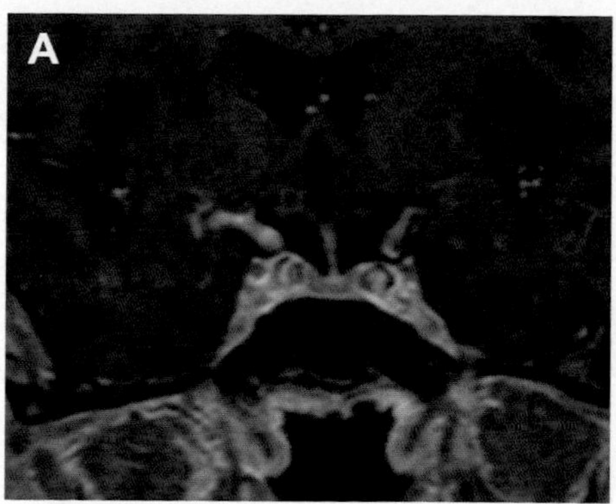

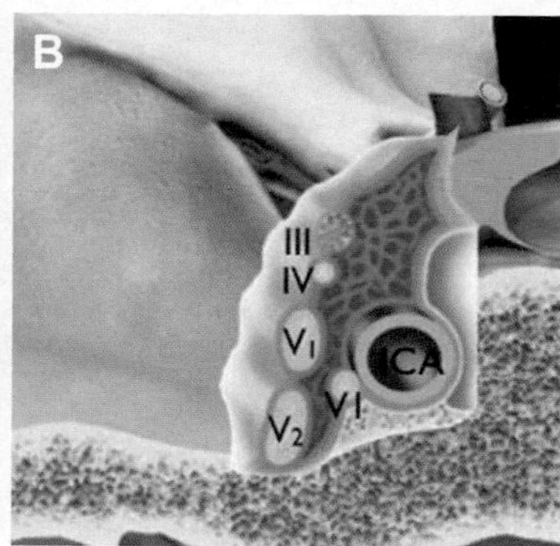

Fig. 4. (*A*) Coronal T1 postgadolinium through the cavernous sinus. The cranial nerves are identified as the foci of nonenhancement within the enhancing cavernous sinus. (*B*). Schematic with cranial nerves labeled lateral to the ICA. (*From* Berkovitz B, Kirsch C, Moxham B, et al. 3D head & neck anatomy with special senses and basic neuroanatomy [DVD]. Primal Pictures; 2007; with permission.)

and *N*eoplastic in determining causes of binocular diplopia.

V: vasculature

In patients who present with a drooping eyelid (ptosis), binocular diplopia, and a poorly reacting pupil, an aneurysm needs to be excluded. A missed aneurysm that may eventually rupture with subarachnoid hemorrhage may have a mortality of up to 50%.[10] The clinical findings of diplopia and ptosis are important clues to the presence of an aneurysm, because CNs III and IV run directly between the PCA and SCA and underneath the posterior communicating artery (Pcom). In addition, these CNs run close together into the cavernous sinus with the ICA located medially to CN VI. Aneurysms compressing the cranial nerves may lead to denervation atrophy of the orbital musculature resulting in a binocular diplopia (**Fig. 5**A–G). Because the pupillary response may be difficult to assess, and loss of CN III results in a ptosis, a good rule to follow is "A new ptosis is a PCom aneurysm until proven otherwise."

In elderly patients or patients with diabetes, strokes or vascular lesions leading to hemorrhage involving the brainstem may present with a diplopia (**Fig. 6**A, B). A computed tomographic (CT) scan is helpful to assess for hemorrhage, and a diffusion weighted imaging (DWI) MR imaging may help delineate new infarcts; vasculature can be assessed either via computed tomographic angiography (CTA) or magnetic resonance angiography (MRA).

In addition to aneurysms at risk for rupture, life-threatening vascular causes that may cause diplopia include vascular malformations, dissections, strokes, and arteritis, such as giant cell arteritis. When viewing the study, double check the course of the CNs III, IV, and VI, and adjacent vessels and nuclei for strokes of the basal midbrain (see **Fig. 6**; **Fig. 7**). Strokes of the midbrain are often associated with other symptoms, including a contralateral hemiplegia due to the adjacent corticospinal tract fibers, or if in the red nucleus, an ipsilateral ophthalmoplegia and contralateral intentional tremor.[3,4]

As a brief review, CNs III, IV, and VI are at risk from an aneurysm from adjacent vessels resulting in a possible denervation atrophy of the corresponding musculature; this means double checking the posterior communicating artery, PCA, SCA, or ICA. In patients with a ptosis with the double vision, pay close attention to the Pcom, as an aneurysm from this vessel may cause a ptosis by the aneurysm compressing the CN III with denervation of the levator palpebrae superiorus and continued action of CN VII on the orbicularis oculi.

In addition to aneurysms, double check the basilar and posterior inferior cerebellar arteries for thrombus or increased attenuation of the vessels on CT and lack of flow on MR imaging, MRA, or CTA. Be on the lookout for dissections, which may lead to a stroke in the pons or midbrain (see **Fig. 7**). If there is abnormal increased attenuation within the basilar artery (thrombus), this may occlude the pontine arterial branches, resulting in a pontine infarct. The visual complex coordination is controlled by thePPRF coordinating CN III and CN VI via ascending fibers of the MLF for lateral gaze. Pontine infarcts in this region may result in paralysis of conjugate lateral gaze. Lesions along the MLF can result in lateral gaze problems and nystagmus due to involvement of vestibular-oculomotor fibers.[2–4,11]

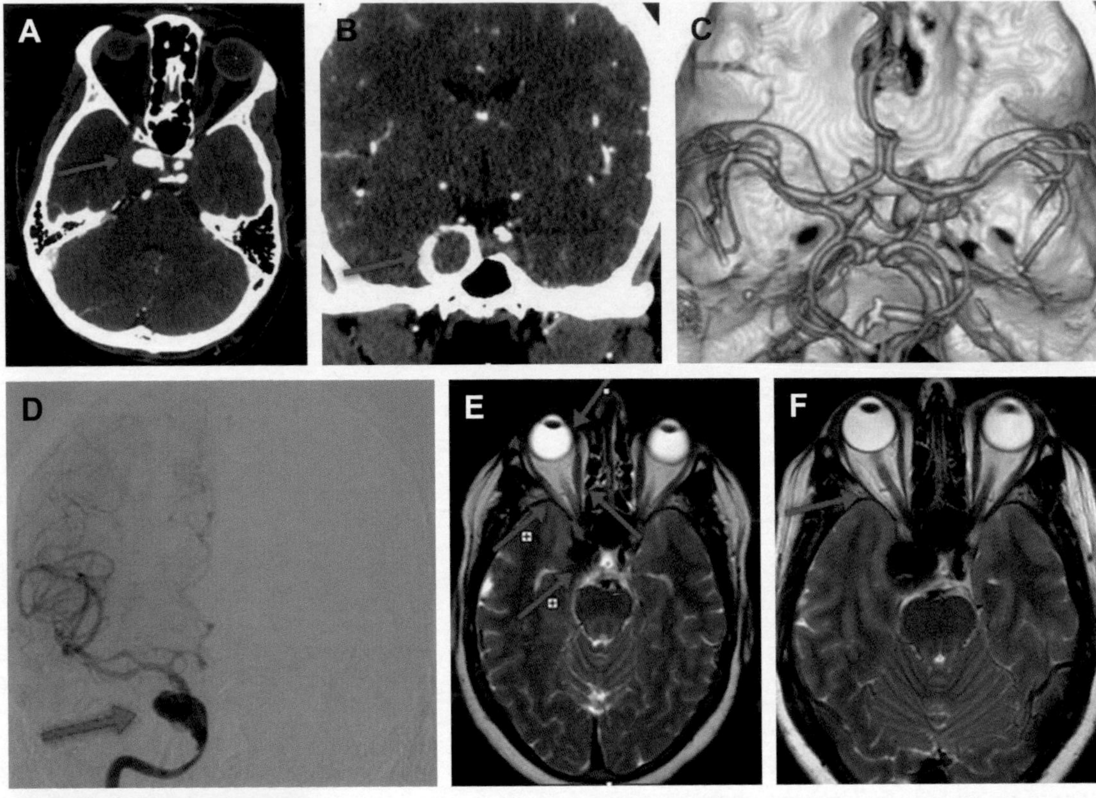

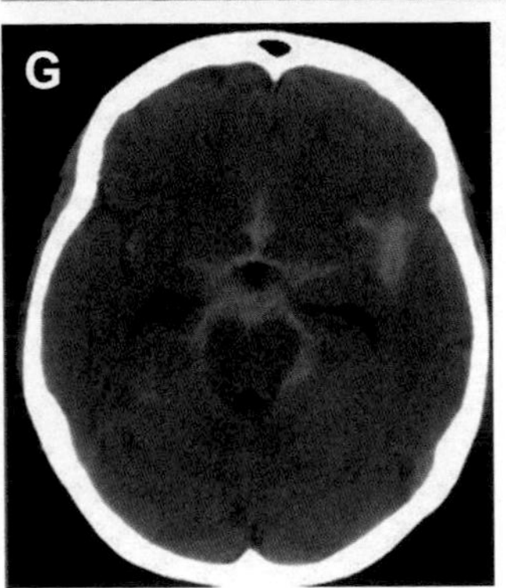

Fig. 5. (*A, B*) Axial and coronal CT scan with contrast demonstrating a large calcified right ICA aneurysm (*arrow*). (*C*) CT angiography 3D reconstruction notes that the right and left sides are reversed, demonstrating the large right ICA aneurysm. (*D*) Cerebral angiography before coiling of the aneurysm (*arrow*). (*E*) Axial T2 MR imaging posterior arrow with + sign, showing ICA aneurysm with decreased T2 signal from hemosiderin and calcification. Anterior arrow with + sign denervation atrophy of the right lateral rectus muscle from compression of CN VI. (*F*) Axial T2 MR imaging, months later after coiling with susceptibility artifact, severe denervation atrophy of the right lateral rectus, with medially deviated right globe (*arrow*). (*G*) Axial CT scan of different patient demonstrating the appearance of subarachnoid hemorrhage.

In binocular diplopia with a small pupil (miosis) and ptosis and anhydrosis (lack of sweating on the same side), be on high alert for Horner syndrome and assess the vessels for a dissection (see **Fig. 7**A, B). Diplopia and ptosis are like the old ads for potato chips, stating, "You can't have just one." If there are multiple findings with diplopia, this is a strong indicator to double check for the underlying abnormality.[2–4,11]

Last, in patients who have experienced a rapid alteration in venous pressure affecting the superior orbital venous vasculature or external bleeds, make sure there are no compressive masses along the orbital cone (**Fig. 8**).

I: inflammatory and infectious causes

Infectious, inflammatory, or neoplastic leptomeningeal processes and increased intracranial pressure can affect cranial nerves as well as temporal lobe uncal herniation, which displaces the cerebral peduncle to the contralateral side, distorting CN III along the tentorial notch. Pay careful attenuation to patients who are at increased risk for infections, including embolic causes in patients who are immunocompromised, on dialysis, or at risk for septic emboli. In dialysis patients who cannot have contrast due to elevated creatinine, a noncontrast MR imaging with a DWI may be useful to help identify abscesses, which demonstrate

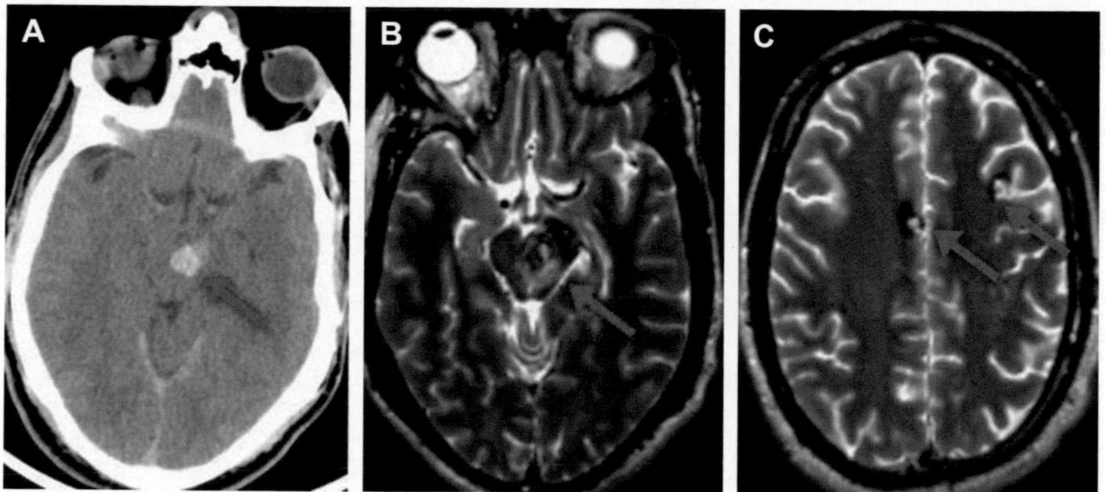

Fig. 6. A 63-year-old man presented with new onset binocular diplopia. (*A*) Axial CT scan with arrow showing intraparenchymal hemorrhage in the midbrain. (*B*) Corresponding axial T2 MR imaging demonstrates lesion with surrounding edema. (*C*) Axial T2 MR imaging of same patient with arrows demonstrating small foci of hyperintense T2 signal with surrounding hemosiderin in patient with multiple cavernous angiomas.

restricted diffusion on the acute diffusion coefficient images (ADC) and bright signal on the DWI, as demonstrated in **Fig. 9**. In patients with sinus infections at risk for extension, look at the cavernous sinus carefully for signs of infection and possible thrombosis, as in **Fig. 10**. Inflammatory causes such as Guillain-Barré or Miller Fisher variants can be life threatening, and additional

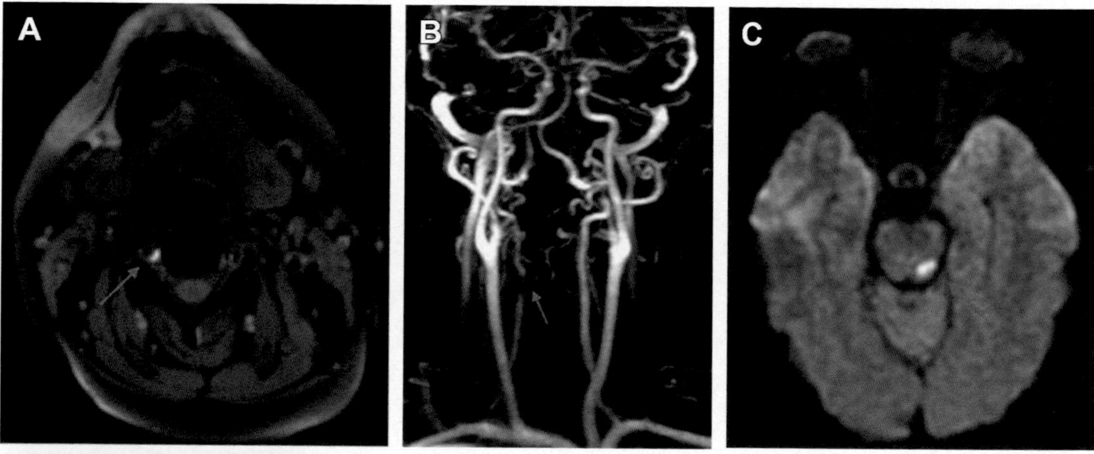

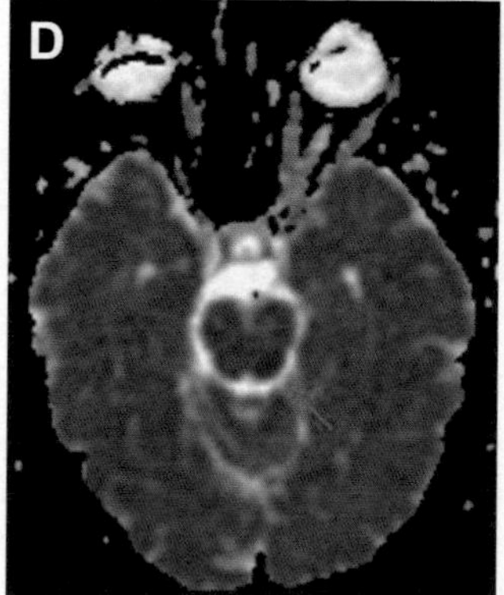

Fig. 7. (*A*) Axial T1 postgadolinium fat-saturated T2 MR imaging with arrow noting right vertebral artery dissection in 42-year-old woman presenting with sudden onset diplopia. (*B*) Postcontrast time-of-flight 3D MRA with arrow pointing to right vertebral artery dissection. (*C, D*) Axial DWI and ADC MR imaging with bright DWI signal and restricted diffusion from acute (*arrow*) stroke in the left inferior colliculus.

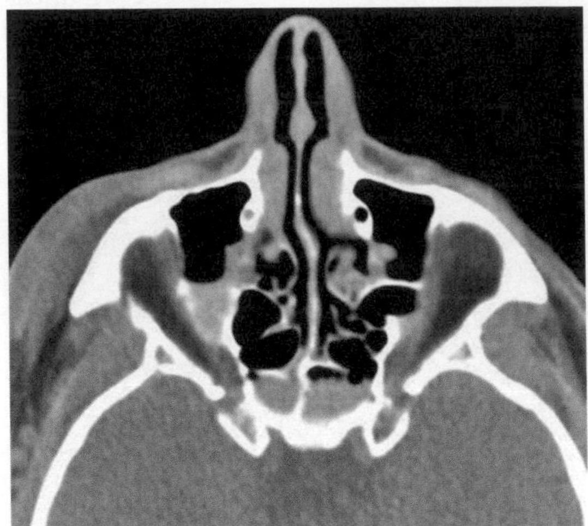

Fig. 8. Traumatic–axial noncontrast CT through the facial bones in a patient status post motor vehicle accident with fracture deformity through the right superior orbital fissure resulting in a binocular diplopia, with hemorrhagic air fluid levels in the sphenoid sinus.

inflammatory changes from demyelination if involving the nuclei will affect the cranial nerves, as in **Fig. 11**. Remember, if ptosis is combined with other deficits, it is like a dangerous bag of potato chips, "you can't have just one"; therefore, look carefully for *I*nvolvement of other ocular findings with the diplopia.[1,3,4,11,12] Demyelinating disease, in particular, may be located at multiple sites, requiring assessment of both the brain and the spinal cord (see **Fig. 11**).

Additional inflammatory causes, including tumefactive inflammatory fibrosis, Tolusa-Hunt, paraneoplastic, or immunoglobulin G (IgG) depositional disease, may involve and affect the cranial nerves with irregular enhancement noted along the cranial nerves on postgadolinium MR imaging, with a resultant binocular diplopia.[13–17]

S: scalp tenderness, skull base, and sphenoid bone

New headache with scalp tenderness in the temporal regions or pain with chewing may be seen with giant cell arteritis. New imaging techniques including CTA and thin postgadolinium contrast MR imaging with fat saturation may demonstrate inflammatory change along the superficial temporal artery, aiding in the diagnosis.[1–3] Because CNs III, IV, and VI extend close together from the cavernous sinus through the superior orbital fissure, trauma through the fissure may damage any of the nerves, resulting in a binocular diplopia. In trauma patients with a binocular diplopia, double check cranial nerves especially at the skull base and superior orbital fissure for adjacent fracture deformities. Skull base fractures may affect CN VI because it lies close to the floor of the posterior cranial fossa. Fractures involving the sphenoid or superior orbital fissure may affect nerves CN III, CN IV, CN IV, or V1[2,5,9,18] (**Fig. 12**).

I: increased intracranial pressure

As the incidence of obesity increases in the general population, so has the prevalence of idiopathic intracranial hypertension or pseudotumor cerebri.[19] Therefore, if a patient with a larger body mass index presents with diplopia, pseudotumor cerebri should be considered because this may cause a binocular diplopia, from a CN IV or CN VI palsy occurring from the nerve being compressed along the petrous temporal ridge. Ancillary radiographic findings suggestive of the diagnosis include a partially empty sella, papilledema that can be assessed on the thin-section T2 images or DWI diffusion sequences, prominent enlarged optic nerve sheathes, and compression and flattening of the transverse sinus on MR imaging as well as skull base erosive changes (see **Fig. 12**). In patients with uncal herniation and severe increased intracranial pressure, this may compress CN III and also result in a blown pupil.[1–3,11]

O: onset of new headache or psychosis

Onset of new headache, that is, worst headache of life, should prompt assessment for subarachnoid hemorrhage (see **Fig. 5**G), or new headaches with scalp tenderness or pain with chewing may be seen with giant cell arteritis, requiring careful double checking of the superficial temporal artery, and may help in aiding in the diagnosis.[1–3] In patients with a new onset psychosis and binocular diplopia, clinicians and radiologists should also exclude NMDA receptor antibody encephalitis, paraneoplastic syndromes, or reactive inflammatory causes, including IgG4 or umefactive fibroinflammatory fibrosis.[11,13,14,20] Remember, a patient does not always need to have teratoma. Therefore, in cases with a negative MR imaging, do not forget about neuroinflammatory syndromes and for clinicians to carefully exclude NMDA receptor antibody encephalitis or any additional immune-related abnormality.[18,20,21]

N: neoplasm

All patients with a history of neoplasm and new onset binocular diplopia should be imaged. Patients with tumors either primary in neurofibromatosis with schwannomas along the nerve or metastatic with leptomeningeal disease, or tumor compressing the nerve, or skull base invasion, require imaging with careful attention to the course of the CN III–VII. *N*eoplasms in the region of the

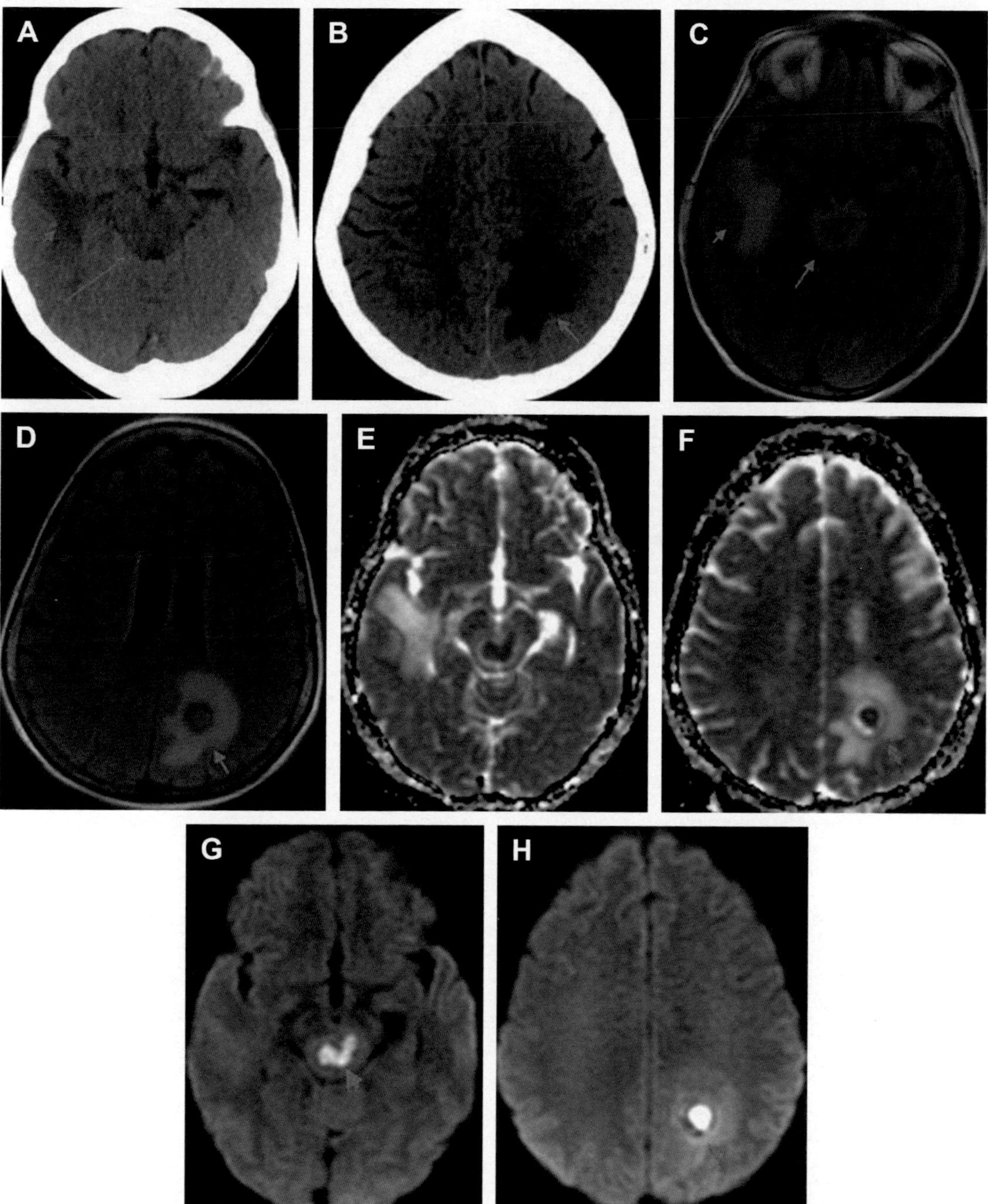

Fig. 9. A 58-year-old woman dialysis patient who presented with binocular diplopia and ophthalmoplegia. Patient could not receive contrast due to elevated creatine and poor renal function. (*A, B*) Axial CT scans at level of cerebral peduncles and left parietal lobe with arrowhead and arrows denoting areas of decreased attenuation consistent with edema. Note the faint rim of increased attenuation from abscess rim within the left parietal edema. (*C, D*) Corresponding axial fluid-attenuated inversion recovery (FLAIR) MR imaging with hyperintense FLAIR signal (edema) surrounding foci of decreased attenuation (abscesses) (*arrow*). (*E–H*) MR imaging, ADC and DWI. Arrows and arrowhead denote restricted diffusion of the abscess within the brainstem and left parietal lobe with dark ADC and hyperintense DWI signal.

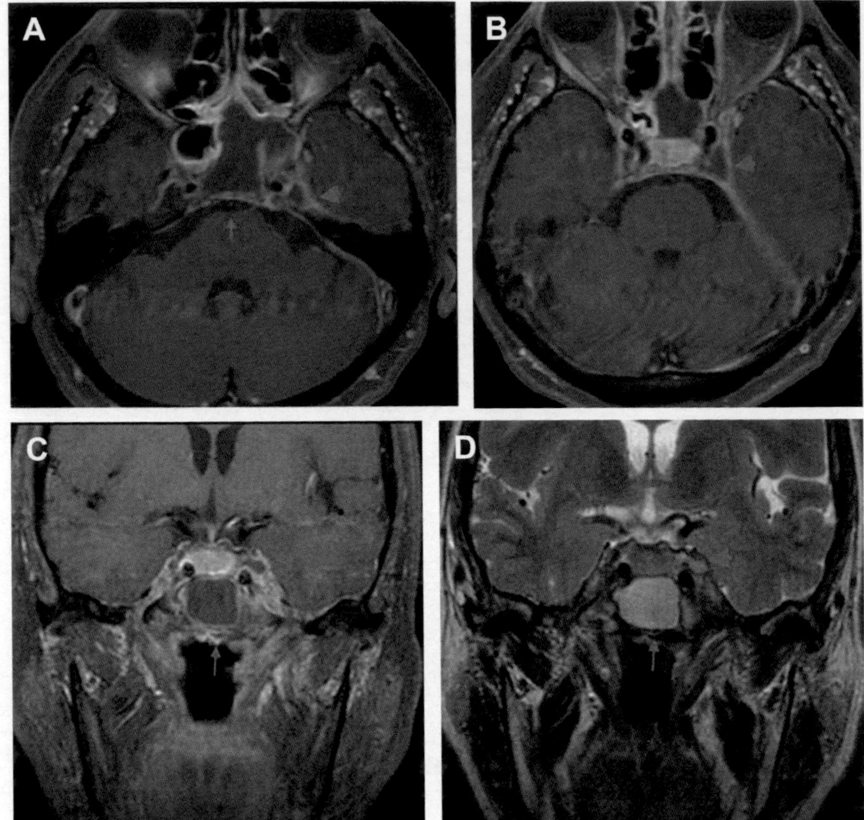

Fig. 10. (*A, B*) Patient with infected sphenoid mucocele presenting with diplopia. Axial postcontrast fat-saturation T1 images through the sphenoid sinus and cavernous sinus with small arrow demarcating sphenoid mucocele and arrowhead demonstrating sinus inflammatory change extending into the left cavernous sinus. (*C*) Coronal postcontrast with fat-saturation arrowhead pointing out small "goldfish"-shaped foci of nonenhancement in the left cavernous sinus consistent with abscess (arrow pointing the mucocele in the sphenoid sinus). (*D*) Coronal T2 series through sella and cavernous sinus arrow pointing to opacified sphenoid sinus with arrowhead demarcating extension into the left cavernous sinus and the "goldfish"-shaped abscess.

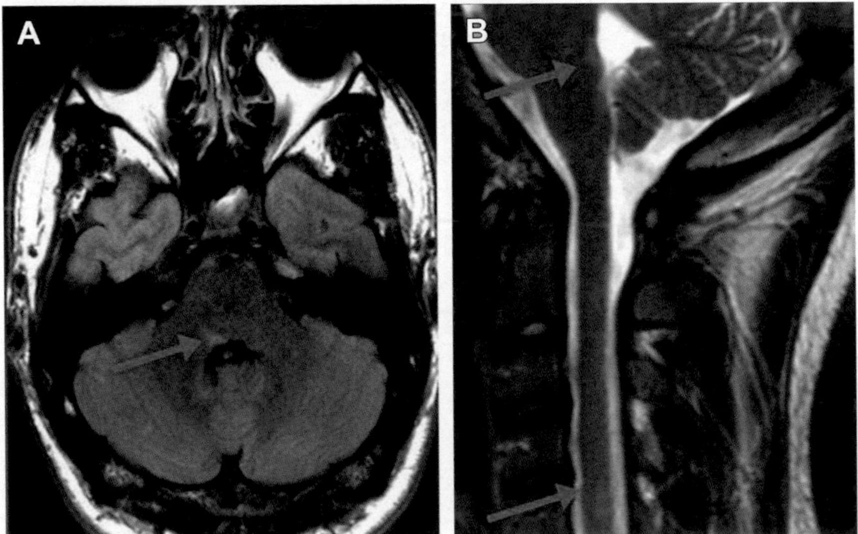

Fig. 11. (*A*) MR imaging brain-axial FLAIR of the brain at the level of the pons. (*B*) Sagittal T2-weighted image of the cervical spine in a 23-year-old man presenting with binocular diplopia involving right CN VI. Arrows denote the FLAIR and T2 hyperintensity at the level of the right CN VI nucleus, just anterior to the fourth ventricle, in patient with demyelinating disease. Second arrow more inferiorly on the T2-weighted MR imaging demonstrates an additional demyelinating plaque in the cervical spinal cord.

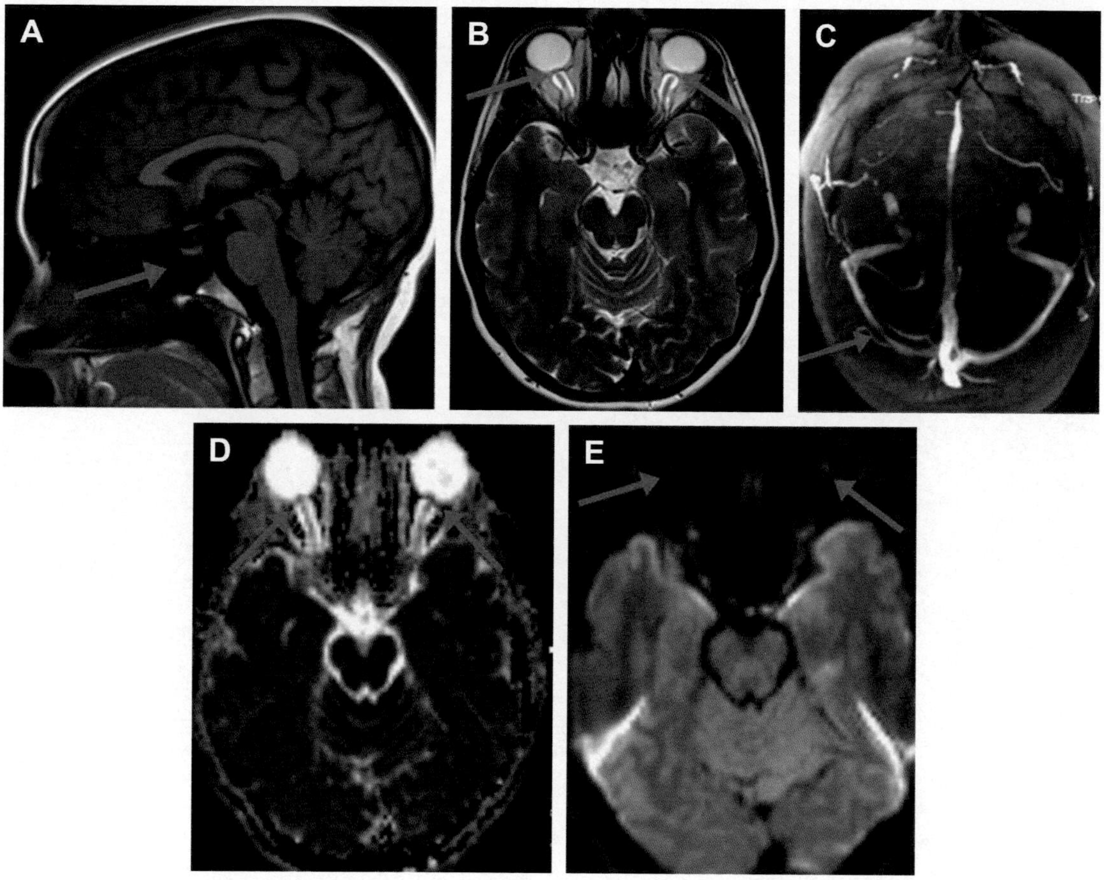

Fig. 12. A 32-year-old woman presented with binocular diplopia, with multiple cranial nerve palsies, with visual loss and headache. Patient underwent a diagnostic lumbar puncture with elevated intracranial pressure diagnosing pseudotumor cerebri or idiopathic increased intracranial hypertension. (*A*) Sagittal T1 MR imaging. Arrow points to a partially empty sella. (*B*) Axial T2 MR imaging. Arrows demarcate enlarged optic nerve sheaths and flattening of the posterior globe margins with papilledema. (*C*) Magnetic resonance venography with arrow pointing to the flattened right transverse sinus. (*D, E*) ADC and DWI images with arrows pointing to the restricted diffusion at the optic nerve heads consistent with papilledema.

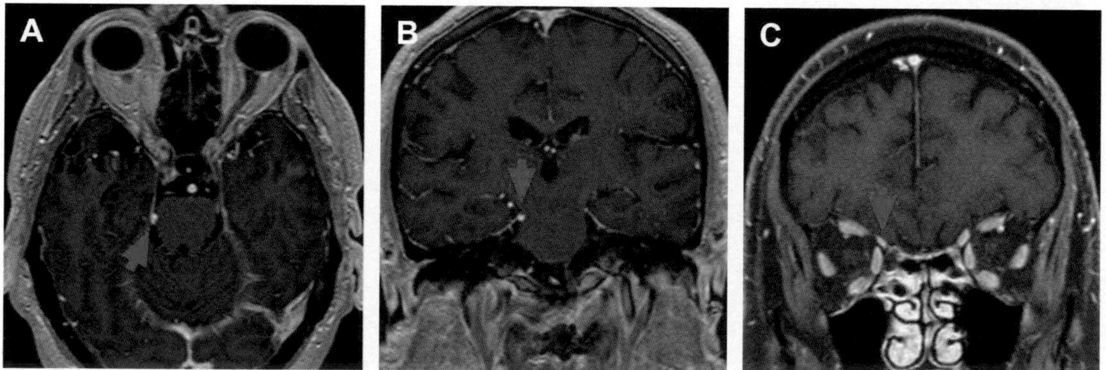

Fig. 13. A 54-year-old man complaining of vertical binocular diplopia, compensating by tilting his head. (*A, B*) Axial and coronal T1 postgadolinium MR imaging with small arrow demarcating meningioma at the right tentorial incisura along the course of the distal right CN IV. (*C*) Coronal T1 postgadolinium MR image with arrow pointing to the decreased size of the right superior oblique muscle.

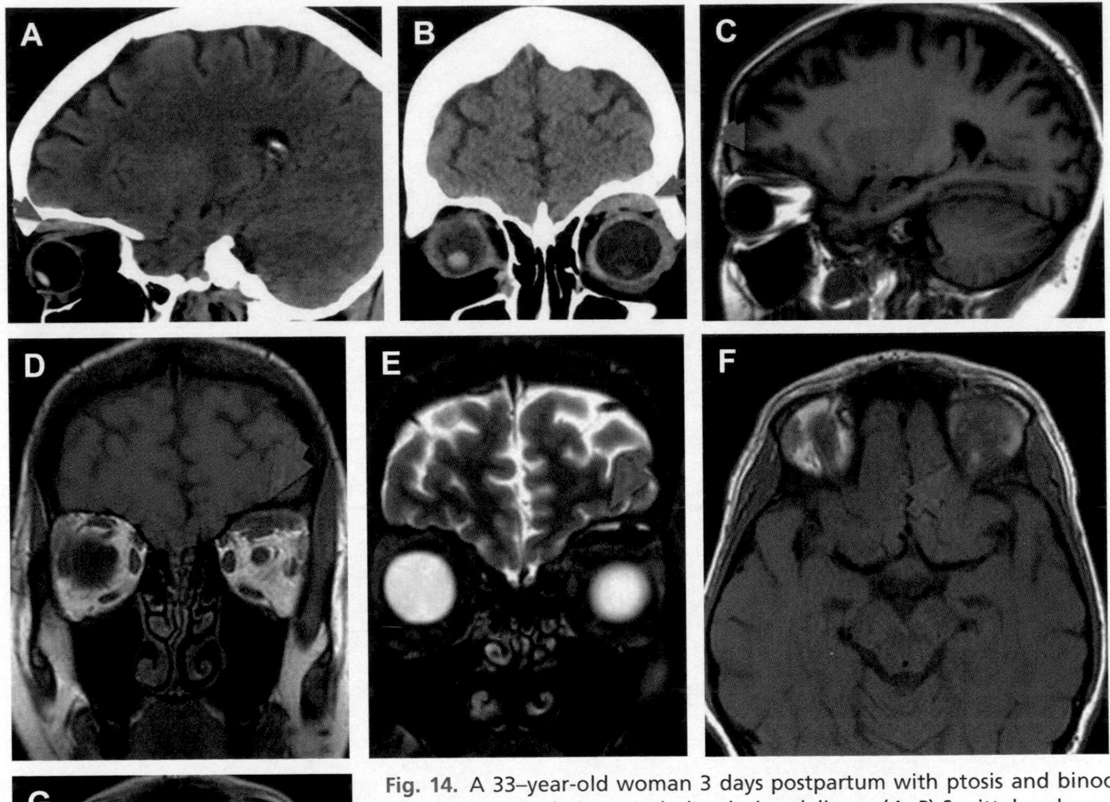

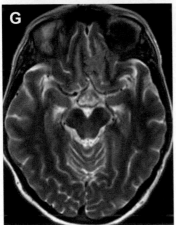

Fig. 14. A 33–year-old woman 3 days postpartum with ptosis and binocular diplopia had strong Valsalva during delivery. (*A, B*) Sagittal and coronal CT scan with small arrow pointing to increased attenuation consistent with hematoma displacing the left levator palpebral and superior rectus muscle inferiorly. (*C–G*) MR imaging of same patient with (*C*) sagittal T1 MR imaging, (*D, E*) coronal T1 -and T2-weighted MR imaging, and (*F, G*) MR imaging. Axial T1- and T2-weighted images with arrows pointing to hematoma with isointensity on T1 and decreased signal on T2 displacing the musculature with resultant ptosis, downward displacement of the globe and inferior gaze deviation.

fourth ventricle can also compress CN VI; often this occurs in conjunction with its neighbor CN VI, resulting in both a diplopia with paralysis of lateral gaze and an ipsilateral paralysis of the muscles of facial expression.[1–3] Even a small tumor results in a diplopia if it affects CN III, IV, or VI, as in **Fig. 13**.

In some patients, the mass that is compressing the nerves or muscles resulting in a diplopia may not necessarily be a tumor; therefore, in any patients who may be at risk for a bleed from either trauma, alterations in pressure, or coagulopathies, double check the surrounding periorbital tissue to make sure that there is no compressive causes (**Fig. 14**).

SUMMARY

In binocular diplopia, patients see double with both eyes open. The differential diagnosis for binocular diplopia is extensive, and because this may be a harbinger of life-threatening abnormality, a careful radiographic assessment is critical. This article presents the anatomy and the course of the CN III, CN

IV, and CN VI, and imaging features of abnormality leading to double vision, at either the level of the brainstem, subarachnoid space, cavernous sinus, superior orbital fissure, and orbit. This article uses the acronym VISION as a reminder to double check for causes, including *V*asculature, Infectious or *I*nflammatory, double checking the *S*calp for giant cell arteritis, and the *S*kull base and *S*uperior orbital fissure in trauma, in patients with a larger body mass index, exclude *I*ncreased *I*ntracranial pressure, and in patients with *O*nset of new or worst headaches, double check for subarachnoid hemorrhage. In patients with binocular diplopia and new *O*nset psychosis, this may be a sign of NMDA receptor antibody encephalitis; although these are often associated with teratomas, a teratoma does not always need to be present. In addition, paraneoplastic syndromes or neuroimmune-mediated abnormality should be excluded. All patients with history of *N*eoplasm, primary or metastatic, require careful neuroimaging. A final good rule of thumb, regardless of the age of any patient, is "If diplopia is progressive, or with symptoms of more than 1, then careful neuroimaging should be done!" Patients with binocular diplopia require a careful physical examination, and radiographic images need careful assessment and double check of the brainstem, course of the cranial nerves, and adjacent vessels, to exclude life-threatening critical abnormality.

REFERENCES

1. Pelak SV. Evaluation of diplopia: an anatomic and systematic approach. Hospital Physician; 2004. p. 16–24.
2. Murchison AP, Gilbert ME, Savino PJ. Neuroimaging and acute ocular motor mononeuropathies: a prospective study. Arch Ophthalmol 2011;129(3):301–5.
3. Tamhankar MA, Volpe NJ. Management of acute cranial nerve 3, 4, and 6 palsies: role of neuroimaging. Curr Opin Ophthalmol 2015;26(6):464–8.
4. Bae YF, Kim JH, Choi BS, et al. Brainstem pathways for horizontal eye movement: pathological correlation with MRI imaging. Radiographics 2013;33:47–59.
5. Wilson-Pauwels L, Akesson EJ, Stewart PA. Cranial nerves: anatomy and clinical comments. Toronto: BC Decker; 1988.
6. Berkovitz B, Kirsch C, Moxham B, et al. 3D head & neck anatomy with special senses and basic neuroanatomy. Primal Pictures; 2007.
7. Kshettry VR. The Dorrello canal—historical developmental controversies in microsurgical anatomy, and clinical implications. Neurosug Focus 2013;34(3):e4.
8. Umansky F, Elidan J, Valarezo A, et al. Dorello's canal: a microanatomical study. J Neurosurg 1991; 75(2):294–8.
9. Kirsch CF. Advances in magnetic resonance imaging of the skull base. Int Arch Otorhinolaryngol 2014;18:127–35.
10. Van Gijn J, Kerr RS, Rinkel GJ. Subarachnoid hemorrhage. Lancet 2007;369(9558):306–18.
11. Karmel M. Deciphering diplopia. Eyenet Magazine 2009.
12. Stalcup ST, Tuan AS, Hesselink JR. Intracranial causes of ophthalmoplegia: the visual reflex pathways. Radiographics 2013;33(5):E153–69.
13. Holodny AI, Kirsch CF, Hameed M, et al. Tumefactive fibroinflammatory lesion of the neck with progressive invasion of the meninges, skull base, orbit, and brain. Am J Neuroradiol 2001;22(5):876–9.
14. Dalmau J, Porta-Etessam J. Paraneoplastic cerebral syndromes with oto-neuro-ophthalomologic manifestations. Rev Neurol 1999;31(12):1213–9.
15. Tan H. Bilateral oculomotor palsy secondary to pseudotumor cerebri. Pediatr Neurol 2010;42(2):141–2.
16. Speer C, Pearlman J, Phillips PH, et al. Fourth cranial nerve palsy in pediatric patients with pseudotumor cerebri. Am J Ophthalmol 1999;127(2):236–7.
17. Krishna R, Kosmorsky GS, Wright KW. Pseudotumor cerebri sine papilledema with unilateral sixth nerve palsy. J neuroophthalmol 1998;18(1):53–5.
18. Dalmau J, Gleichman AJ, Hughes EG, et al. Anti-NMDA-receptor encephalitis: case series and analysis of the effects of antibodies. Lancet Neurol 2008;7(12):1091–8.
19. Hamdallah IN, Shamseddeen HN, Getty JLZ, et al. Greater than expected prevalence of pseudotumor cerebri: a prospective study. Surg Obes Relat Dis 2013;9(1):77–82.
20. Taraschenko O, Zimmerman EA, Bunch ME, et al. Anti-NMDA receptor encephalitis associated with atrial fibrillation and hearing loss. Neurol Neuroimmunol Neuroinflamm 2014;1(3):e24.
21. Cahalan S. Brain on fire: my month of madness. Simon and Schuster; 2013.

Imaging of the Sella and Parasellar Region

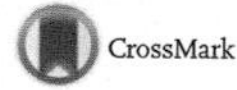

John L. Go, MD*, Anandh G. Rajamohan, MD

KEYWORDS

• Pituitary adenoma • MR imaging • Cavernous carotid fistula • Aneurysm • Apoplexy • Tolosa-Hunt syndrome

KEY POINTS

- Tumor and tumor-like conditions may involve the sellar and parasellar region.
- In suspected lesions of the sellar and parasellar region, dedicated MR imaging of the sellar region should be used.
- Vascular lesions, such as an aneurysms, may involve the stellar region. CT or MR angiography should be performed if suspected.

INTRODUCTION

The sella and parasellar region is a unique region of the skull base situated directly posterior to the anterior skull base in the central region of the skull base inferiorly. Centered within the sphenoid bone, this region may truly represent the center of the central skull base. Given the location of the pituitary gland in this region, small lesions in this location may have major physiologic effects on the human body. This article reviews the anatomy, embryology, and pathologic processes that occur in this region as well as optimum imaging techniques.

ANATOMY AND EMBRYOLOGY

The sellar region is located posterior to the anterior skull base in the central aspect of the skull base. The alisphenoid and basisphenoid components of the sphenoid bone form this region. The planum sphenoidale, which joins the two ethmoid bones, forms a flat surface along the posterior aspect of the anterior skull base (**Fig. 1**). Along the posterior margin of the planum sphenoidale is the limbus and a groove for the optic chiasm, the chiasmatic groove. The sella begins along the posterior margin of the chiasmatic groove, the tuberculum sellae, which is the anterior lip of the sella with the paired anterior clinoid processes laterally. Most of the sella is the sella turcica (Latin for Turkish saddle). The posterior lip of the sella turcica is the dorsum sellae, with the posterior clinoid processes laterally. Situated within the sella turcica is the pituitary gland. Situated above the sella is the hypothalamic region and the anteroinferior aspect of the third ventricle. Extending inferiorly from the hypothalamus is the infundibular stalk, representing the axons whose cell bodies reside in the hypothalamic region from the tuber cinereum. The infundibular stalk passes through a reflection of dura that covers the superior aspect of the sella, the diaphragma sellae, and becomes the pars nervosa component of the pituitary gland.[1]

The pituitary gland is composed of the adenohypophysis and the neurohypophysis. The embryologic notochord, which is the remnant neural tube, is the precursor for the nucleus pulposus in

Division of Neuroradiology, Department of Radiology, Keck School of Medicine, University of Southern California, 1200 North State Street, Room 3740A, Los Angeles, CA 90033, USA
* Corresponding author. Los Angeles County Medical Center, University of Southern California, 1200 North State Street, Room 3740A, Los Angeles, CA 90033.
E-mail address: jlgo@med.usc.edu

Radiol Clin N Am 55 (2017) 83–101
http://dx.doi.org/10.1016/j.rcl.2016.09.002
0033-8389/17/© 2016 Elsevier Inc. All rights reserved.

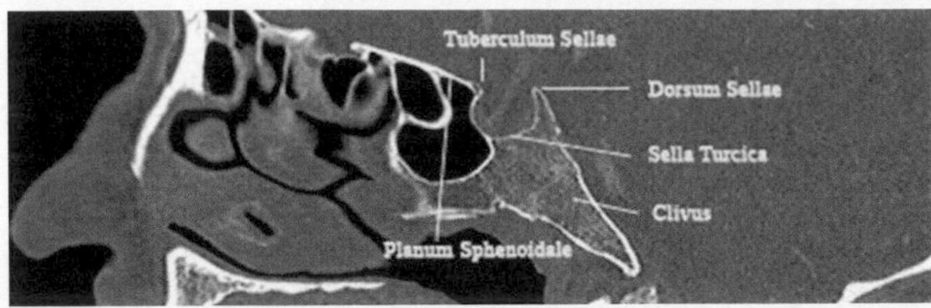

Fig. 1. Sagittal computed tomography (CT) anatomy of the sella.

the spine. The superior continuation of the notochord at the skull base is through the midline aspect of the clivus extending superiorly to the dorsum sellae. During the fourth week of gestation, the notochord is situated anterior to the midclivus and is contact with the posterior central aspect of the pharynx. As the notochord migrates posteriorly to the primordial clivus, a small portion of the pharynx, the Rathke pouch, extends posteriorly and becomes the adenohypophysis of the pituitary gland. The passage of this tissue is through a primordial canal called the craniopharyngeal canal, which eventually involutes but may rarely be seen as a normal variant as a channel through the clivus to the sellar region.[2,3]

Axons from the cell bodies in the hypothalamic region extend inferiorly to form the infundibular stalk and the pars nervosa. The two components meet to form the pituitary gland within the sellar turcica. Between the adenohypophysis and the neurohypophysis is the pars intermedia.

The parasellar region is composed of the cavernous sinus and Meckel cave, which is located posterior and inferior. The Meckel cave is an anterior extension of the subarachnoid space through which the trigeminal nerve (cranial nerve V) enters by way of the porus trigeminus. The trigeminal (gasserian) ganglion is situated within the Meckel cave, from which the three major divisions of cranial nerve V arise: V1 (ophthalmic division), V2 (maxillary division), and V3 (mandibular division). The cavernous sinus (**Fig. 2**), a major venous sinus, is formed by the periosteal and meningeal layers of dura along its medial and lateral wall, thus formed by four layers of dura. Housed within the two layers of dura laterally are cranial nerves III, IV, V1, and V2. These cranial nerves are thus interdural in location.[4]

Traveling within the cavernous sinus is the cavernous segment of the internal carotid artery, as well as cranial nerve VI. Extending from the cavernous sinus anteriorly are the superior and inferior ophthalmic veins. The clival plexus extends from the cavernous sinus posteriorly and lies posterior to the clivus. Intersinus communication between the two cavernous sinuses is also present, which may drain posterior to the dura behind the clivus. The sphenoparietal sinus extends from the inferior aspect of the cavernous sinus and drains laterally along the greater wing of the sphenoid posteriorly. The superior and inferior petrosal sinuses also emanate from the inferior aspect of the cavernous sinus.

Arterial branches of the cavernous internal carotid artery include the meningohypophyseal trunk from the posterior genu of the internal carotid artery, the McConnell arteries from the transverse segment of the cavernous carotid medially to provide arterial blood flow to the pituitary gland, as well as the inferolateral trunk laterally from the transverse segment. The inferior hypophyseal artery, arising from the meningohypophyseal trunk, supplies blood to the neurohypophysis and the infundibular stalk. Although there are arterial branches to the pituitary gland, these only provide 20% to 25% of blood flow to the pituitary gland. Most of the blood flow to the gland is through a portal venous system with arterial feeders from the superior hypophyseal artery, which extend to the hypothalamic region. The portal venous system extends from the hypothalamic region to the pituitary gland along the infundibular stalk.

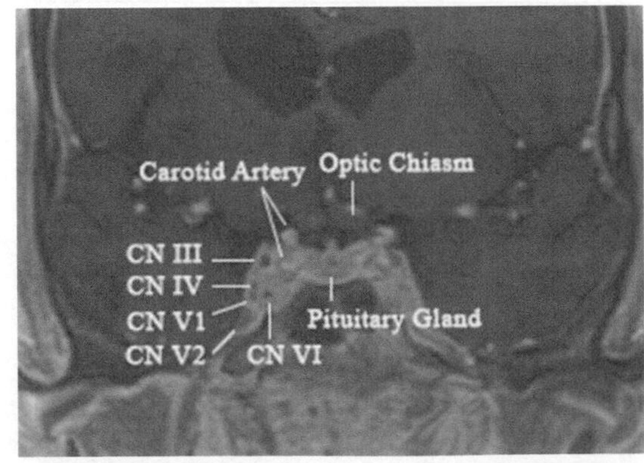

Fig. 2. Coronal postcontrast MR imaging anatomy through the cavernous sinus and sella. CN, cranial nerve.

Because this is a portal venous system, there is a lack of a blood-brain barrier and the infundibular stalk enhances on postcontrast images.[5]

The anterior lobe of the pituitary gland is composed of the pars tuberalis, pars intermedia, and pars distalis. The pars distalis forms the bulk of the intrasellar component of the pituitary gland. Three types of cells are located within the pars distalis: acidophil cells, which secrete somatotrophic and lactotroph hormones (LHs); basophil cells, which secrete adrenocorticotrophic hormones (ACTHs), thyrotrophic stimulating hormones, follicle stimulating hormones, interstitial cell stimulating hormone, LH, and melanocyte stimulating hormone; and chromophobe cells, whose significance is uncertain at this time. The pars tuberalis forms the median eminence of the gland and a small portion of the anterior infundibulum. The pars intermedia is situated between the pars distalis and the posterior neurohypophysis. The pars nervosa, which contains the axons from the hypothalamic region, contains vasopressin (antidiuretic hormone [ADH]) and oxytocin.

Situated above the sella is the suprasellar cistern, which includes the circle of Willis, the anterior inferior third ventricle and hypothalamic region, the optic pathway, the columns of the fornix, and mammillary bodies.

IMAGING

The optimum imaging of the sella and parasellar region is with magnetic resonance (MR) imaging. Computed tomography (CT) imaging is complementary to MR imaging for the depiction of bony changes, including remodeling or frank bone destruction. Although lesions of the sella and parasellar region may initially be discovered on routine CT of the head or sinus, further analysis and better tissue characterization is performed on MR imaging. If MR imaging is contraindicated, thin-section imaging of the sella is performed by a volumetric acquisition in the axial plane with submillimeter slices on multidetector CT followed by reconstruction in all three planes with a slice thickness of up to 1 mm. Coronal and sagittal planes are the optimum planes to examine the sella and parasellar region. Contrast should be used on all dedicated sella studies. Assessment of the lateral scout localizer should also be performed to determine the presence of bony remodeling of the sella turcica.[6]

On MR imaging, a dedicated sella protocol should be performed. Precontrast thin-section T1-weighted coronal and sagittal images of the sella region are performed as well as T2-weighted coronal with fat saturation. Whole-brain axial fluid-attenuated inversion recovery (FLAIR), gradient echo, and diffusion-weighted images are then performed. After the administration of contrast, postcontrast, thin-section T1-weighted coronal and sagittal images are then performed of the sellar region. At our institution, dynamic contrast-enhanced MR in the coronal plane using a power injector with saline chase is performed initially with dynamic first-pass gadolinium images obtained sequentially in the coronal plane. Either three or four sequential coronal images are obtained using a fast T1-weighted sequence in the coronal plane for the first 10 to 20 seconds to obtain first-pass gadolinium images through the sellar region in the setting of suspected de novo pituitary adenomas (**Table 1**).[2,7,8]

Table 1
Typical sellar protocol. For the dynamic postcontrast images, power injector is used with dual chamber containing 10–15 mL of contrast and 20 mL of saline

Sequence	Plane of Scan	TR/TE (ms)	Flip Angle (Degrees)/ETL	Slice Thickness (mm)	Gap (mm)	Matrix Size
FSE T2 weighted	Coronal	2925/112	180/15	2	0.5	256 × 256
SE T1 weighted	Coronal	500/10	90	2	0.5	192 × 192
DCE T1 weighted	Coronal	525/min	180/4	4	0	384 × 192
T1-weighted postcontrast FS	Coronal	600/min	90	2	0.5	256 × 192
T1-weighted postcontrast FS	Sagittal	500/min	90	3	0	256 × 192

On injection using a flow rate of 3 mL/s of contrast followed by saline, DCE T1-weighted images obtained every 20 seconds for a total number of 15 phases.

Abbreviations: DCE, dynamic contrast enhancement; ETL, echo train length; FS, fat saturated; FSE, fast spin echo; SE, spin echo; TE, echo time; TR, repetition time.

The normal pituitary gland is isointense to gray matter signal intensity on both T1-weighted and T2-weighted images. The posterior pituitary is typically hyperintense in signal intensity on T1-weighted images and isointense to hypointense on the T2-weighted images. Although the cause of the increased signal intensity on T1-weighted images is controversial, this may be caused by secretory granules associated with ADH.[9] On postcontrast imaging, there is homogeneous moderate to avid enhancement of the anterior lobe of the pituitary gland. Enhancement of the posterior pituitary may be difficult to ascertain because it is already hyperintense on precontrast T1-weighted images. On dynamic images, because most of the blood flow to the gland is through the portal venous system, progressive and rapid enhancement can be seen dynamically after contrast is seen in the infundibular stalk. Contrast-related venous enhancement of the cavernous sinuses is also seen on the postcontrast images. The superior border of the gland is concave or transverse in position and the infundibular stalk is typically in a midline position.

DISORDERS

General

A host of pathologic processes may involve the sellar and parasellar region and it is beyond the scope of this article to review all entities. This article includes tumor and tumor-like conditions, vascular lesions, and congenital/developmental lesions. Because the cavernous sinus is formed by dura, dural-based processes are also briefly discussed.

TUMOR AND TUMOR-LIKE CONDITIONS

Pituitary Adenoma

Pituitary adenoma is the most common tumor of the sellar region and comprises up to 80% of all tumors in this location. These tumors are World Health Organization (WHO) grade I tumors and malignant transformation is rare. From 14% to 27% of cases are asymptomatic and are incidentally picked up on imaging. These tumors may be categorized as microadenomas (<10 mm in greatest dimension) or macroadenomas (≥10 mm). These tumors may also be classified as either functioning (secreting hormones) or nonfunctioning tumors. The most common functioning adenomas are prolactin-secreting adenomas. These functioning adenomas are typically seen when the prolactin level is greater than 200 ng/mL, whereas cavernous sinus involvement is seen with prolactin levels greater than 1000 ng/mL. The modified Kovacs and Horvath classification is used to classify adenomas based on cell type (acidophil, basophil, or chromophobe cells) and hormones produced by the tumor.

On MR imaging, pituitary adenomas typically show hypointense or isointense signal intensity relative to the remainder of the gland on the precontrast T1-weighted sequences and isointense signal with the brain cortex on T2-weighted sequences. On postcontrast images performed within 20 minutes of injection, these masses show a decreased degree of enhancement compared with the avidly enhancing pituitary gland (**Fig. 3**).[2,7,8,10–14]

During dynamic imaging of the pituitary gland, microadenomas show a lack of or delayed enhancement compared with the rapid and avid enhancement of the pituitary gland, presenting as hypoenhancing lesions. During recirculation, contrast diffuses within the tumor from the remaining aspect of the gland and the tumor may not be visualized. Dynamic imaging may increase the sensitivity of depicting small pituitary microadenomas from the postcontrast studies.[2,7,8]

Secondary signs of a pituitary adenoma are a convex superior border of the gland and displacement of the infundibular stalk away from the side of the tumor. Adenomas may also show cystic change, calcification, and hemorrhage. The cystic component of the lesion may show variable signal intensity on MR imaging because of the presence of protein or blood products. Non-functioning pituitary adenomas may present with visual disturbances or cranial neuropathy caused by suprasellar or parasellar involvement.

Prolactinomas tend to occur in the lateral or posterior aspect of the anterior lobe. Growth hormone–producing adenomas tend to occur in the lateral or anterior aspect of the anterior lobe. ACTH-producing adenomas tend to lie within the central posterior aspect of the anterior lobe adjacent to the posterior lobe.

Adenomas may extend superiorly into the suprasellar cistern, laterally into the cavernous sinus and parasellar region, posteriorly into the clivus, inferiorly into the nasopharynx and nasal cavity, or a combination of these (**Fig. 4**). Lateral extension from the sella into the cavernous sinus should be determined because this determines surgical resectability. It is common for these tumors to laterally displace the medial wall of the cavernous sinus dura and displace the cavernous carotid artery. True cavernous sinus invasion should be considered if the normal hypointense signal intensity of the dura on T1-weighted and T2-weighted images is not well visualized or the tumor makes a claw sign with the cavernous carotid artery, which indicates cavernous sinus invasion.

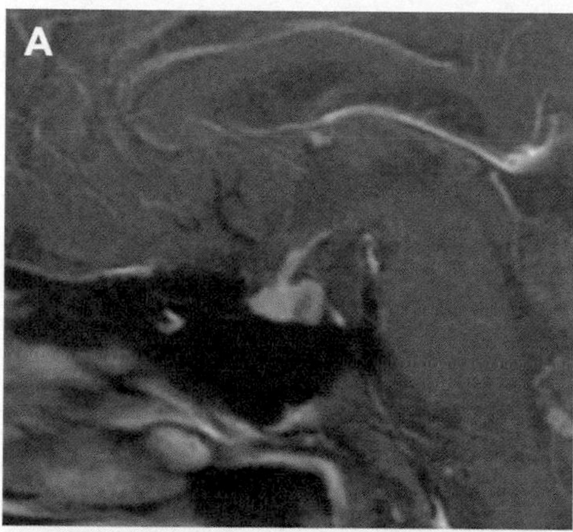

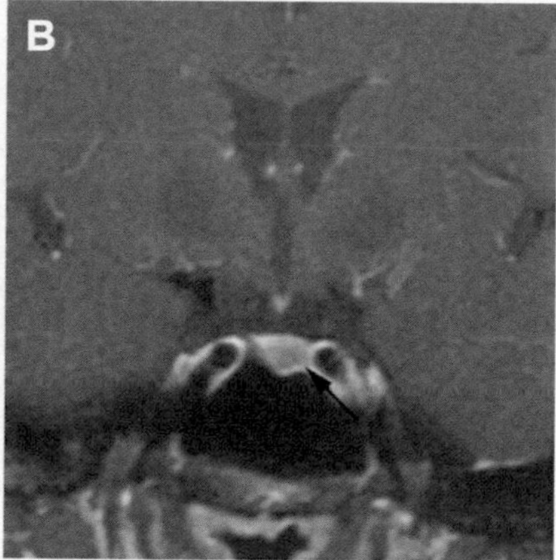

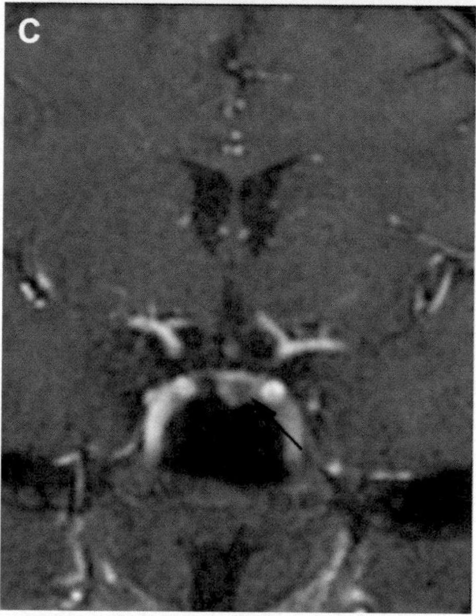

Fig. 3. Pituitary microadenoma. Sagittal (*A*) and coronal (*B*) postcontrast T1-weighted imaging (T1WI) shows a lesion in the posterior aspect of the pituitary gland measuring less than 1 cm. (*C*) Dynamic contrast-enhanced images confirm that the microadenoma hypoenhances relative to the surrounding normal pituitary tissue.

Postsurgical imaging of the sellar region for the determination of residual or recurrent tumor may at times be challenging. Because of the presence of fat packing at the operative site in patients who have undergone a transsphenoidal approach, precontrast T1-weighted imaging (T1WI) should be performed without fat saturation. Postcontrast T1WI should be performed with fat saturation.

MENINGIOMA

Meningiomas are the most common extra-axial tumors and occur in the suprasellar and parasellar regions in 5% to 10% of cases. Arising from meningothelial cells of the dura, these dural-based masses are typically isointense to gray matter on T1WI and T2-weighted imaging (T2WI). After the administration of gadolinium, these masses show homogeneous moderate to avid enhancement. A dural tail may be present, although this is not pathognomonic for meningioma, because this may be seen in other dural-based conditions. Thirty percent of meningiomas may also show diffusion restriction and calcification is common in up to 50% of meningiomas.

Meningiomas that are located superior to the sellar region may show a normal pituitary gland within the sella turcica (**Fig. 5**). However, extensive central skull base meningiomas that involve the sella and parasellar regions may not show a normal pituitary gland.

On CT, these masses are hyperdense on noncontrast examination. Meningiomas are named by their location (ie, planum sphenoidale, tuberculum sellae, diaphragma sella, dorsum sellae, anterior clinoid, posterior clinoid, or cavernous sinus meningiomas). Parasellar meningiomas tend to displace and not encircle or encase the cavernous segment

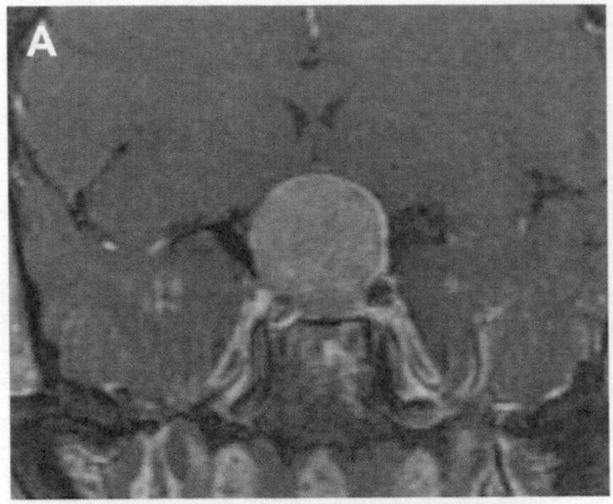

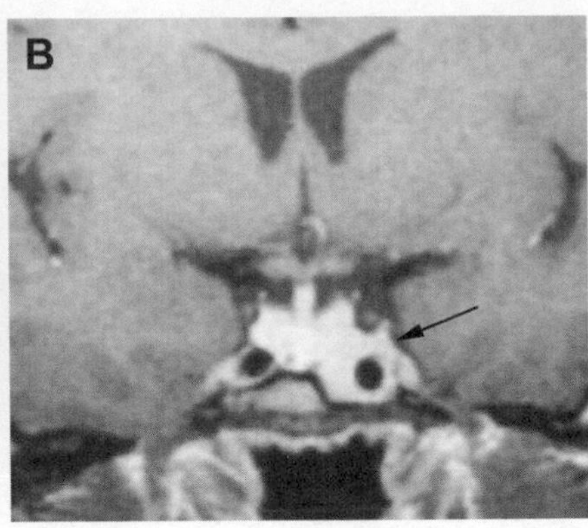

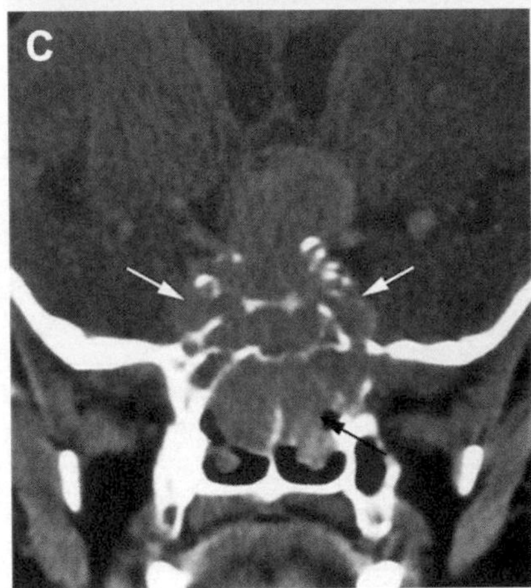

Fig. 4. Pituitary macroadenoma. (*A*) This macroadenoma shows extension superiorly to the suprasellar cistern where it compresses the optic chiasm. There was no cavernous sinus invasion. (*B*) Coronal postcontrast T1WI shows a different macroadenoma that invades into the adjacent left cavernous sinus. Note there is no narrowing of the left internal carotid artery. (*C*) There is invasion of both cavernous sinuses (*white arrows*) by this macroadenoma along with superior extension into the suprasellar cistern and inferior extension into the nasal cavity (*black arrow*) shown on coronal CT.

of the internal carotid artery, a differentiating point with pituitary macroadenoma, which may encircle/encase the cavernous carotid artery.

CRANIOPHARYNGIOMA

Craniopharyngiomas are nonglial tumors that arise from the stratified squamous epithelium of the Rathke pouch remnant and are the most common nonglial tumors of childhood. There is a bimodal peak of occurrence, with the first occurring in the second decade of life and the second peak in the fourth to fifth decade. There are two histologic subtypes: the adamantinomatous type and the papillary type. In the first peak, occurring in childhood, these tumors are most commonly the adamantinomatous type and tend to be complex with a solid and cystic component. The cystic component may show peripheral rim calcification. Seventy-five percent of these tumors are purely suprasellar, 5% are intrasellar, and 20% have both a sellar and suprasellar component. The lesions that occur in the second peak typically are solid masses and are of the papillary type. These masses may show calcification. On MR imaging, the cystic component may show variable signal intensity because of the protein content within the cyst. The solid component is fairly nonspecific with intermediate signal intensity on T1WI and isointense to hyperintense signal intensity on T2WI (**Fig. 6**). Surrounding hyperintense signal intensity on T2WI in the adjacent brain parenchyma may be seen.[15–17]

METASTATIC DISEASE

Metastatic disease to the pituitary is an uncommon occurrence and occurs in less than 5% of patients. The most common metastases to the pituitary gland are from lung and breast cancer (**Fig. 7**). Although these may be clinically silent lesions, patients may also present with endocrinopathy, visual disturbances caused by suprasellar extension, or cranial neuropathy caused by parasellar involvement. There is also a suggestion of preferential infundibular and posterior pituitary involvement because of the arterial feeders to these locations. Metastasis to the pituitary gland may mimic a pituitary adenoma. Rapid growth and associated bone destruction typically suggest metastatic disease.[18–20]

ORIGIN OF THE PRIMARY NEOPLASM IN CASES OF PITUITARY METASTASIS

Primary Site	%
Breast	39.7
Lung	23.7
Prostate	5.0
Kidney	2.6
Skin (melanoma)	2.4
Colon	2.4
Thyroid	2.1
Stomach	1.8
Pancreas	1.3
Pharynx	1.3
Endometrium	1.3
Leukemia	1.3
Bladder	1.1
Liver	1.1
Cervix	1.1
Undetermined	3.1

From Komininos J, Vlassopoulou V, Protopapa D, et al. Tumors metastatic to the pituitary gland: case report and literature review. J Clin Endocrinol Metab 2004;89(2):574–80.

PITUICYTOMA/GRANULAR CELL MYOBLASTOMA

Pituicytoma is a WHO grade I spindle cell noninfiltrating glial tumor arising from the neurohypophysis. These masses have also been called granular cell myoblastoma, infundibuloma, or pilocytic astrocytoma of the suprasellar region and may present as a sellar or suprasellar mass. The lesions may arise from the hypothalamic region, infundibular stalks, or present as a mass from the posterior lobe in the pituitary gland. The lesions are typically isointense to gray matter on T1WI, heterogeneously isointense to hyperintense on T2WI, and show heterogeneous moderate enhancement on postcontrast images (**Fig. 8**). These tumors are rare, with 31 cases reported in the literature, and have only been described in adults, with a male/female ratio of 1.6:1.[21–24]

LYMPHOCYTIC HYPOPHYSITIS

Lymphocytic hypophysitis represents a nonspecific inflammatory process associated with the hypothalamic region and infundibular stalk, and may progress to the pituitary gland. The normal infundibular stalk is widened, measuring greater than 2 mm in width with associated enhancement of the hypothalamic region (**Fig. 9**). On T2WI, this process is isointense to hypointense to gray matter signal intensity. There may be associated enhancement of the adjacent dura and the sphenoid sinuses. Although most common in postpartum women, this may also be seen in middle aged men and represents an underlying autoimmune process because it may be associated with Hashimoto thyroiditis. Patients may present with diabetes insipidus or panhypopituitarism. Patients typically respond to steroid therapy and hormonal replacement therapy.[25–31]

PITUITARY HYPERPLASIA

Pituitary size is typically measured in the craniocaudal dimension. Normally pituitary size may vary with the upper limits of normal of 6 mm in children, 8 mm in men and postmenopausal women, 10 mm in young menstruating women, and up to 12 mm in pregnant women. Enlargement of the pituitary may be seen in patients with hypothyroidism or Addison disease, in whom persistent stimulation of the pituitary gland results from absence of a negative feedback loop from the end organs to limit production of hormones. The pituitary gland shows increased size and homogeneous enhancement, which may extend into the suprasellar region (**Fig. 10**). On correction of the endocrinopathy, the pituitary gland may return to normal size.[32,33]

HAMARTOMA OF THE TUBER CINEREUM

The tuber cinereum is located in the inferior posterior aspect of the hypothalamus anterior to the mammillary bodies and is best depicted on a sagittal T1WI (**Fig. 11**). Hamartoma of the tuber cinereum represents disorganized microglia and is associated with the hypothalamus and may extend inferiorly to involve the infundibular stalk and pituitary gland. Because this represents disorganized brain tissue, these lesions typically do not show cystic change, calcification, hemorrhage, or enhancement. Patients typically present with precocious puberty and gelastic seizures (uncontrollable bouts of laughing). Because of their typical presentation and location, these are typically pathognomonic lesions. On MR imaging, these lesions are isointense to gray matter signal intensity on T1WI and T2WI and are of variable size, measuring up to 4 cm at the time of presentation.

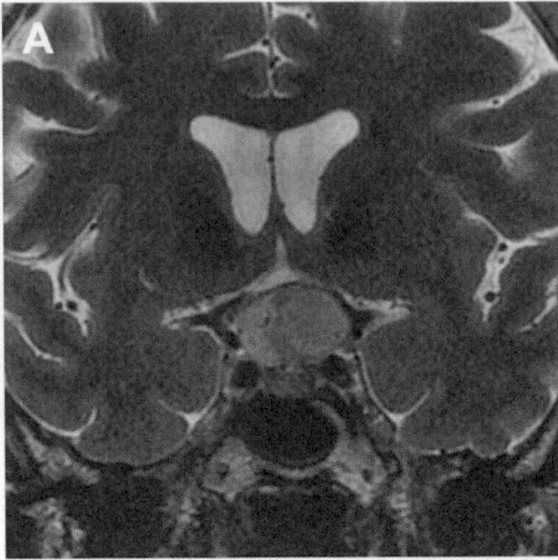

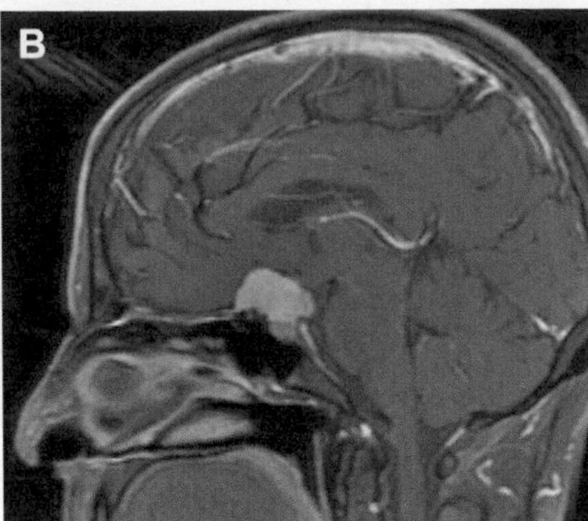

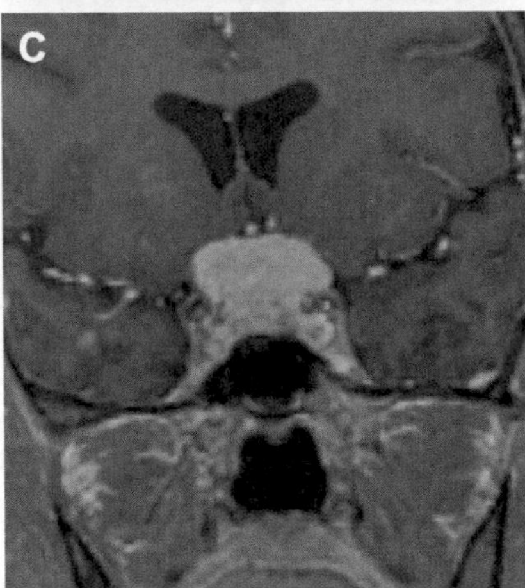

Fig. 5. Planum sphenoidale meningioma. (*A*) A suprasellar mass can be seen splaying the circle of Willis arteries on coronal T2WI. The mass is hyperintense relative to the normal pituitary gland. (*B*) On sagittal postcontrast T1WI the mass can be seen along the planum sphenoidale to the tuberculum sellae with extension to the suprasellar cistern. The pituitary gland can be seen inferior to the tumor. (*C*) The meningioma shows fairly homogeneous enhancement and partially extends into the superior aspect of the sella.

PITUITARY APOPLEXY/PITUITARY INFARCT/ EMPTY SELLA

Pituitary apoplexy is a clinical syndrome of acute change in mental status, nausea, vomiting, ophthalmoplegia, cranial neuropathy, and acute endocrinologic abnormalities caused by rapid expansion of a lesion in the sella/suprasellar region because of hemorrhage (**Fig. 12**). The most common cause is acute hemorrhage within a pituitary adenoma, but acute hemorrhage within a Rathke cleft cyst or other tumor in this location with rapid expansion and mass effect on the optic pathway, hypothalamic region, or parasellar region is the causative factor. Infarction of the pituitary gland may also occur in Sheehan syndrome in postpartum women and presents with apoplexy.

On MR imaging, acute fluid-fluid level within the pituitary gland or within the lesion representing acute hemorrhage as well as associated mass effect is present. Associated blooming on gradient echo imaging may also be present. On CT, a mass or mass-like lesion with hyperdensity may be seen. Associated dural reaction with enhancement on MR may be present.[34–37]

In the chronic state, the pituitary gland may be absent, with an empty sella and the presence of panhypopituitarism. The presence of an empty sella with expansion of the sella turcica may be seen in empty sella syndrome or in patients with increased intracranial pressure, such as in pseudotumor cerebri.

VASCULAR LESIONS

Aneurysm

Aneurysm in the sellar or suprasellar region may mimic a mass, especially on a noncontrast study. These aneurysms may arise from the cavernous carotid artery or from the supraclinoid internal carotid artery. On rare occasions a purely intrasellar aneurysm may be present and can present with hyperprolactinemia. Because of long-standing compression of the pituitary gland, these patients occasionally present with panhypopituitarism. Peripheral rim calcification may be present to

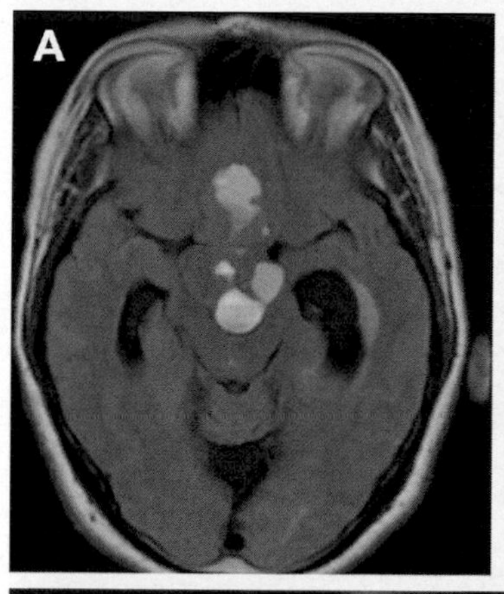

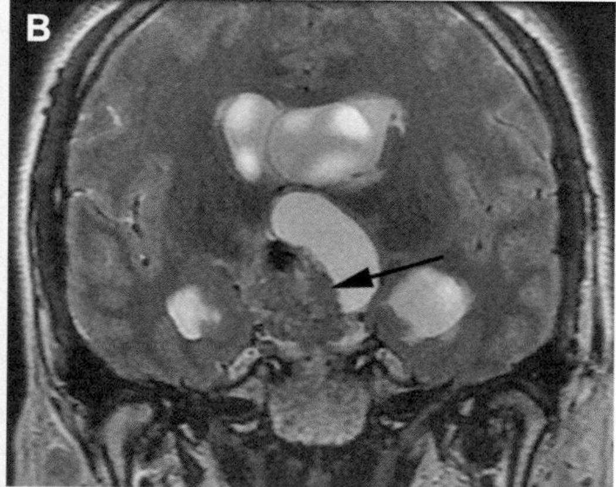

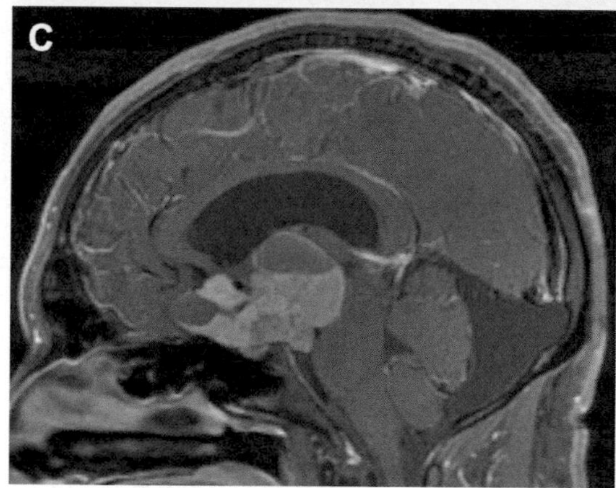

Fig. 6. Craniopharyngioma. (*A*) There is a suprasellar mass containing multiple cystic spaces with fluid-fluid levels. (*B*) Coronal T2WI shows that the mass also has a sizable solid component (*black arrow*) in addition to the cystic areas. Note the hydrocephalus caused by the mass. (*C*) The solid components show enhancement in this cystic and solid craniopharyngioma.

suggest an aneurysm. On MR imaging, an aneurysm should show a signal flow void with phase-encoding artifact present (**Fig. 13**). Partially thrombosed aneurysm may show alteration of signal intensity on T1WI and T2WI because of the presence of clot. A swirl sign, representing slower turbulent flow with contrast-related enhancement, may be present to also suggest the presence of aneurysm. CT angiography, MR angiography, or catheter angiography may be needed to fully characterize the aneurysm and determine its point of origin.[38,39]

ARTERIOVENOUS FISTULA

Cavernous carotid arteriovenous fistulae are covered elsewhere in this issue (See Gaurav Jindal and colleagues' article "Imaging Evaluation and Treatment of Vascular Lesions at the Skull Base," in this issue.).

CONGENITAL/DEVELOPMENTAL LESIONS

Ectopic Pituitary

Failure of descent of the neurohypophysis into the sellar region results in an ectopic position of the posterior pituitary gland in the suprasellar cistern (**Fig. 14**). The pituitary gland is hypoplastic in appearance with absence of the infundibular stalk. The posterior pituitary bright spot is located in a midline position superior to the sella typically at the level of the tuber cinereum or a truncated infundibular stalk. Because of the small sella turcica, there may be medialization of the cavernous carotid arteries.[40–44]

RATHKE CLEFT CYST

Rathke cleft cysts arise from the remnant of Rathke pouch during development of the pituitary gland. The remnant of Rathke pouch represents the pars intermedia located between the pars distalis and the pars nervosa. These cysts may lie within the sella, extend into the suprasellar cistern, or present purely as suprasellar cysts, but are always located inferior to the optic chiasm. The wall of the cyst is composed of stratified epithelial cells. On CT imaging, these cysts are typically hypoattenuating and may show calcification associated with the wall. On MR imaging, the signal intensity may be variable because of the presence of

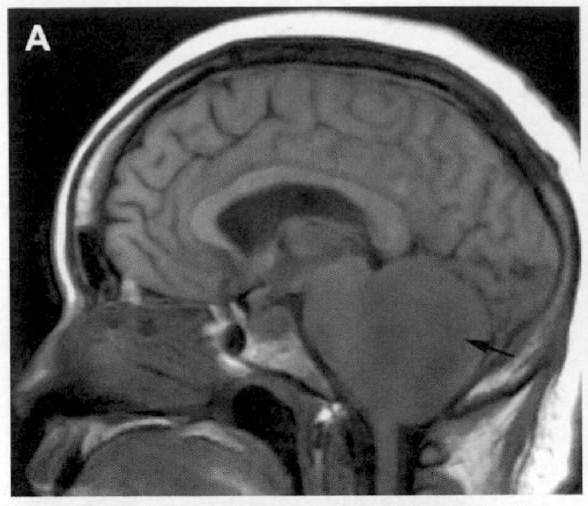

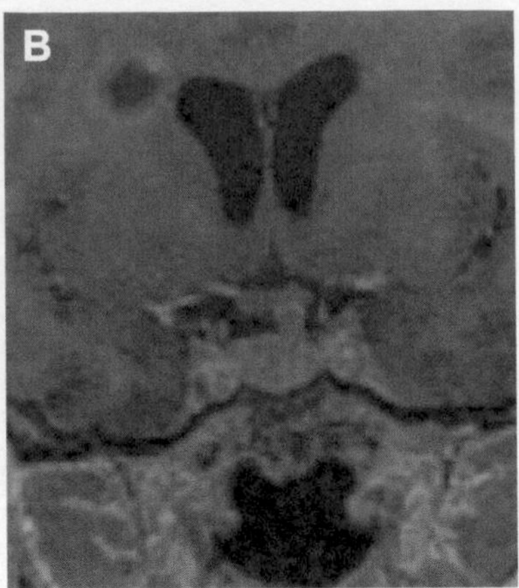

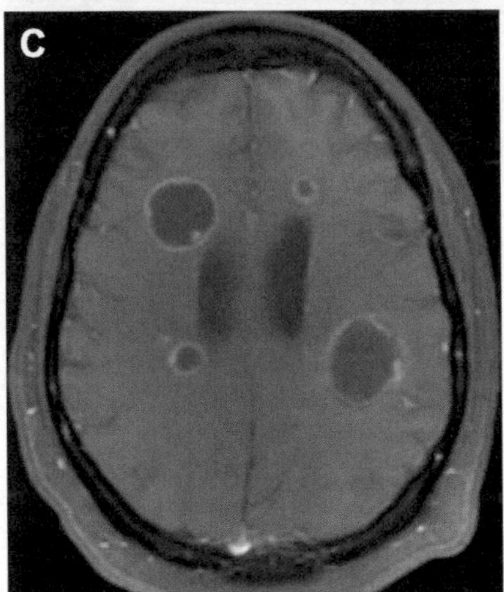

Fig. 7. Metastatic disease to the pituitary gland. (*A*) Sagittal noncontrast T1WI shows mass-like change to the pituitary gland. There was also mass effect in the cerebellum (*black arrow*) effacing the fourth ventricle. (*B*) The entire gland and stalk were replaced with abnormal enhancement and expansile change. (*C*) Additional ring-enhancing masses could be seen elsewhere in the brain. The pituitary lesion was confirmed to be a breast cancer metastasis.

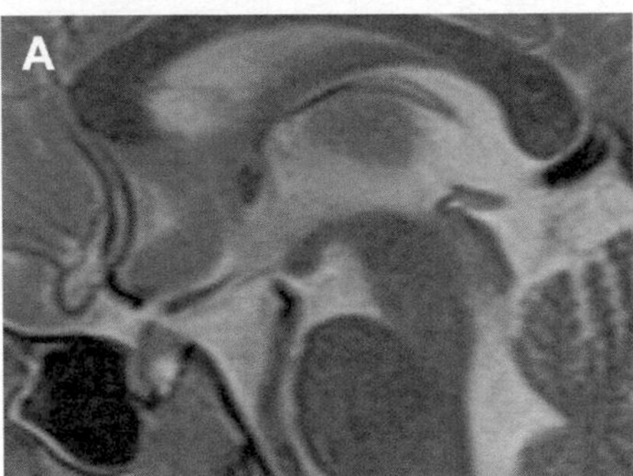

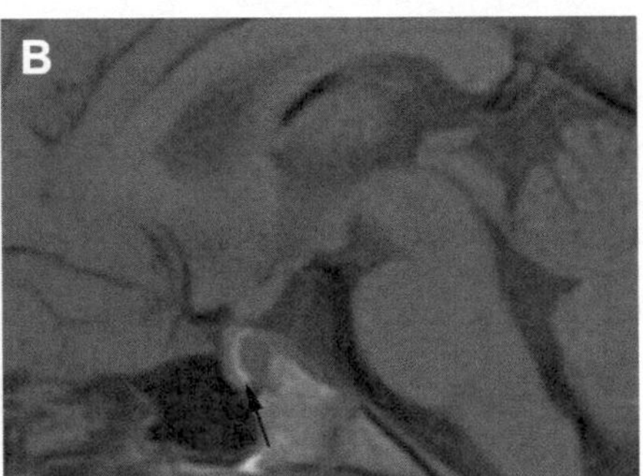

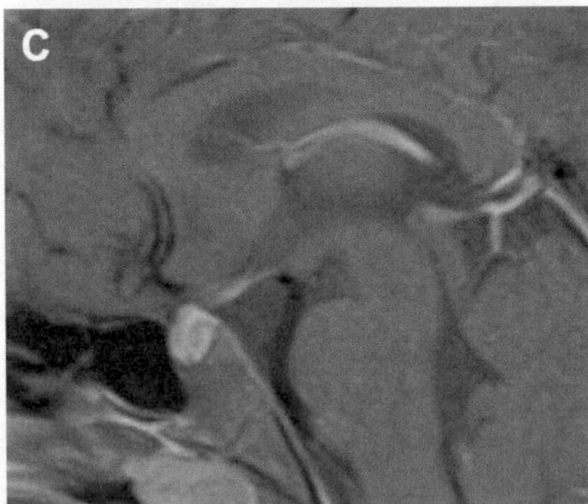

Fig. 8. Pituicytoma. Sagittal T2WI (*A*) and T1WI (*B*) reveal a mass in the posterior aspect of the sella. Note the pituitary bright spot being displaced anteriorly (*black arrow*). (*C*) The mass enhances following contrast administration and looks similar to the anterior pituitary gland.

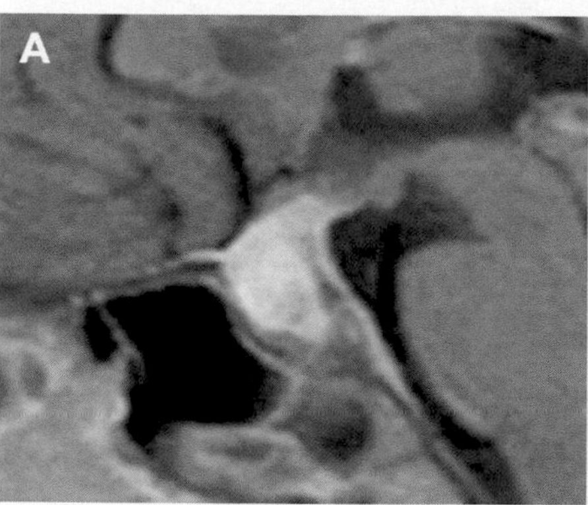

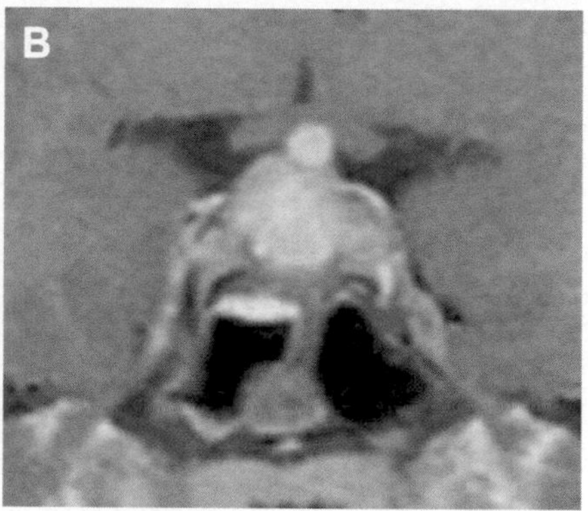

Fig. 9. Lymphocytic hypophysitis. (*A, B*) There is mass-like enhancement and enlargement of the pituitary gland and infundibulum. Both the anterior and posterior pituitary gland were involved in this case of lymphocytic infundibular panhypophysitis.

protein within the cyst (**Fig. 15**). A fluid-debris level may be seen. In the event of hemorrhage, fluid-fluid levels may be present. There may be thin-walled enhancement associated with the cyst and there should be no solid component to the lesion.[45–47]

ECTODERMAL INCLUSION CYSTS

Dermoids, epidermoids, teratomas, and lipomas may be seen in the suprasellar, sellar, and parasellar region. Arising from ectodermal rests, epidermoids are typically heterogeneously hypoattenuating lesions on noncontrast CT. On MR imaging, these lesions are heterogeneously hypointense on T2WI, heterogeneously hyperintense on T2WI, and do not show enhancement. Dermoids may contain fat and thus show hyperintense signal intensity on T1WI and T2WI (**Fig. 16**). Teratomas may also contain hair, sweat glands, and teeth, and thus may show variable signal intensity on MR imaging because of the solid nature of some of these components. Calcification/ossification may aid in the diagnosis of a teratoma. Epidermoids and teratomas tend to be in a midline position, whereas dermoids are parasellar in location. Lipomas, which arise from the meninx primitiva, pathognomonically show fat attenuation on CT and fat signal intensity on MR imaging without enhancement or other components. These lesions may occur in the suprasellar cistern on in the cavernous sinus.[9,48–54]

ARACHNOID CYST

From 10% to 15% of arachnoid cysts may arise in the suprasellar cistern or be situated within the sella. These cysts are homogeneously

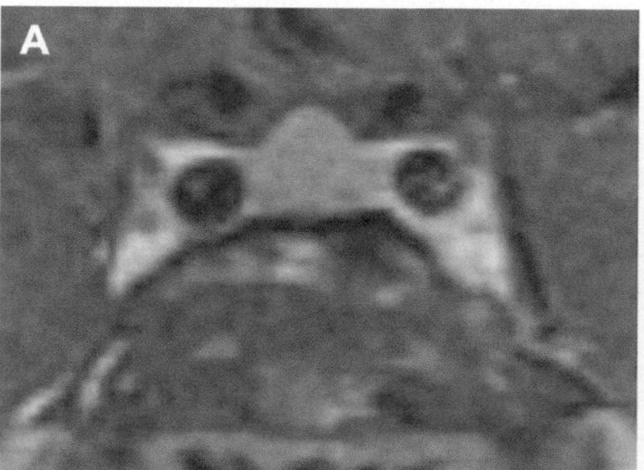

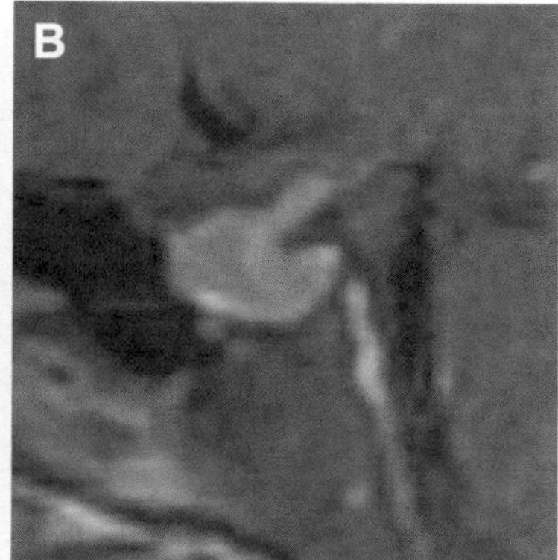

Fig. 10. Pituitary hyperplasia. (*A*) Coronal postcontrast T1WI shows a symmetrically enlarged pituitary gland. (*B*) On sagittal sequences, note the convex superior border of the anterior pituitary gland. This appearance is characteristic in pituitary hyperplasia.

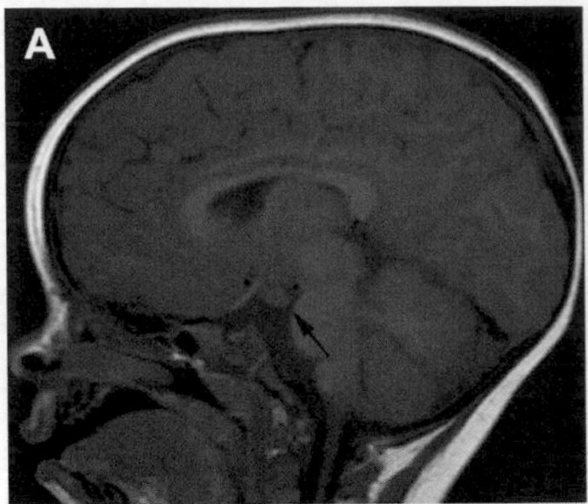

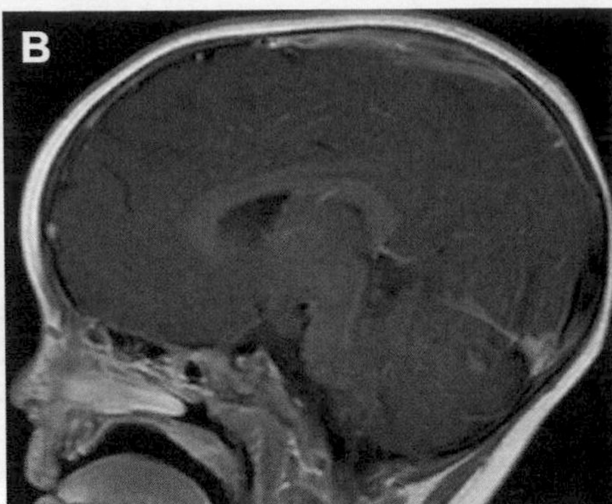

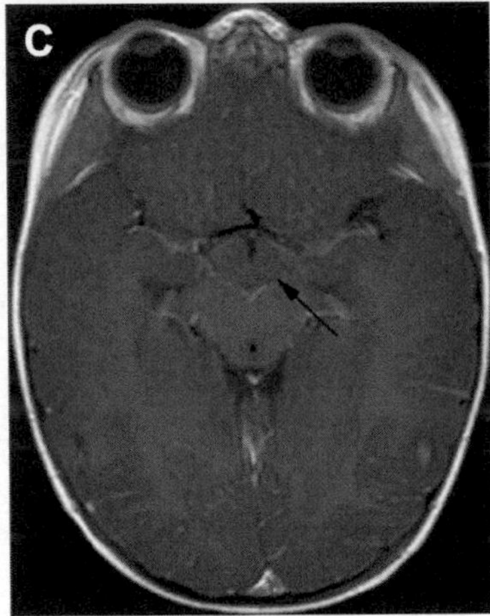

Fig. 11. Hypothalamic hamartoma. (*A*) A mass (*black arrow*) can be seen involving the tuber cinereum in this child experiencing gelastic seizures. Sagittal (*B*) and axial (*C*) postcontrast T1WI show the lesion following signal similar to gray matter without hyperenhancement characteristic of a hypothalamic hamartoma.

hypoattenuating on noncontrast CT and are equal to cerebrospinal fluid (CSF) signal intensity on T1WI and T2WI (**Fig. 17**). These lesions do not enhance and are diffusion negative. Expansion of the sellar turcica is typically seen and may be mistaken for empty sella. A thin wall may be seen, which distinguishes this entity from empty sella.[55–57]

PARASELLAR LESIONS

Schwannoma

Nerve sheath tumors may arise from cranial nerves III, IV, V, and VI. The most common schwannoma arising in the cavernous sinus is from cranial nerve V. On MR imaging, nerve sheath tumors are isointense to gray matter on T1WI and heterogeneously hyperintense on T2WI (**Fig. 18**). These lesions follow the course of the nerve. The other major diagnostic consideration for a parasellar mass is a meningioma. Distinguishing features for meningioma include presence of dural tail and broad-based origin along the dural surface, as well as intermediate signal intensity of these lesions on T2WI. Meningiomas also show homogeneous moderate to avid enhancement on postcontrast images, whereas schwannomas show a heterogeneous moderate degree of enhancement. Associated hypoesthesia or anesthesia associated with the affected nerve is seen with schwannoma.[57–61]

Hemangioma

Cavernous sinus hemangiomas are not true tumors but represent venous vascular malformations. Although these lesions are typically isointense to gray matter on T1WI, they are markedly hyperintense in signal intensity on T2WI, which aids in making this diagnosis (**Fig. 19**). On postcontrast images, these lesions may show variable patterns of enhancement. These lesions are typically nonsurgical, and, if suspected, a tagged red cell nuclear medicine study may be performed because these lesions show persistent activity on the delayed blood pool images.[62–66]

DURAL-BASED LESIONS

Dural-based processes may involve the parasellar region, including tuberculosis, fungal infection, and sarcoidosis. The differential diagnosis of

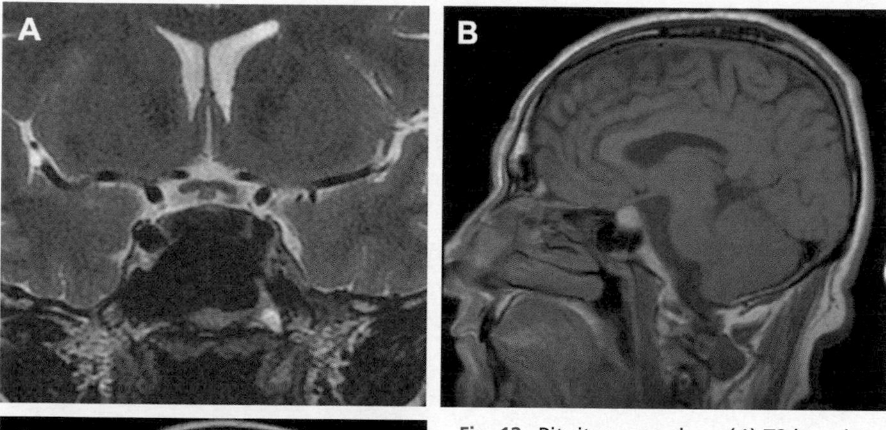

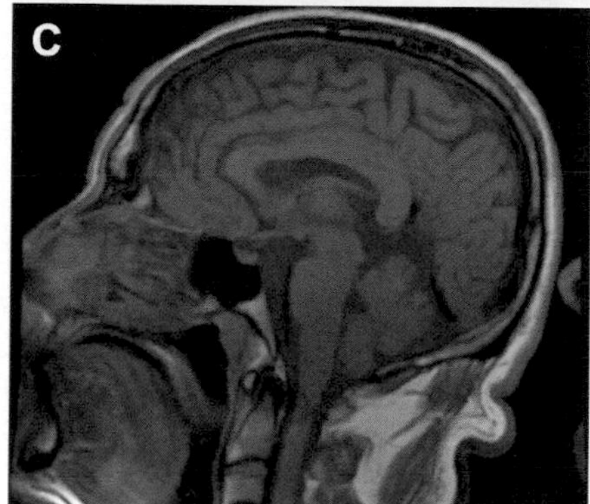

Fig. 12. Pituitary apoplexy. (*A*) T2 hypointense changes can be seen centrally within the pituitary gland on coronal T2WI. (*B*) Sagittal T1WI shows corresponding T1 hyperintense change compatible with blood products. (*C*) A follow-up scan done 1 year later shows resolution of the blood products.

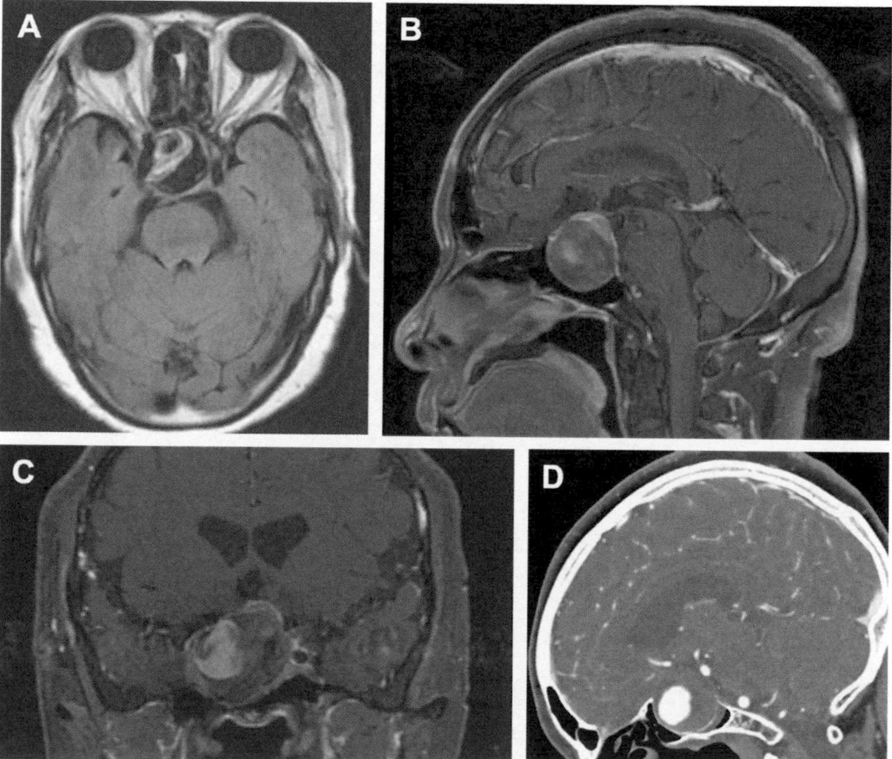

Fig. 13. Sellar aneurysm. (*A*) Axial T2-FLAIR through the sella shows a round mass with heterogeneous signal showing a swirl sign. (*B*) Sagittal postcontrast T1WI shows the mass expanding the sella and compressing the optic chiasm with areas of both hyperintense and hypointense signal. (*C*) Pulsation artifact can be seen along the phase-encoding direction, classic for aneurysm. (*D*) The presence of an internal carotid artery aneurysm from the cavernous segment was confirmed on CT angiogram.

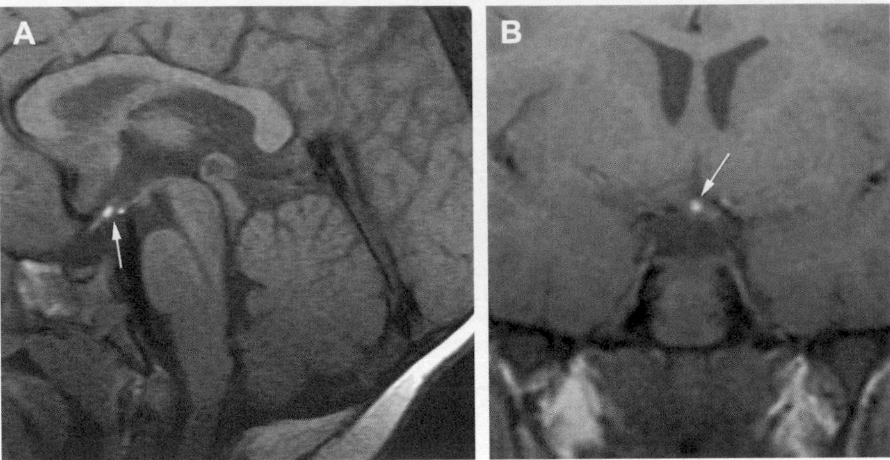

Fig. 14. Ectopic posterior pituitary gland. Sagittal (*A*) and coronal (*B*) T1WI through the sella shows abnormal position of the posterior pituitary bright spot (*white arrows*), which can be seen located more superiorly with small size of the gland.

pachymeningeal enhancement should include these entities as well as metastatic disease and lymphoma. The diagnosis is typically made by lumbar puncture and CSF analysis. One entity to consider in the setting of dural enhancement is dural-based pseudotumor. This disorder is self-limiting and represents the presence of a polymorphic collection of lymphocytes and associated fibrosis. Involvement of the cavernous sinus may result in painful proptosis, headache, and multiple

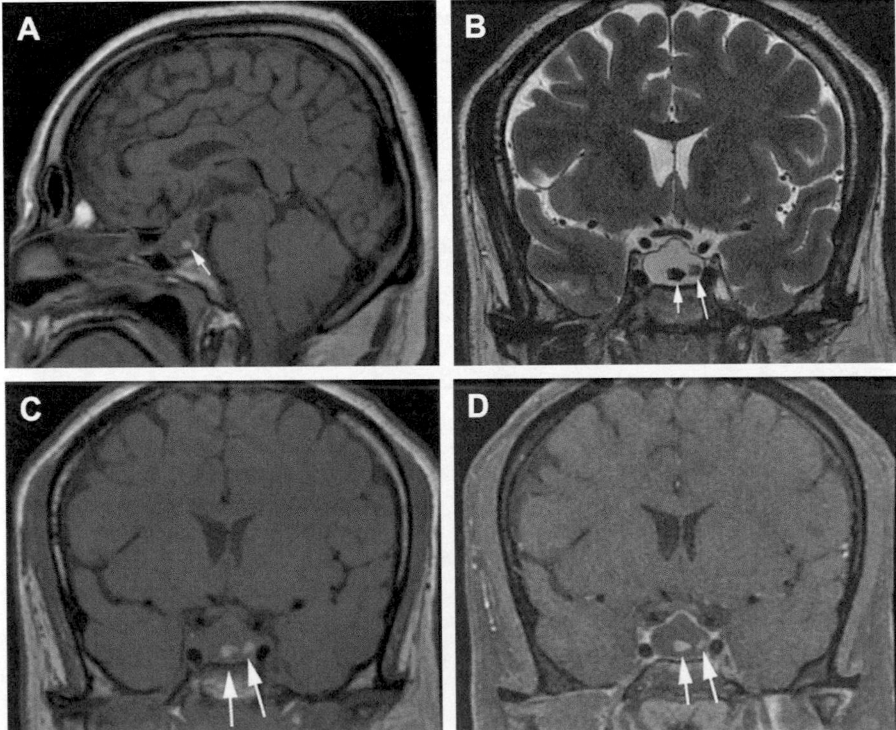

Fig. 15. Rathke cleft cyst. (*A–D*) Sagittal T1WI (*A*) shows a primarily hypointense expansile cystic lesion occupying the sella. T1 hyperintense T2 hypointense nodules (*white arrows*) can be seen within the cystic portion of the lesion, classic for Rathke cleft cyst. Only a thin wall of enhancement could be seen following contrast administration (*D*).

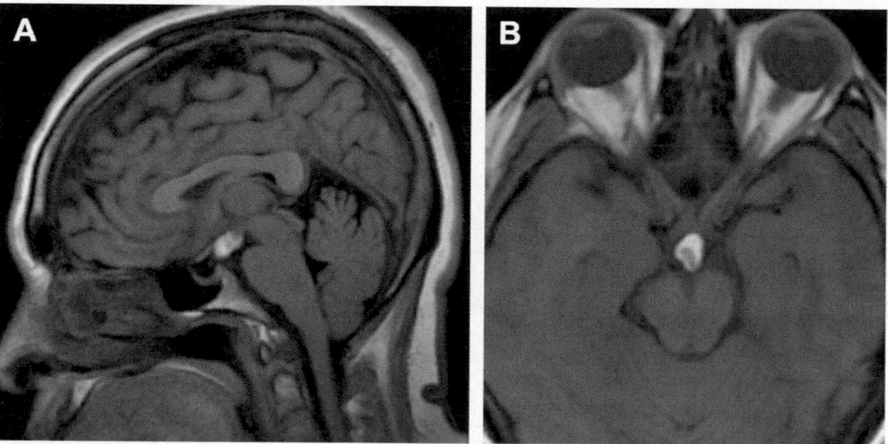

Fig. 16. Dermoid cyst. (*A*) Sagittal T1WI shows a lobulated hyperintense mass in the suprasellar cistern along the undersurface of the hypothalamus. (*B*) The mass follows primarily fat signal intensity but there are also some hypointense contents suggesting this was not a simple lipoma but a dermoid cyst.

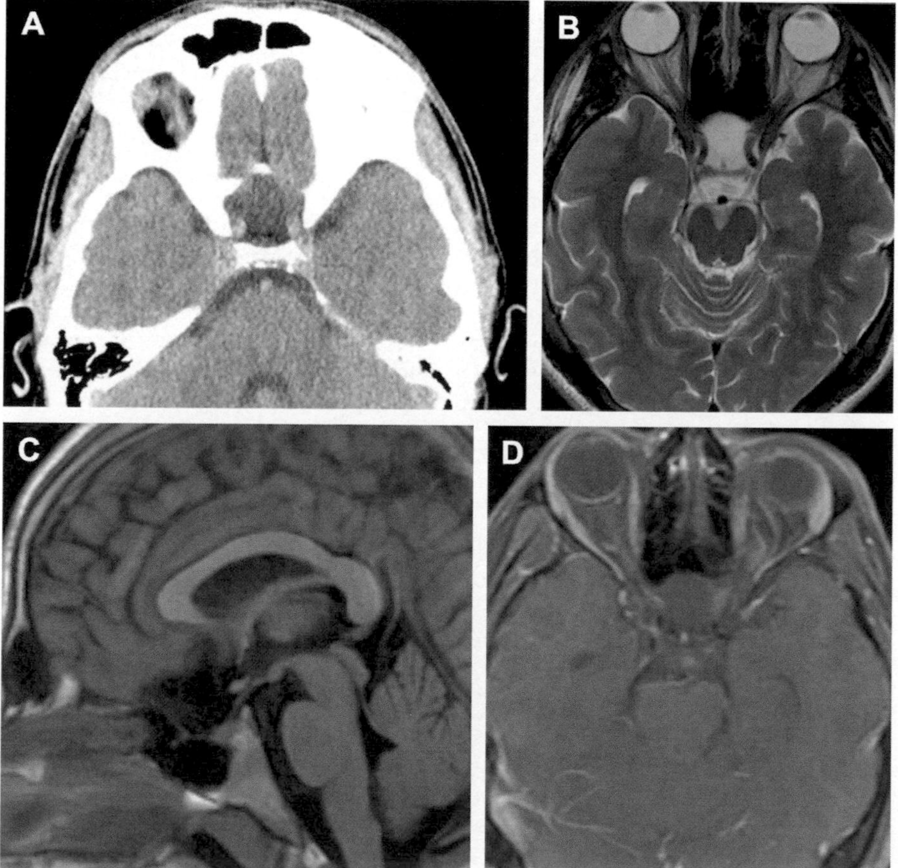

Fig. 17. Arachnoid cyst. (*A*) Axial noncontrast CT image through the suprasellar region shows a CSF attenuation structure. (*B*) This structure follows CSF intensity on T2WI and all other sequences. (*C*) The arachnoid cyst extends down into the sella, which is expanded. The pituitary gland is normal. (*D*) There is no associated enhancement on postcontrast T1WI.

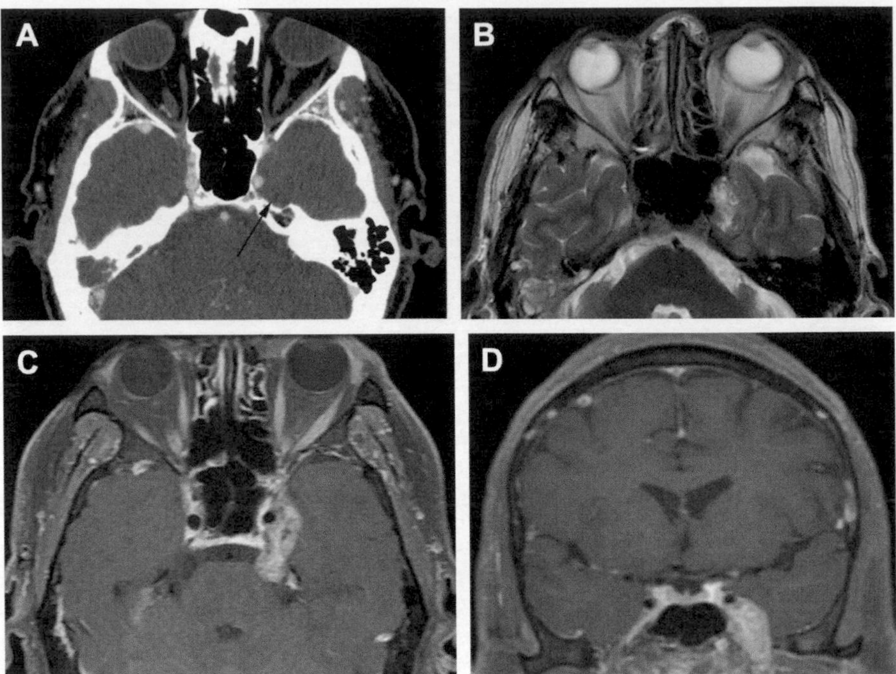

Fig. 18. Schwannoma. (*A*) Axial postcontrast CT image through cavernous sinus shows an expansile lesion adjacent to the left cavernous carotid artery with subtle osseous remodeling of the left petrous apex (*black arrow*). (*B*) The mass shows T2 hyperintense change. (*C, D*) An enhancing lesion can be seen following the left trigeminal nerve consistent with schwannoma.

cranial neuropathy (cranial nerves III, IV, V, and/or VI), and the clinical syndrome is called Tolosa-Hunt syndrome (**Fig. 20**). On MR imaging, this is seen as asymmetric enlargement and enhancement of the cavernous sinus. On T2WI, this mass is isointense to hypointense to gray matter signal intensity and shows diffusion abnormality. Typically, this process is responsive to steroid therapy. Although this process may be indistinguishable from meningioma, lymphoma, or granulomatous process, the acute nature of the process should suggest this entity as a consideration.[67–73]

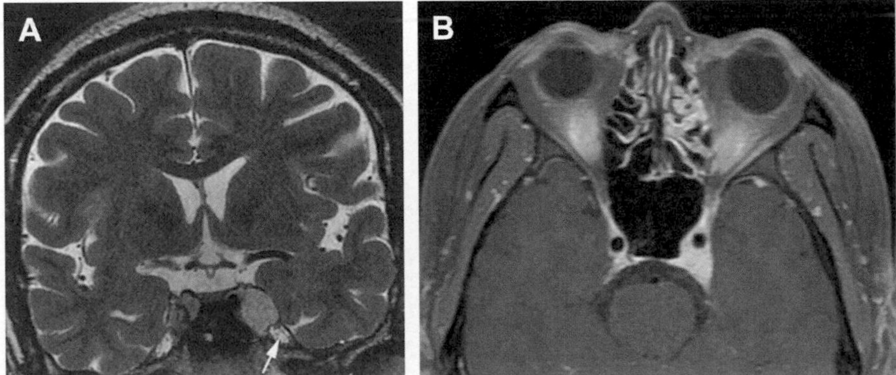

Fig. 19. Cavernous sinus hemangioma. (*A*) There is a T2 hyperintense mass filling and expanding the left cavernous sinus. The mass is distinct from the adjacent Meckel cave (*white arrow*) located more inferiorly. (*B*) Postcontrast T1WI shows uniform enhancement and enlargement of the left cavernous sinus consistent with the underlying cavernous sinus hemangioma.

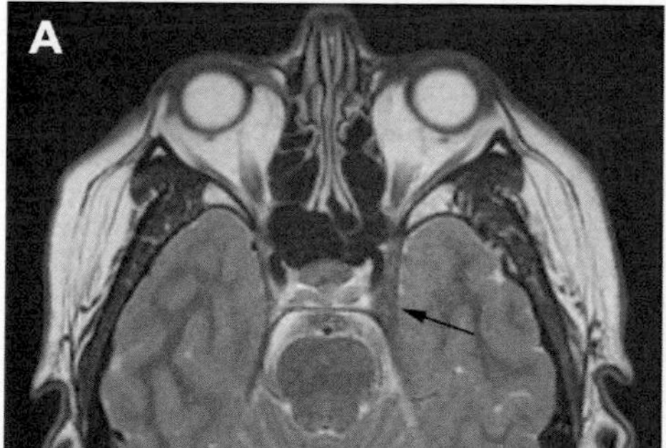

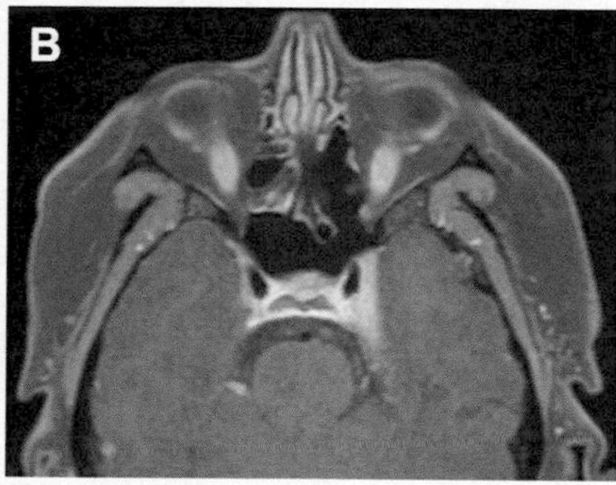

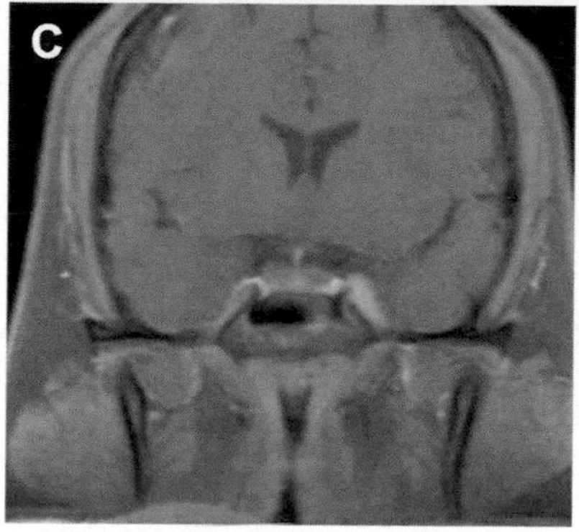

Fig. 20. Tolosa-Hunt syndrome. (*A*) There is asymmetric T2 hypointense change within the left cavernous sinus (*black arrow*). (*B, C*) This area of abnormal signal shows enhancement on postcontrast T1WI. This patient was experiencing painful ophthalmoplegia consistent with Tolosa-Hunt syndrome.

SUMMARY

A host of pathologic processes may involve the sellar and parasellar region. Although pituitary adenoma and meningioma are the most common pathologic processes to involve the sellar region and schwannoma and meningioma in the parasellar region, this article discusses the most common tumor and tumor-like conditions, vascular lesions, and congenital/developmental processes that involve this area.

REFERENCES

1. Borges A. Skull base tumors. Part I: imaging technique, anatomy and anterior skull. Eur J Radiol 2008;66(3):338–47.
2. Elster AD. Modern imaging of the pituitary. Radiology 1993;187:1–14.
3. Delman BN, Fatterpaker GM, Law M, et al. Neuroimaging for the pediatric endocrinologist. Pediatr Endocrinol Rev 2008;5(Suppl 2):708–19.
4. Casselman J, Mermuys K, Delanote J, et al. MRI of the cranial nerves – more than meets the eye: technical considerations and advanced anatomy. Neuroimaging Clin North Am 2008;18(2):197–231.
5. Cheng Y, Zhang H, Su L, et al. Anatomical study of cavernous segment of the internal carotid artery and its relationship to the structures in sella region. J Craniofac Surg 2013;24(2):622–5.
6. Miki Y, Kanagaki M, Takahashi JA, et al. Dynamic pituitary MRI has high sensitivity and specificity for the diagnosis of mild Cushing's syndrome and should be part of the initial workup. Horm Metab Res 2007;39:451–6.
7. Pisaneschi M, Kapoor G. Imaging the sella and parasellar region. Neuroimaging Clin North Am 2005;15:203–19.
8. Friedman TC, Zuckerbraun E, Lee ML, et al. Dynamic pituitary MRI has high sensitivity and specificity for the diagnosis of mild Cushing's syndrome and should be part of the initial workup. Horm Metab Res 2007;39:451–6.
9. Bonneville F, Cattin F, Marsot-Dupuch K, et al. T1 signal hyperintensity in the sellar region: spectrum of findings. Radiographics 2006;26(1):93–113.
10. Bonneville JF, Bonneville F, Cattin F. Magnetic resonance imaging of pituitary adenomas. Eur Radiol 2005;15:543–8.
11. Rumboldt Z. Pituitary adenomas. Top Magn Reson Imaging 2005;16:277–88.
12. Sonksen P, Sonksen C. Pituitary incidentaloma. Clin Endocrinol (Oxf) 2008;69(2):180.
13. Kumar J, Kumar A, Sharma R, et al. Magnetic resonance imaging of sellar and suprasellar pathology: a pictorial review. Curr Probl Diagn Radiol 2007;36(6):227–36.
14. Rao VJ, James RA, Mitra D. Imaging characteristics of common suprasellar lesions with emphasis on MRI findings. Clin Radiol 2008;63(8):939–47.

15. Garre ML, Cama A. Craniopharyngioma: modern concepts in pathogenesis and treatment. Curr Opin Pediatr 2007;19(4):471–9.
16. Nielsen EH, Feldt-Rasmussen U, Poulsgaard L, et al. Incidence of craniopharyngioma in Denmark (n = 189) and estimated world incidence of craniopharyngioma in children and adults. J Neurooncol 2011;104:755–63.
17. Keil MF, Stratakis CA. Pituitary tumors in childhood: update to diagnosis, treatment, and molecular genetics. Expert Rev Neurother 2008;8(4):563–74.
18. He W, Chen F, Dalm B, et al. Metastatic involvement of the pituitary gland: a systematic review with pooled individual patient data analysis. Pituitary 2015;18(1):159–68.
19. Komininos J, Vlassopoulou V, Protopapa D, et al. Tumors metastatic to the pituitary gland: case report and literature review. J Clin Endocrinol Metab 2004;89(2):574–80.
20. Skarin A. Diabetes insipidus as the initial manifestation of non-small lung cancer. J Clin Oncol 2002; 20(23):4597–602.
21. Chu J, Yang Z, Meng Q, et al. Pituicytoma: case report and literature review. Br J Radiol 2011; 84(999):e55–7.
22. Brat DJ, Scheithauer BW, Fuller GN, et al. Newly codified glial neoplasms of the 2007 WHO classification of tumors of the central nervous system: angiocentric glioma, pilomyxoid astrocytoma and pituicytoma. Brain Pathol 2007;17:319–24.
23. Brat DJ, Scheithauer BW, Staugaitis SM, et al. Pituicytoma: a distinctive low-grade glioma of the neurohypophysis. Am J Surg Pathol 2000;24:362–8.
24. Gibbs WN, Monuki ES, Linskey ME, et al. Pituicytoma: diagnostic features on selective carotid angiography and MR imaging. AJNR Am J Neuroradiol 2006;27:1639–42.
25. Ngaosuwan K, Trongwongsa T, Shuangshoti S. Clinical course of IgG4-related hypophysitis presenting with focal seizure and relapsing lymphocytic hypophysitis. BMC Endocr Disord 2015;29:15–64.
26. Chrisoulidou A, Boudina M, Karavitaki N, et al. Pituitary disorders in pregnancy. Hormones (Athens) 2015;14(1):70–90.
27. Imber BS, Lee HS, Kunwar S, et al. Hypophysitis: a single-center case series. Pituitary 2015;18(5): 630–41.
28. Takahashi Y. Autoimmune hypophysitis: new developments. Handb Clin Neurol 2014;124:417–22.
29. Lupi I, Manetti L, Raffaelli V, et al. Diagnosis and treatment of autoimmune hypophysitis: a short review. J Endocrinol Invest 2011;34(8):e245–52.
30. Foyouzi N. Lymphocytic adenohypophysitis. Obstet Gynecol Surv 2011;66(2):109–13.
31. Lury KM. Inflammatory and infectious processes involving the pituitary gland. Top Magn Reson Imaging 2005;16(4):301–6.
32. Winters SJ, Vitaz T, Nowacki MR, et al. Addison's disease and pituitary enlargement. Am J Med Sci 2015;349(6):526–9.
33. Neves CP, Massolt ET, Peters RP, et al. Pituitary hyperplasia: an uncommon presentation of a common disease. Endocrinol Diabetes Metab Case Rep 2015;2015:150056.
34. Ahmed M, Rifai A, Al-Jurf M, et al. Classical pituitary apoplexy presentation and a follow-up of 13 patients. Horm Res 1989;31:125–32.
35. Bills DC, Meyer FB, Laws ER Jr, et al. A retrospective analysis of pituitary apoplexy. Neurosurgery 1993; 33:602–9.
36. Mohr G, Hardy J. Hemorrhage, necrosis and apoplexy in pituitary adenomas. Surg Neurol 1982; 18:181–9.
37. Nawar RN, Abdel-Mannan D, Selman WR, et al. Pituitary tumor apoplexy: a review. J Intensive Care Med 2008;23(2):75–90.
38. Faje AT, Tritos NA. Cavernous carotid artery aneurysm, a rare cause of intrasellar mass and hyperprolactinemia. J Clin Endocrinol Metab 2012;97(3):723–4.
39. Heshmati HM, Fatourechi V, Dagam SA, et al. Hypopituitarism caused by intrasellar aneurysms. Mayo Clin Proc 2001;76(8):789–93.
40. Ören NC, Cagiltay E, Akay F, et al. Panhypopituitarism with ectopic posterior pituitary lobe, heterotopia, polymicrogyria, corpus callosum dysgenesis, and optic chiasm/nerve hypoplasia: is that an undefined neuronal migration syndrome? AJNR Am J Neuroradiol 2015;36(5):E33–5.
41. Mahomed N, Motshudi T. The ectopic posterior pituitary gland. S Afr J Surg 2013;51(4):148.
42. Grech R, Galvin L, Looby S, et al. Teaching neuroimages: ectopic posterior pituitary. Neurology 2013; 81(16):e121–2.
43. Lacovazzo D, Lugli F, Giampietro A. Ectopic posterior pituitary causing hyperprolactinemia. Endocrine 2012;42(2):449–50.
44. Di Lorgi N, Secco A, Napoli F, et al. Developmental abnormalities of the posterior pituitary gland. Endocr Dev 2009;14:83–94.
45. Yang CX, Feng M, Liu XH, et al. Symptomatic Rathke's cleft cyst with rapid enlargement masquerading as Rathke's cleft cyst apoplexy. Chin Med J (Engl) 2016;129(16):2009–10.
46. Rasmussen Z, Abode-Iyamah KO, Kirby P, et al. Rathke's cleft cyst: a case report of recurrence and spontaneous involution. J Clin Neurosci 2016;32:122–5.
47. Park M, Lee SK, Choi J, et al. Differentiation between cystic pituitary adenomas and Rathke cleft cysts: a diagnostic model using MRI. AJNR Am J Neuroradiol 2015;36(10):1866–73.
48. Tan LA, Kasliwal MK, Harbhajanka A, et al. Hyperdense suprasellar mass: an unusual radiological presentation of intracranial dermoid cyst. J Clin Neurosci 2015;22(7):1208–10.

49. Abele TA, Yetkin ZF, Raisanen JM, et al. Non-pituitary origin sellar tumors mimicking pituitary macroadenomas. Clin Radiol 2012;67(8):821–7.
50. Tuna H, Torun AN, Erdogran A. Intrasellar epidermoid cyst presenting as pituitary apoplexy. J Clin Neurosci 2008;15(10):1154–6.
51. Shaw AS, Connor SE. Parasellar epidermoid cyst rupturing into the nasopharynx. J Laryngol Otol 2005;119(2):140–3.
52. Sweiss RB, Shweikeh F, Sweiss FB, et al. Suprasellar mature cystic teratoma: an unusual location for an uncommon tumor. Case Rep Neurol Med 2013; 2013:180497.
53. Liu Z, Lv X, Wang W, et al. Imaging characteristics of primary intracranial teratoma. Acta Radiol 2014; 55(7):874–81.
54. West BJ, Moskowitz H. Non-midline intracranial lipoma misdiagnosed as meningioma: case report. Conn Med 2007;71(5):285–9.
55. Park KH, Gwak HS, Hong EK, et al. Inflamed symptomatic sellar arachnoid cyst: case report. Brain Tumor Res Treat 2013;1(1):28–31.
56. Dubuisson AS, Stevenaert A, Martin DH, et al. Intrasellar arachnoid cysts. Neurosurgery 2007;61(3): 505–13.
57. Johnsen DE, Woodruff WW, Allen IS, et al. MR imaging of the sellar and juxtasellar regions. Radiographics 1991;11(5):727–58.
58. Skolnik AD, Loevner LA, Sampathu DM, et al. Cranial nerve schwannomas: diagnostic imaging approach. Radiographics 2016;19:150199.
59. Zhang L, Yang Y, Xu S, et al. Trigeminal schwannomas: a report of 42 cases and review of the relevant surgical approaches. Clin Neurol Neurosurg 2009; 111(3):261–9.
60. Lo PA, Harper CG, Besser M. Intracavernous schwannoma of the abducens nerve: a review of the clinical features, radiology and pathology of an unusual case. J Clin Neurosci 2001;8(4):357–60.
61. El-Kalliny M, Van Loveren H, Keller JT, et al. Tumors of the lateral wall of the cavernous sinus. J Neurosurg 1992;77(4):508–14.
62. Lanotte M, Giordana MT, Forni C, et al. Schwannoma of the cavernous sinus. Case report and review of the literature. J Neurosurg Sci 1992;36(4):233–8.
63. Wang Y, Li P, Zhang XJ, et al. Gamma knife surgery for cavernous sinus hemanginoma: a report of 32 cases. World Neurosurg 2016. [Epub ahead of print].
64. Tang X, Wu H, Wang B, et al. A new classification and clinical results of Gamma Knife radiosurgery for cavernous sinus hemangiomas: a report of 53 cases. Acta Neurochir (Wien) 2015;157(6):961–9 [discussion: 969].
65. Hasiloglu ZI, Asik M, Kizilkilic O, et al. Cavernous hemangioma of the cavernous sinus misdiagnosed as a meningioma; a case report and MR imaging findings. Clin Imaging 2013;37(4):744–6.
66. Yin YH, Yu XG, Xu BN, et al. Surgical management of large and giant cavernous sinus hemangiomas. J Clin Neurosci 2013;20(1):128–33.
67. Jinhu Y, Jianping D, Xin L, et al. Dynamic enhancement features of cavernous sinus cavernous hemangiomas on conventional contrast-enhanced MR imaging. AJNR Am J Neuroradiol 2008;29(3): 577–81.
68. Pérez CA, Evangelista M. Evaluation and management of Tolosa-Hunt syndrome in children: a clinical update. Pediatr Neurol 2016;62:18–26.
69. Guedes BV, da Rocha AJ, Zuppani HB, et al. A case review of the MRI features in alternating Tolosa-Hunt syndrome. Cephalalgia 2010;30(9):1133–6.
70. Jain R, Sawhney S, Koul RL, et al. Tolosa-Hunt syndrome: MRI appearances. J Med Imaging Radiat Oncol 2008;52(5):447–51.
71. Colnaghi S, Versino M, Marchioni E, et al. ICHD-II diagnostic criteria for Tolosa-Hunt syndrome in idiopathic inflammatory syndromes of the orbit and/or the cavernous sinus. Cephalalgia 2008; 28(6):577–84.
72. Johnston JL. Parasellar syndromes. Curr Neurol Neurosci Rep 2002;2(5):423–31.
73. Hunt WE, Brightman RP. The Tolosa-Hunt syndrome: a problem in differential diagnosis. Acta Neurochir Suppl (Wien) 1988;42:248–52.

Imaging of the Posterior Skull Base

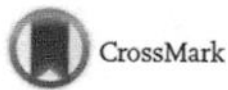

Joici Job, MD, Barton F. Branstetter IV, MD*

KEYWORDS

• Skull base • Cranial nerves • Foramen magnum • Jugular fossa

KEY POINTS

- A dedicated skull base protocol is critical to evaluation of poster skull base anomalies.
- Knowledge of normal lower cranial nerve anatomy allows proper radiologic assessment of posterior fossa pathology.
- Disease of the posterior skull base often presents with symptoms from progression into surrounding regions.

INTRODUCTION

Accurate detection of underlying pathology involving the posterior skull base requires an understanding of normal and normal variant anatomy, especially the course of the lower cranial nerves (CNs), IX through XII. This helps identify and classify common clinical presentations based on location of pathologic involvement.

Posterior skull base pathology can be grouped into 4 major categories: trauma/acquired, neoplastic, infectious, and vascular. This article is organized in accordance with this scheme. Abnormalities of the posterior skull base frequent present with extension of pathology beyond the skull base, both intracranially and caudally, to involve the suprahyoid neck.

Imaging protocols for the posterior skull base should be tailored to the individual patient to optimize characterization of the abnormality and provide relevant information for treatment planning.

PROTOCOLS

At the authors' institution, every skull base MRI is individually tailored to the patient based on prior imaging and clinical history. The key piece of information provided to the technologists is the anatomic extent of imaging. This allows using smaller fields of view and reducing overall imaging time. The default pulse sequences for the skull base protocol are

Full brain
- T1-weighted sagittal
- Diffusion-weighted imaging axial
- Fluid-attenuated inversion recovery (FLAIR) axial

Skull base region of interest
- T1-weighted axial and coronal
- T2-weighted (fat saturated) axial and coronal
- Contrast-enhanced T1-weighted (fat saturated) axial and coronal
- 3-D spoiled gradient (acquired in axial with sagittal and coronal reformatted images)

Some considerations for further tailoring posterior skull base protocols include

- Neurovascular compression: 3-plane thin-section steady-state free-precession imaging (SSFP) to delineate lower CN course and better characterize the culprit vessel (artery/vein), point of contact, and/or deformity.
- Contrast-enhanced FLAIR sequences to improve sensitivity for leptomeningeal disease

Department of Radiology, University of Pittsburgh Medical Center, University of Pittsburgh, 200 Lothrop Street, Pittsburgh, PA 15213, USA
* Corresponding author.
E-mail address: branbf@UPMC.EDU

Radiol Clin N Am 55 (2017) 103–121
http://dx.doi.org/10.1016/j.rcl.2016.08.002
0033-8389/17/© 2016 Elsevier Inc. All rights reserved.

- Contrast-enhanced SSFP sequences to characterize CN involvement (particularly useful when there is extension of disease into the cavernous sinuses.)
- Automated volume measurements on both CT and MRI are useful on serial follow-ups in the post-treatment setting.
- In addition to standard coronal and sagittal reconstructions in bony and soft tissue algorithms, 3-D surface rendering can be helpful for surgical planning on CT. For example, when Eagle syndrome is suspected, these reconstructions may better delineate the course of the styloid process relative to the faucial tonsil.[1]

POSTERIOR SKULL BASE ANATOMY AND EMBRYOLOGY

The clivus forms the anterior aspect of the posterior skull base from fusion of the basisphenoid and basiocciput at the spheno-occipital synchondrosis (**Fig. 1**). The craniocaudal extent of the posterior skull base is from the foramen magnum inferordorsally to the dorsum sellae superoventrally.[2] The laterosuperior portion of the posterior skull base is formed by the posterior surface of the petrous portion of the temporal bone and the mastoid portion of the temporal bone.[3]

The condylar portion of the occipital bone forms the lateral posterior skull base inferiorly. The junction between the petrous portions of the temporal bone and the occipital bone is the petroccipital suture/fissure[4] (see **Fig. 1**). The posterior portion of the posterior skull base is formed by the occipital bone. The petrous ridge of the temporal bone divides the central skull base from the posterior skull base and is the attachment for the fixed edge of the tentorium cerebelli.[5]

Embryologically, there are 4 major ossification centers form the foramen magnum: the supraoccipital, basioccipital, and paired exoccipital. Although the posterior skull base is nearly completely ossified by birth, the intraoccipital, petroccipital, and occipitomastoid sutures do not fuse until later in adulthood[6] (see **Fig. 1**).

Important Posterior Skull Base Foramina

The jugular foramen is located between the petrous portion of temporal bone (otic capsule developmentally) and the basioccipital plate and bordered anteromedially by the petroclival fissure and posterolaterally by the occipitomastoid suture. The long axis of the jugular foramen takes an oblique course running posterolateral to anteromedial. The right jugular foramen is larger than the left 68% of the time.[4]

The jugular foramen is separated from the carotid canal by the caroticojugular spine and inferomedially from the hypoglossal canal by the jugular tubercle. The intrajugular process divides the foramen into the posterolateral sigmoid and anteromedial petrosal portions of jugular foramen. Classically, the smaller anteromedial petrosal portion, also known as pars nervosa, transmits the inferior petrosal sinus and the glossopharyngeal (CN IX) nerve with its tympanic branch (Jacobson nerve). The larger posterolateral sigmoid portion, also known as pars vascularis, transmits the sigmoid sinus, forms inferiorly as the jugular

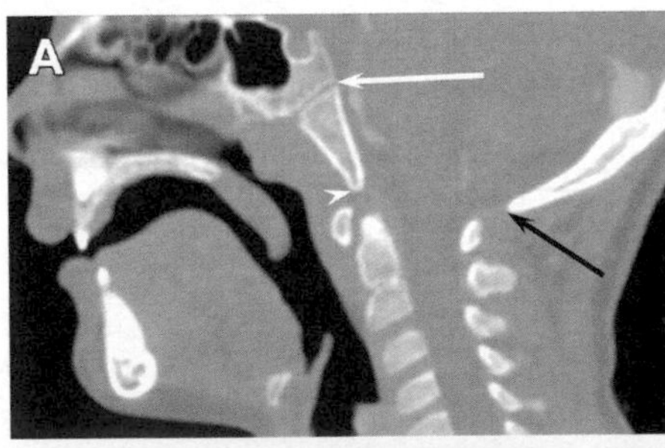

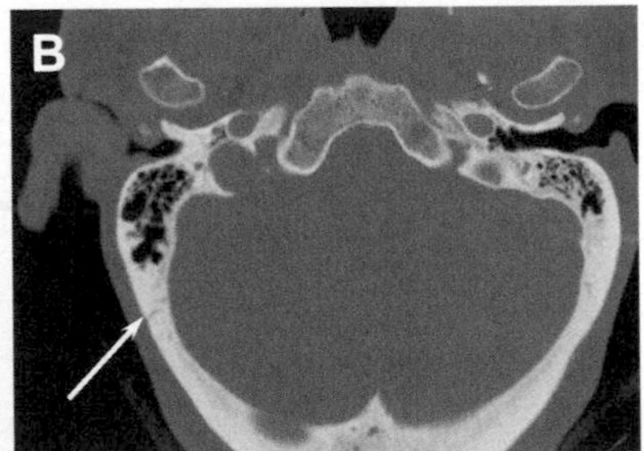

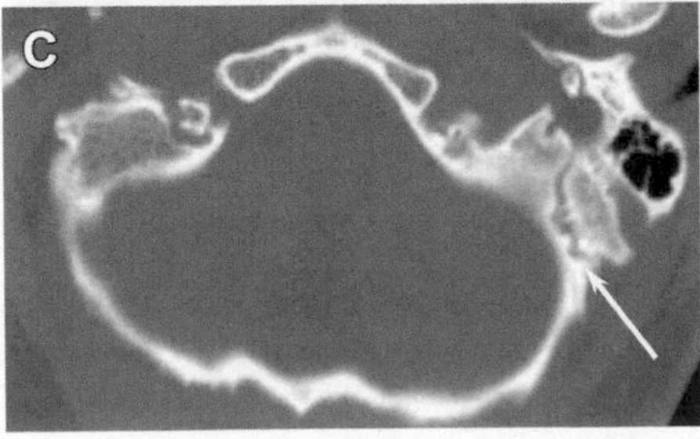

Fig. 1. Posterior skull base landmarks. (*A*) Normal posterior fossa anatomy. Sagittal CT images in a child demonstrates normal suture between unfused basisphenoid and basiocciput–spheno-occipital synchondrosis (*white arrow*). This fuses to form the clivus. Basion (*arrowhead*). Opisthion (*black arrow*). (*B*) Normal partially fused occipitomastoid suture in an adult (*arrow*). (*C*) Normal unfused occipitomastoid suture in a child (*arrow*).

bulb, and transmits the meningeal branches of the ascending pharyngeal and occipital arteries, along with the vagus (X) nerve with its auricular branch (Arnold nerve) and the accessory (XI) nerve.[6] The vagus (X) and accessory (XI) nerves, however, may travel through the pars nervosa instead of the pars vascularis.[4] The petrosal portion also receives venous tributaries from the hypoglossal canal, petroclival fissure, and vertebral venous plexus.[4]

The hypoglossal canal is located between the occipital condyle inferiorly and the jugular tubercle superolaterally.[7] The proximal portion may be divided by fibrous septa that separate the 2 roots of the hypoglossal nerve, which merge as the nerve emerges from the skull base.[8] A single hypoglossal canal occurs in 84% of cases, whereas a bipartitioned hypoglossal canal occurs in 13.5%, and a tripartitioned canal in 2.1%[9,10] (**Fig. 2**).

The foramen magnum is formed entirely within the occipital bone and is oval in shape with a longer anteroposterior dimension. The anterior margin is the basion and the posterior margin is the opisthion. Its contents include the spinal roots of the accessory nerve as they course upward from the cervical spine before heading toward the jugular bulb, the vertebral arteries, and the anterior and posterior spinal arteries.[2]

Other Posterior Skull Base Anatomic Considerations

The undersurface of the mastoid portion of the temporal bone contains the mastoid process, which is a lateral bony projection that provides attachment for the sternocleidomastoid, splenius capitis, posterior belly of digastric, and longissimus capitis muscles[8] (**Fig. 3**).

There is a groove along the medial margin of mastoid process, the mastoid notch, on which the posterior belly of the digastric muscle attaches, and posterior and medial to this is the occipital groove, which is traversed by the occipital artery (see **Fig. 3**).[8] This keeps the fairly constant relationship of the occipital artery coursing along medial margin of posterior belly of digastric muscle.

Posterior to these structures is the mastoid foramen, which is at the intersection of the temporal and occipital bones and carries mastoid emissary vein to the sigmoid sinus and a tiny branch of the occipital artery, called posterior meningeal artery traverse.[8]

There are 2 pertinent clinical scenarios to consider when these transosseous vascular channels are enlarged on a routine temporal bone CT:

- The first is an underlying abnormal high-flow vascular abnormality, such as dural arteriovenous fistula, which often has arterial supply from the occipital artery in the posterior fossa.
- The second is to notify the surgeon in a preoperative setting, to avoid inadvertent vascular injury intraoperatively.

The squamosal portion of the occipital bone contains the sagittal sulcus for the superior sagittal sinus and falx cerebri, internal occipital crest for attachment of the falx cerebelli (see **Fig. 3**), and the transverse groove for the transverse sinuses.[8] The lower surface of the basiocciput contains the

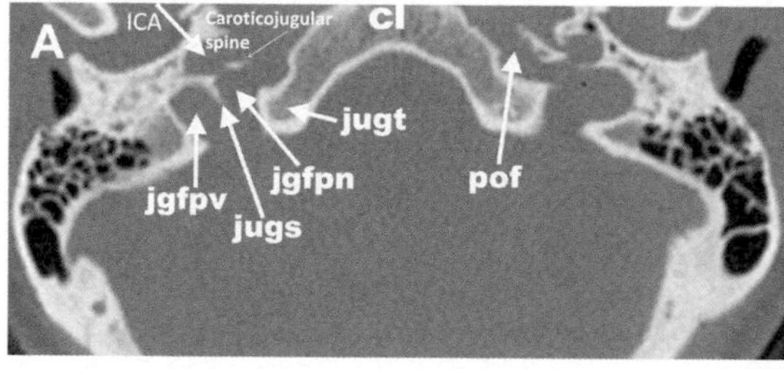

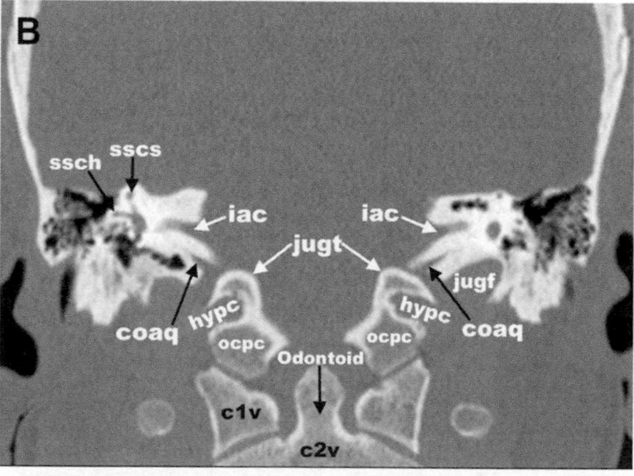

Fig. 2. Normal CT anatomy of the jugular region. Axial CT (*A*) and coronal CT (*B*) demonstrate normal bony anatomy and relationships. cl, clivus; c1v, C1 vertebra; c2v, c2 vertebra; coaq, cochlear aqueduct; hypc, hypoglossalcanal; iac, internal auditory canal; ICA, vertical segment of petrous ICA; jgfpn, pars nervosa of jugular foramen; jgfpv, pars vascularis of jugular foramen; jugf, jugular foramen; jugs, jugular spine; jugt, jugular tubercle; ocpc, occipital condyle; ssch, horizontal sumicircular canal; sscs, superior semicircular canal. (*Courtesy of* Neil Borden, MD, Pittsburgh, PA.)

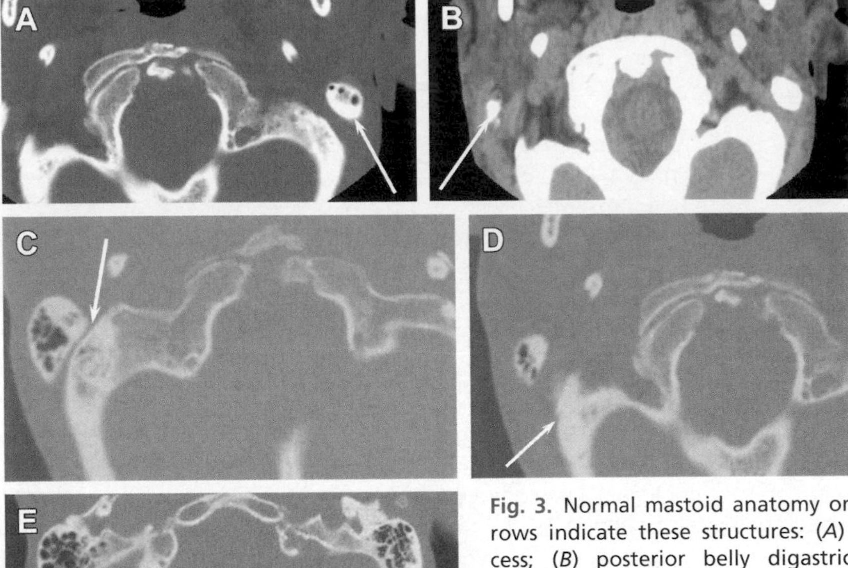

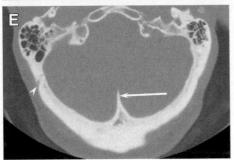

Fig. 3. Normal mastoid anatomy on axial CT. Arrows indicate these structures: (*A*) mastoid process; (*B*) posterior belly digastric muscle; (*C*) mastoid notch; and (*D*) groove for occipital artery. (*E*) Channel for mastoid emissary veins (*arrowhead*) and internal occipital crest (*arrow*).

midline pharyngeal tubercle on which the fibrous raphe of the pharynx attaches[8] (**Fig. 4**). The condylar canal and fossa just posterior to the occipital condyles receive the posterior margin of the superior facet of the atlas and an emissary vein from the transverse sinus. The upper portion of the basiocciput contains the groove for the inferior petrosal sinus[8] (see **Fig. 4**).

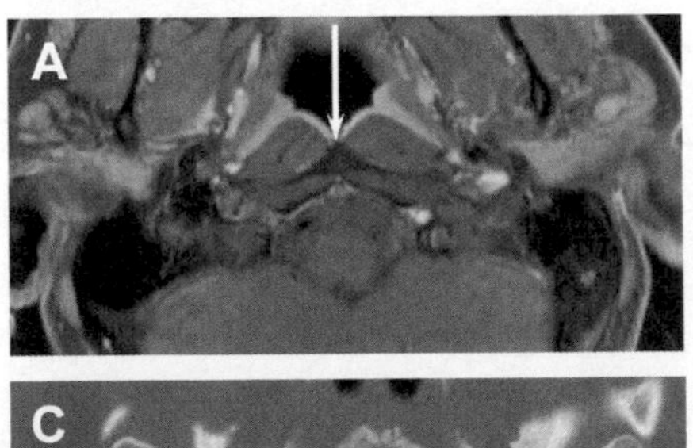

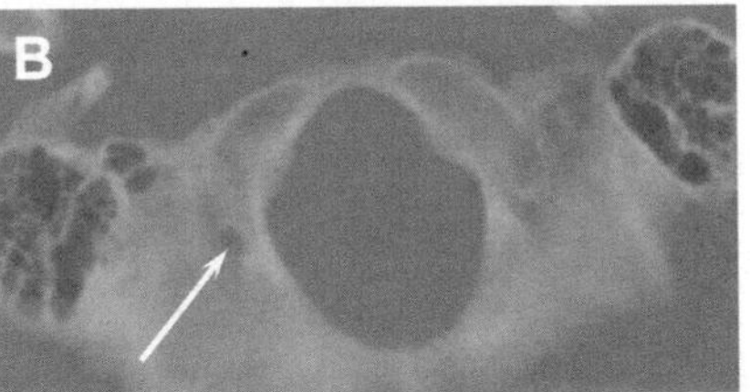

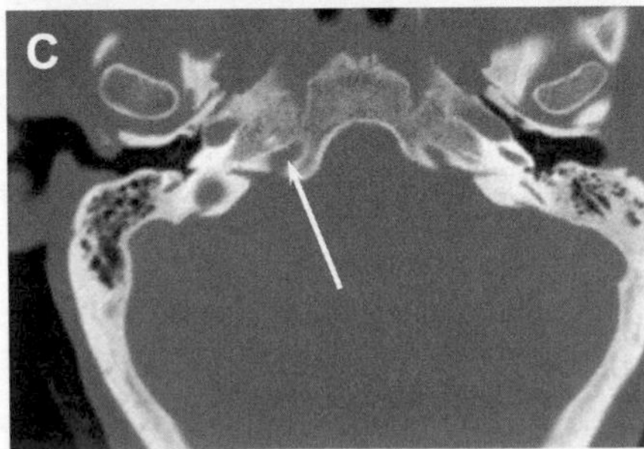

Fig. 4. Basioccipital anatomy. (*A*) Axial contrast-enhanced T1-weighted at the level of the nasopharynx, with arrow delineating pharyngeal tubercle. (*B*) Axial bone-window CT, with arrow indicating condylar canal. (*C*) Axial CT demonstrating normal groove for inferior petrosal sinus (*arrow*) as it drains into pars nervosa of jugular foramen.

SPACE-SPECIFIC SYNDROMES OF THE POSTERIOR SKULL BASE

Vernet syndrome, also known as jugular foramen syndrome, results from a constellation of CN palsies of CN IX–XI due to compression from jugular foramen lesions.[11–13]

The most common lesions involving the jugular foramen are glomus jugulare paraganglioma, schwannoma, and meningioma, of which paragangliomas makes up 80% of primary neoplasms.[6]

The classic hypervascular glomus jugulare paraganglioma, with multiple flow voids, may be multicentric in 5% to 10% of cases and even more frequently when associated with familial paraganglioma, multiple endocrine neoplasia syndrome type 1, or neurofibromatosis type 1.[14]

If there are multiple soft tissue lesions that enhance poorly on CT, neurofibromas are a consideration, and clinical history and other stigmata of neurofibromatosis should be sought for confirmation (**Fig. 5**).

Interpretation tip: If there is a lesion involving the posterior skull base, which extends into/from suprahyoid neck, it can be rapidly localized to within the carotid sheath by identifying the internal carotid artery (ICA), internal jugular vein (IJ), and styloid process. If the lesion displaces the internal carotid anteriorly and splays it apart from adjacent jugular vein, it arises from within the carotid sheath. This narrows down the primary differential considerations to paragangliomas versus nerve sheath tumors (most commonly vagal schwannomas).

Depending on the extent of the lesion, rare cases of Collet-Sicard syndrome can also develop, which is Vernet syndrome with additional CN XII palsy, or Villaret syndrome, which is Collet-Sicard syndrome with ipsilateral Horner syndrome.[15]

CRANIAL NERVE IX

The glossopharyngeal nerve is a complex mixed nerve with motor, sensory, and autonomic functions. There are 4 major nuclei in the medulla associated with CN IX functions, including[16]

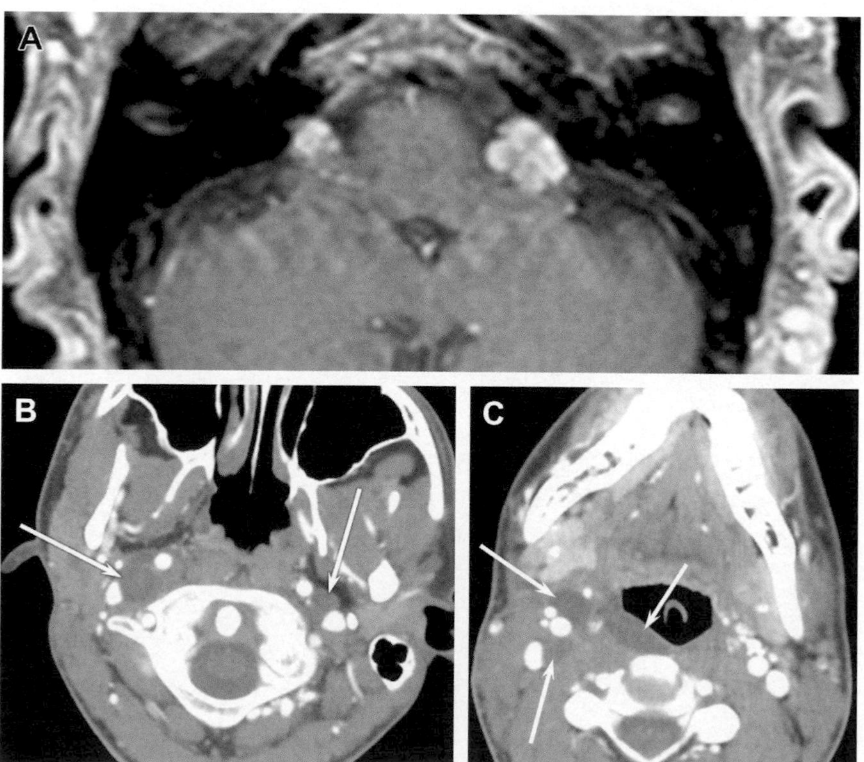

Fig. 5. Neurofibromas of the lower CNs. (*A*) Axial-enhanced T1-weighted image shows bilateral enhancing masses along the expected course of the lower CNs. (*B*) Axial-enhanced CT shows bilateral nonenhancing masses (*arrows*) at the expected location of the vagus nerves. (*C*) Axial-enhanced CT shows plexiform configuration to a nonenhancing mass (*arrows*) with involvement of the carotid and retropharyngeal spaces.

1. Nucleus ambiguous/motor nucleus: at the level of the floor of fourth ventricle, in the bulbar triangle, where special visceral efferent motor fibers arise to innervate the third pharyngeal arch and stylopharyngeus muscle
2. Inferior salivatory nucleus: responsible for general visceral efferent and parasympathetic innervation, with pathway through tympanic canaliculus
3. Solitary nucleus: responsible for special visceral afferent (taste from posterior third of tongue) at the superior aspect of nucleus and general visceral afferent (sensory receptors at the carotid body [which measures CO_2] and carotid sinus [which measures blood pressure]) at the caudal aspect of the nucleus
4. Spinal trigeminal nucleus: responsible for general somatic afferent (GSA) (sensory information of from pharynx, tongue base soft palate, and tympanic membrane)

CN IX exits from the retroolivary sulcus/postolivary sulcus and heads toward the pars nervosa of the jugular foramen.

On the routine axial plane, the cisternal segment of CN IX exits just inferior to the level of the flocculus at the level of upper medulla, where there is still a pronounced lateral contour[17] (**Fig. 6**).

The cisternal segment of CN IX is also smaller in size than its neighboring, more caudal, CN X, where the lateral contour of the medulla is more rounded.

Dysphagia and loss of sensation of posterior third of tongue (unilateral) are common symptoms with pathology affecting CN IX. Glossopharyngeal neuralgia, with symptoms of severe unilateral pharyngeal pain, is infrequent. In the setting of neurovascular compression as the cause of symptoms, the most common culprit vessel is posterior inferior cerebellar artery (PICA), followed by the vertebral artery, followed by anterior inferior cerebellar artery.[18,19]

Extracranially, CN IX's superior and inferior nuclei lie at the level of the skull base or, more precisely, in pars nervosa of the jugular foramen, where the sensory fibers of CN IX arise. Specifically, the petrosal fossula is where the more conspicuous inferior ganglion of CN IX resides and is lateral to the inferior petrosal sinus within pars nervosa.[16]

At the level of the carotid space, the nerve usually heads posterolateral to ICA in the carotid sheath, courses along the stylopharyngeus muscle (which it innervates), along pharyngeal constrictors, and across the base of tongue. It has nerve branches along the styloglossus muscle, crossing the ascending palatine artery, and innervating the inferior aspect of palatine tonsil.[16] This explains why a medialized position of styloid process has a higher likelihood of being symptomatic in Eagle syndrome, even if there is not extensive ossification of stylohyoid ligament (**Fig. 7**).

Jacobson nerve has collateral branches that communicate between CNs IX, VII, and V3.[16] It carries sensory information from the middle ear and contributes parasympathetic fibers as it courses from the superior aspect of the petrosal fossula toward the caroticojugular spine through the inferior tympanic canaliculus (**Fig. 8**) into the middle ear to the cochlear promontory, where it divides into 6 branches innervating mucosal membranes surrounding the round and oval windows, eustachian tube, and caroticotympanic nerve. These anastomose with pericarotid sympathetics and the deep greater and lesser petrosal nerves, which in turn anastomose with the superficial greater petrosal nerve to form the pterygoid nerve.[16] Also, the superficial and deep lesser petrosal nerves anastomose and head to the otic ganglion at the level of foramen ovale and the

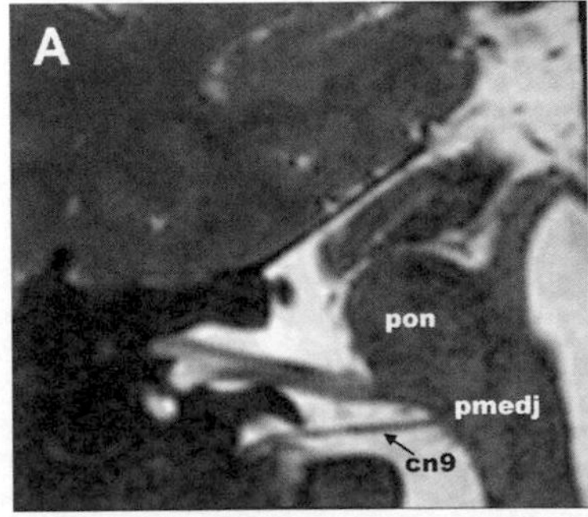

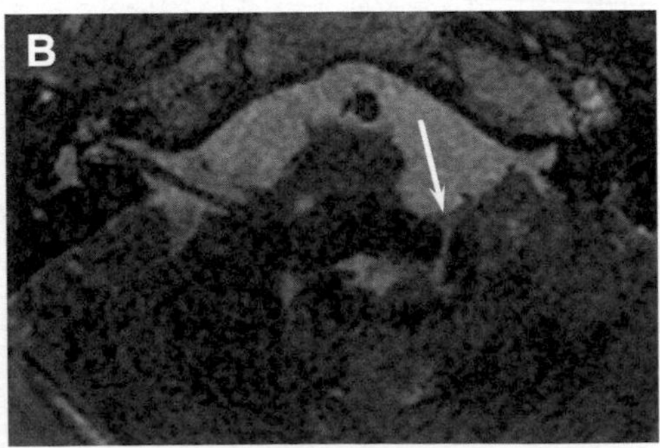

Fig. 6. Anatomy of CN IX. (*A*) Sagittal oblique SSFP sequence through the pons (pon) and pontomedullary junction (pmedj), with arrow indicating cisternal segment of CN IX (cn9). (*B*) Axial oblique SSFP image at the level of cisternal segment of left CN IX to illustrate the pronounced lateral contour of the superior medulla (*arrow*) as a useful landmark in this plane. (*Courtesy of* [*A*] Dr Neil Borden.)

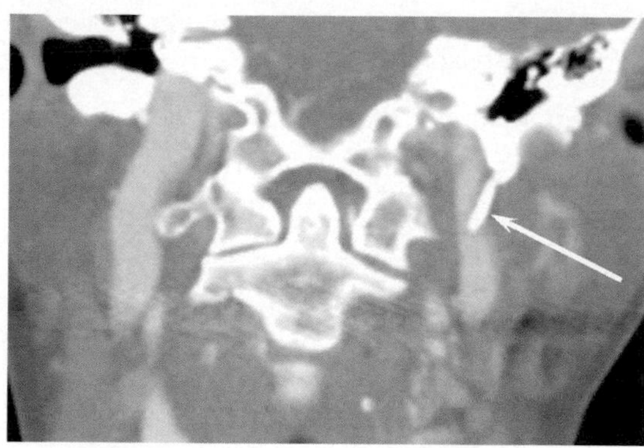

Fig. 7. Eagle syndrome. Coronal reformatted CT. A medialized styloid process (*arrow*) may cause glossopharyngeal neuralgia even without excessive ossification.

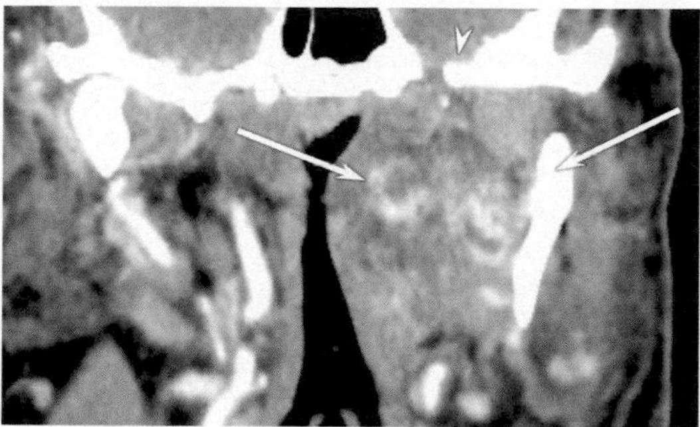

Fig. 9. Coronal CT reformat in a patient with recurrent pleomorphic adenoma demonstrates multispatial recurrent tumor (*arrows*), which involves the parotid and masticator spaces, just caudal to the level of foramen ovale (*arrowhead*) in a patient with Frey syndrome.

central skull base. From here, the otic ganglion, arises the secretory autonomic function of CN IX, which innervates the parotid gland via CN V's auriculotemporal branch.[16]

This parasympathetic pathway explains Frey syndrome, which is a potential postoperative complication from inadvertent severance and regeneration of the auriculotemporal nerve, as it innervates sweat glands in addition to parotid salivary gland, with symptoms of gustatory sweating (**Fig. 9**).

Understanding the course of Jacobson nerve is helpful when assessing the middle ear component of glomus jugulotympanicum, and glomus tympanicum tumors, as they follow branches of Jacobson nerve that form the tympanic plexus as they cross the cochlear promontory.

Glomus tumors are covered in greater detail by Jindal and colleagues (See, "Imaging Evaluation and Treatment of Vascular Lesions at the Skull Base," in this issue.).

The presence of characteristic bony hyperostosis on CT and MRI in addition to dural-based enhancement helps distinguish skull base meningioma from other pathology. Furthermore, these lesions arise from the skull base, outside the carotid sheath, and do not splay apart the IJ and ICA. If skull base meningiomas are extremely vascular, pretreatment embolization may be required prior to surgical resection.

Using bone changes to differentiate vascular lesions of the jugular bulb

- Glomus tumors cause permeative erosion.
- Schwannomas cause smooth remodeling.
- Meningiomas cause hyperostosis.

Lastly, metastases should always be considered in adults with aggressive lesions involving the skull base.

This anatomy is also key in assessing referred pain from extracranial pathology, commonly

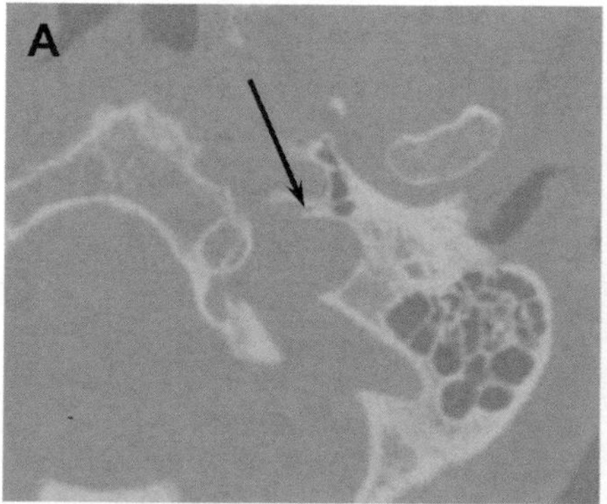

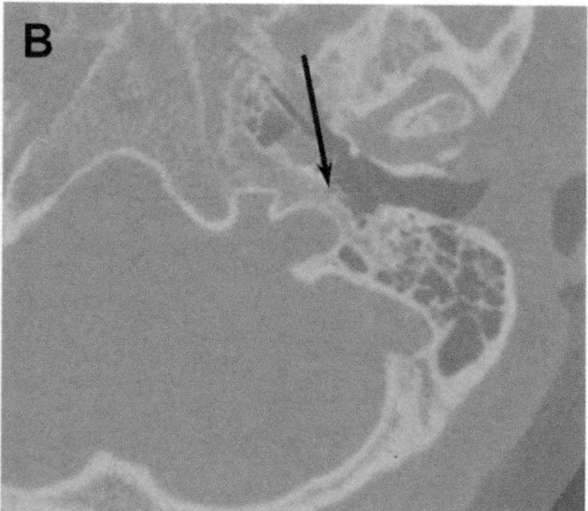

Fig. 8. Jacobson nerve. Axial CT images through the temporal bone show (*A*) inferior aspect of petrosal fossula (*arrow*) in the pars nervosa at site of the origin of Jacobson nerve as it heads toward the middle ear cavity. It is adjacent to the caroticojugular spine at this level. (*B*) Superior aspect of petrosal fossula (*arrow*) and site of origin of normal, nonenlarged inferior tympanic canaliculus, for CN IX branch–Jacobson nerve as it heads into middle ear cavity.

secondary otalgia in patients with oropharyngeal cancer as primary. Malignancies anywhere along the course of CN IX can present as otalgia and a similar principle applies to CNs V, VII, IX, and X, given considerable overlap in innervation of pharynx.[20] If no cause for otalgia is found after assessing the periauricular soft tissues, dedicated imaging of the neck should be obtained to exclude referred/secondary pain.

CRANIAL NERVE X

Function

The vagus nerve is the longest CN and is a mixed nerve, including sensory, special sensory, motor, and parasympathetic functions. It supplies sensory innervation to the middle ear, pharynx, external ear, and tympanic membrane; taste and sensation to the posterior third of the tongue in combination with CN IX; parasympathetic innervation to the aerodigestive tract; motor innervation to the laryngeal and pharyngeal constrictors and uvula; and viscerosensory innervation to the cervical, thoracic, and abdominal fibers as well as to the carotid and aortic bodies.[21]

Anatomy

With much overlap with CN IX, the intra-axial segment of the vagal nerve arises from nuclei in the medulla, dorsal to the inferior olivary nucleus, including

- Nucleus ambiguous (motor)
- Solitary tract nucleus (visceral afferents including taste)
- Dorsal or posterior motor nucleus X (visceral motor parasympathetic)
- Spinal tract and nucleus of the trigeminal nerve (sensory to the ear)

Nerve fibers exit the medulla in the postolivary sulcus to form the cisternal segment, with fibers coursing inferiorly through the medullary cistern, between CN IX and the cranial portion of CN XI (**Fig. 10**). The vagus nerve next enters the jugular foramen (its skull base segment), usually immediately posterior to the jugular spine in the pars vascularis.[2] The superior (jugular) ganglion is located in the jugular foramen, containing parasympathetic and sympathetic fibers and gives off the auricular branch of CN X.

The inferior (nodose) ganglion is located below the jugular foramen (approximately 1–2 cm).[22] Although glomus vagale tumors may arise at either the nodose ganglion or the jugular bulb, they usually tend to be centered around the nodose ganglion.[22]

The extracranial segment of CN X exits the jugular foramen into the carotid sheath, lying posterior to the internal and common carotid arteries and medial to the IJ. This relationship of the vagus nerve within the carotid sheath is helpful because mass effect from CN X pathology results in anterior displacement of ICA and lateral splaying of IJ.

In the jugular foramen, branches of CN X supply the dura of the posterior fossa (meningeal branch), external ear, and external auditory canal (auricular branch or Arnold nerve). Arnold nerve is an anastamotic branch between CN X and CN VII and arises from the superior ganglion of vagus nerve, extends into the mastoid canaliculus to anastomose with the mastoid segment of facial nerve, and extends into the tympanomastoid suture to innervate parts of tympanic membrane and skin of external

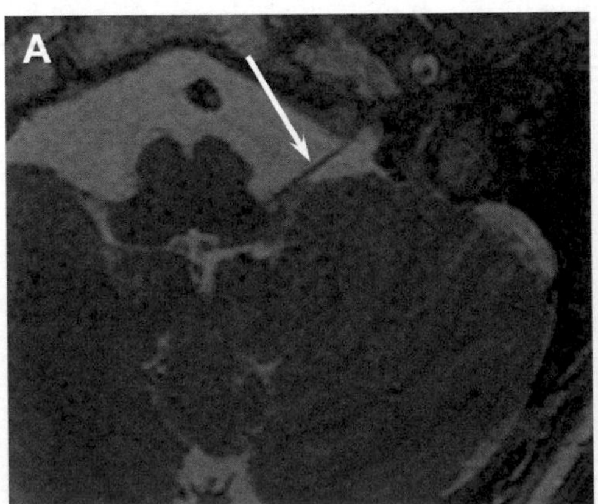

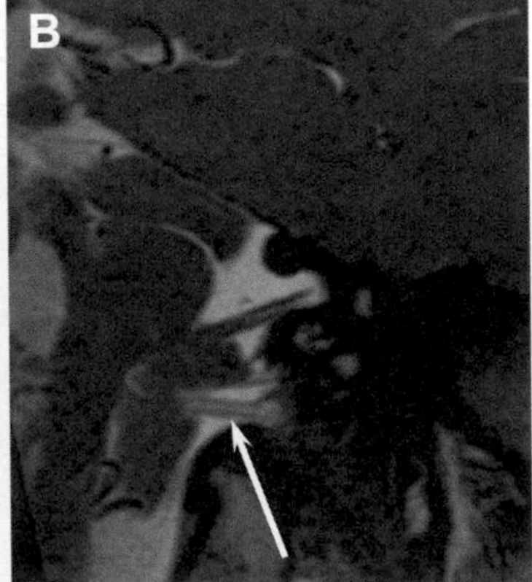

Fig. 10. Normal intracranial course of CN X. (*A*) Axial and (*B*) coronal oblique SSFP images show the vagus nerve (*arrow*), where it crosses the lateral cerebellomedullary cistern and approaches the jugular foramen. CN X is larger than CN IX (see **Fig. 7**), has 2 roots (best seen in [*B*]), and exits slightly caudal to CN IX.

auditory canal[23] (**Fig. 11**). Branches innervating the palate and pharynx, as well as branches to the carotid plexus, arise from the inferior ganglion.[24]

The superior laryngeal nerve on both sides arise just inferior to the inferior ganglion, bifurcating at the hyoid into an internal branch (which pierces the thyrohyoid membrane), carrying sensory and parasympathetic innervation to the larynx, and the external branch, carrying motor to the cricothyroid and inferior pharyngeal constrictor. Similar to the glossopharyngeal nerve, this accounts for referred pain from pharyngeal pathology presenting as otalgia. Inferior to the superior laryngeal nerve, the superior and inferior branches of the cardiac nerve arise, communicating with sympathetic fibers.[23]

The inferior (or recurrent) laryngeal nerve arises near the thoracic inlet on both sides. On the right, it loops behind the subclavian artery, coursing superiorly in the tracheoesophageal groove. On the left, it loops under the aortic arch, posterior to the ligamentum arteriosum, and then follows a similar course. On both sides, it passes under the posterior suspensory ligament extending from the cricoid to the first tracheal rings, entering the larynx at the level of the cricoarytenoid joint. The recurrent laryngeal nerve supplies all of the intrinsic laryngeal musculature, except the cricothyroid muscle.[4]

The vagus nerve also innervates the cardiac plexus, pulmonary plexus, esophagus, stomach, celiac plexus, solid organs, and intestines.[4]

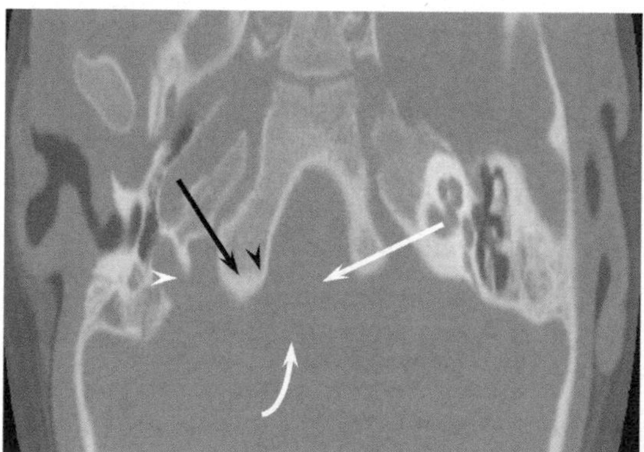

Fig. 11. Arnold nerve. Axial CT with several adjoining anatomic structures labeled. White arrow, minor contour irregularity along pars vascularis of jugular foramen at the expected site of mastoid canaliculus; white arrowhead, tympanomastoid suture along posterior wall of external auditory canal, carrying Arnold nerve; black arrowhead, vertical/mastoid segment of facial nerve canal; curved arrow, anterior portion of occipitomastoid suture (unfused because the patient is a child); black arrow, chorda tympani.

Pathology and Localization

If the vagus nerve is involved in association with CN IX, XI or XII, imaging should focus on the medulla, premedullary cistern, and jugular foramen, where a single lesion can easily involve multiple nerves.

Infarct of the lateral medulla (usually PICA occlusion) is known to cause lateral medullary, or Wallenberg, syndrome. In addition to the classic loss of pain and temperature sensation on the contralateral body and ipsilateral face, there is ipsilateral pharyngeal and palatal hemiparalysis, decreased pharyngeal gag reflex, and ipsilateral vocal cord paralysis due to involvement of the vagal nerve nuclei. These clinical findings, along with vertigo, help differentiate Wallenberg syndrome from lateral pontine syndrome, usually caused by anterior inferior cerebellar artery occlusion (**Fig. 12**).

Lesions that extend into cerebellomedullary cistern include meningiomas, schwannomas, arachnoid cysts, and epidermoid tumors and can involve CN X in addition to neighboring lower CNs. If large enough, they may extent into the cerebellopontine cistern with mass effect on CNs VII and VIII (**Fig. 13**).

In addition to multiple lower CN neuropathies, lesions at the level of the jugular foramen/skull base may present as a painless submucosal neck mass or as symptoms secondary to eustachian tube dysfunction from local mass effect.

The 2 most common tumors in the carotid sheath below the skull base are schwannomas and glomus vagale tumors. Suprahyoid vagal schwannomas are the most common carotid space schwannomas and, unlike glomus vagale tumors, gross total resection can occasionally be achieved without sacrificing the nerve. Larger lesions may have intratumoral nonenhancing regions (**Fig. 14**). Vagal schwannomas can be

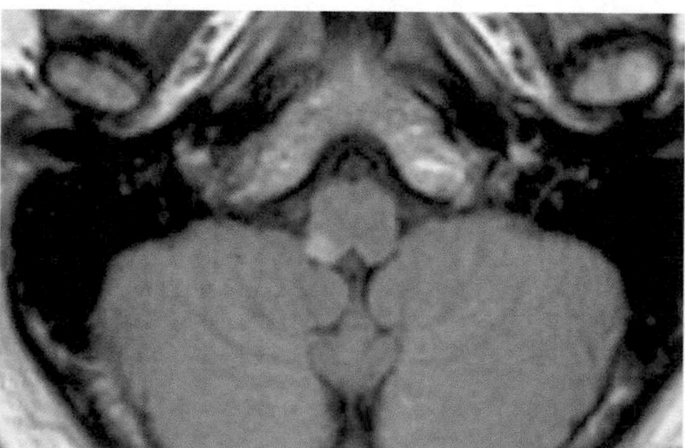

Fig. 12. Lateral medullary syndrome. FLAIR image demonstrates acute infarct involving the right dorsal-lateral medulla.

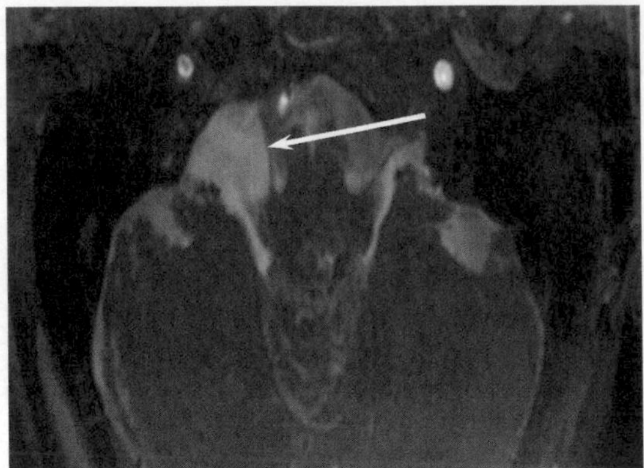

Fig. 13. Axial SSFP image demonstrates an arachnoid cyst in the lateral medullary cistern causing medial and ventral displacement of lower CNs IX and X (*arrow*).

distinguished from other pathology in this region by

- Localizing pathology to the carotid sheath in the suprahyoid neck by noticing anterior displacement of the ICA and splaying from the IJ. Specifically, other pathology in the suprahyoid neck, including sympathetic chain schwannoma (which is medial to and will not splay apart ICA and IJ as it is along the medial margin of carotid sheath), and pathology arising from masticator space, parotid space, and prestyloid parapharyngeal space will not anteriorly displace ICA or splay apart ICA and IJ.
- Superomedial course of lesion toward brainstem
- Smooth osseous margins on CT (**Fig. 15**)
- Heterogeneous enhancement on MR, without large flow voids

Paralysis of the constrictor muscles of the pharynx as well as vocal cord paralysis supports a cause of vagal neuropathy proximal/cranial to the origin of the recurrent laryngeal nerve. The findings of ipsilateral oropharyngeal dilation and thinning of the pharyngeal constrictors, as well as contralateral uvular deviation, support involvement at the level of the pharyngeal plexus origin[25] and should prompt investigation with MRI of the brainstem and skull base.

Isolated vocal cord paralysis (without other findings of CN X pathology) places the level of the pathology below the hyoid.[17] An ipsilateral thyroid mass associated with unilateral vocal cord palsy is considered a worrisome feature by imaging and warrants follow-up and tissue sampling of dominant thyroid nodule.[26,27]

Imaging Protocol for Hoarseness

When there is a known laryngeal primary, CT neck should be centered at the level of true vocal cords, with thin cuts and reconstructions to optimally characterize extent of local and regional disease. Split bolusing of contrast may be considered to optimize characterization of mucosal lesions.

When there is vocal cord paralysis as a presenting symptom, with unknown pathology, caudal extent of imaging field of view should cover the subclavian artery if the right side is symptomatic and should cover the aortopulmonary window if the left is symptomatic, with imaging acquired during quiet respiration.

CRANIAL NERVE XI

CN XI is a pure motor nerve, innervating the trapezius and sternocleidomastoid muscles. Gray's *Anatomy of the Human Body*[28] and other historical texts describe a "Cranial part" and a "Spinal part" to the nerve. The cranial part arises from the nucleus ambiguus and exits into the postolivary sulcus, just below the vagus nerve. This component joins the vagus nerve at the inferior ganglion, becoming inseparable from the vagus more inferiorly. Most

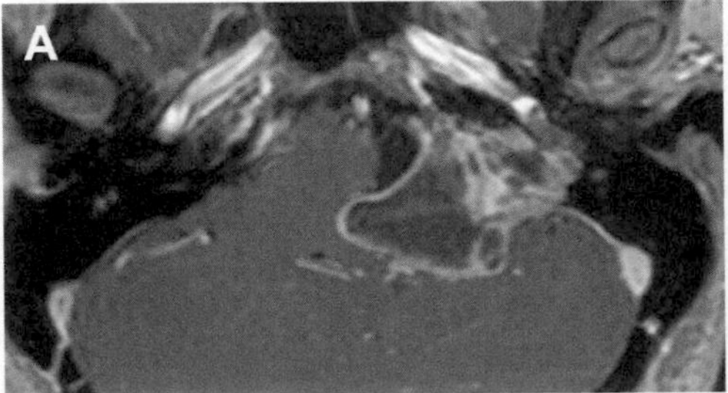

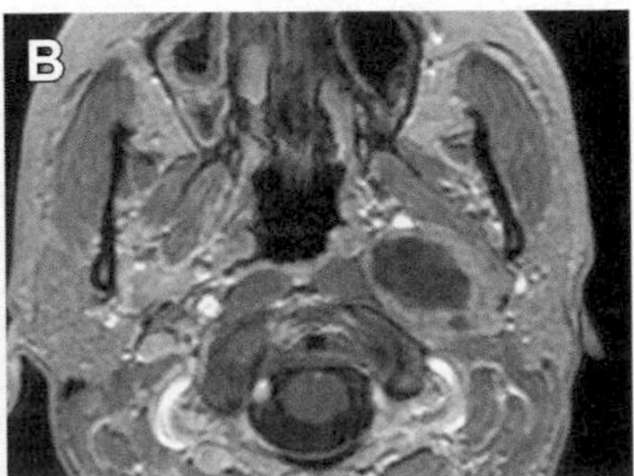

Fig. 14. Vagus schwannoma. Postcontrast axial MRI in the (*A*) lateral medullary cistern and (*B*) upper neck demonstrate a heterogeneously enhancing mass with imaging characteristics similar to a vestibular schwannoma, but a more inferior location and involvement of the jugular bulb. (*B*) Extension into the carotid sheath is common for lesions that arise in the jugular bulb.

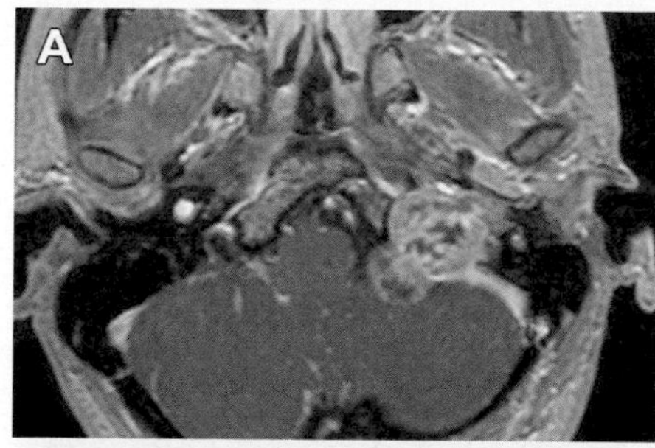

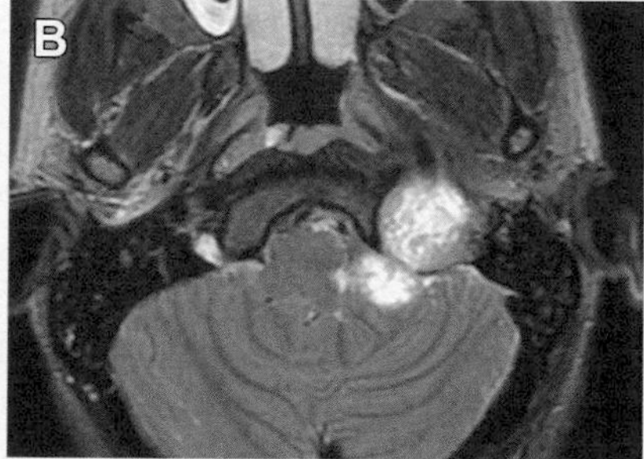

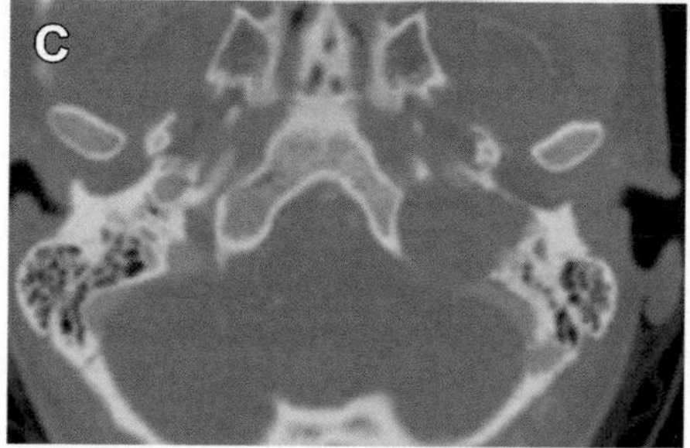

Fig. 15. Vagus schwannoma. (*A*) T1-weighted, (*B*) T1-weighted, and (*C*) CT images demonstrate a heterogeneously enhancing mass with heterogeneous T2-weighted signal centered in the jugular fossa. The CT shows the smooth pattern of remodeling that is, typical of schwannomas that extend through the skull base.

modern investigators consider this cranial part and medial branch a component of the vagus nerve and the spinal part alone to be CN XI.[29–40]

The spinal part arises from motor fibers of the spinal nucleus, which extends from C1 to C5 as a column of cells posterior to the anterior horn called the spinal accessory nucleus. Fibers arise from the lateral margin of the cervical cord, between the anterior and posterior spine rootlets, and run superiorly through foramen magnum, laterally over the condyle into the pars vascularis of the jugular foramen.

The spinal accessory nerve exits the jugular foramen with the vagus nerve and the posterior meningeal artery into the carotid space. It courses along inferior border of the digastric muscle to reach the deep margin of sternocleidomastoid muscle approximately 4 cm below the mastoid bone. After receiving anastomotic branches from cervical C3 to C5 nerves, it terminates along the undersurface of the trapezius muscle.

The most common cause of isolated CN XI palsy is injury during a surgical neck dissection and presents clinically as inability to shrug the shoulder. Radiographically, it can be appreciated as atrophy of the sternocleidomastoid and trapezius and, eventually, compensatory hypertrophy of the levator scapulae, which should not be mistake for a neck mass (**Fig. 16**).

Imaging for potential cause of CN XI palsy when associated with other lower CN palsies should focus on the brainstem and jugular foramen as well as the craniocervical junction (**Fig. 17**).

CRANIAL NERVE XII

The hypoglossal nerve has a purely motor function, innervating intrinsic and a majority of the extrinsic tongue musculature (the exception being the palatoglossus muscle, which is innervated by the vagus nerve).

The hypoglossal nerve can be divided into 5 segments: medullary, cisternal, skull base, carotid space, and sublingual.

The medullary segment of the hypoglossal nerve originates from the hypoglossal nucleus within the medulla and extends through the medulla

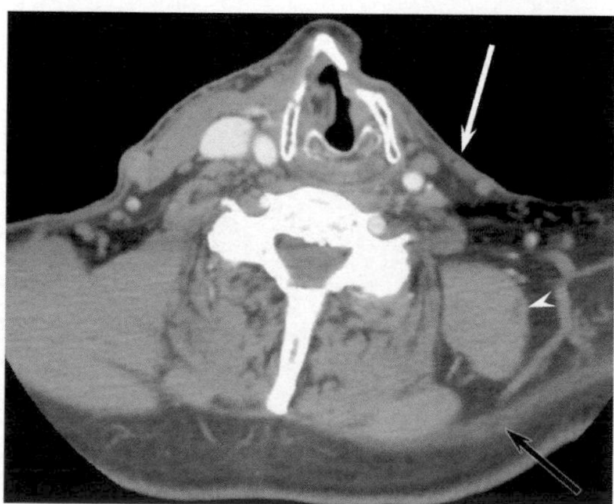

Fig. 16. CN XI palsy. The sternocleidomastoid muscle (*white arrow*) and the trapezius muscle (*black arrow*) are atrophied, whereas the levator scapulae muscle (*arrowhead*) is hypertrophied to compensate.

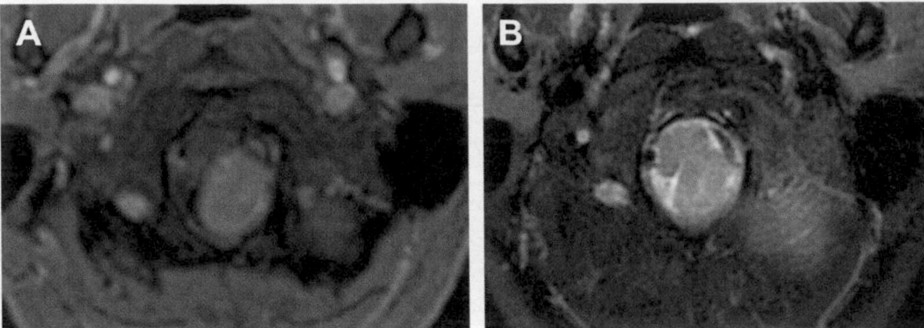

Fig. 17. Schwannoma of CN XI. Axial (*A*) T1-weighted and (*B*) T2-weighted images show a uniformly enhancing lesion arising in the posterolateral foramen magnum with T2-weighted signal isointense to the brainstem. The tumor forms sharp angles with underlying bone, unlike the more common meningioma.

oblongata in a paramedian location. The nerve fibers (approximately 10–12) have the most anterior point of exit from the medulla relative to the other lower CNs, in the preolivary sulcus, posterolateral to the vertebral artery. The vertebral arteries then course caudal to the inferior most nerve roots within the premedullary cistern, before CN XII exits the posterior skull base via the hypoglossal canal (**Fig. 18**). Emerging from the hypoglossal canal, the hypoglossal nerve enters the carotid space where it courses inferiorly and passes between the ICA and IJ, superficial to the vagus nerve, to the level of the angle of the mandible, making a large curve. Near the level of the carotid bifurcation, the nerve loops anteriorly around the root of the occipital artery, inferior to the posterior belly of the digastric muscle. At the level of the hyoid bone, the nerve crosses the lingual artery and curves anteriorly along the surface of the hyoglossus muscle, lateral to the lingual artery within the sublingual space. As it travels further anteriorly, the hypoglossal nerve lies on the surface and pierces the genioglossus muscle (**Fig. 19**).

The cervical portions of the nerve expose it to injury during neck surgeries, despite its lack of primary innervation in the neck.

During its course, it gives off multiple branches, notably meningeal branch, anastomotic branches with the superior cervical sympathetic ganglion, cervical plexus, and inferior ganglion of vagus nerve. Anastamoses with C1–C3 and CN XII descending branch form ansa cervalis and there are minor branches, which communicate with V3 and the lingual nerve.[16]

Damage to the hypoglossal nerve is uncommon as an isolated CN palsy. Possible causes include tumors and penetrating traumatic injury. If the clinical symptoms are accompanied by acute pain, a possible cause may be dissection of the ICA (**Fig. 20**).

Although the tongue usually atrophies on the side ipsilateral to the lesion, supranuclear disease affecting CN XII results in paralysis of the tongue contralateral to the side of the lesion. Deviation of the tongue occurs away from the side of the lesion in supranuclear pathology.

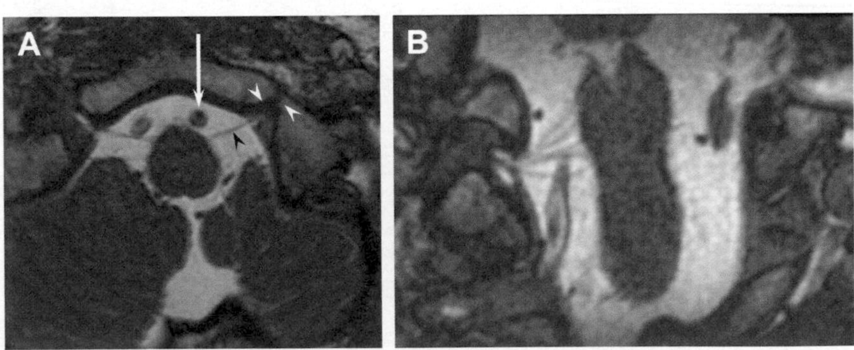

Fig. 18. Cisternal course of hypoglossal nerve. (*A*) Axial SSFP MRI shows the oblique course of the hypoglossal nerve (*black arrowhead*) as it crosses the lateral cerebellomedullary cistern toward the hypoglossal canal (*white arrowheads*). The vertebral artery (*arrow*) is anterior to the nerve. (*B*) Coronal SSFP image reveals the numerous nerve rootlets that compose right CN XII.

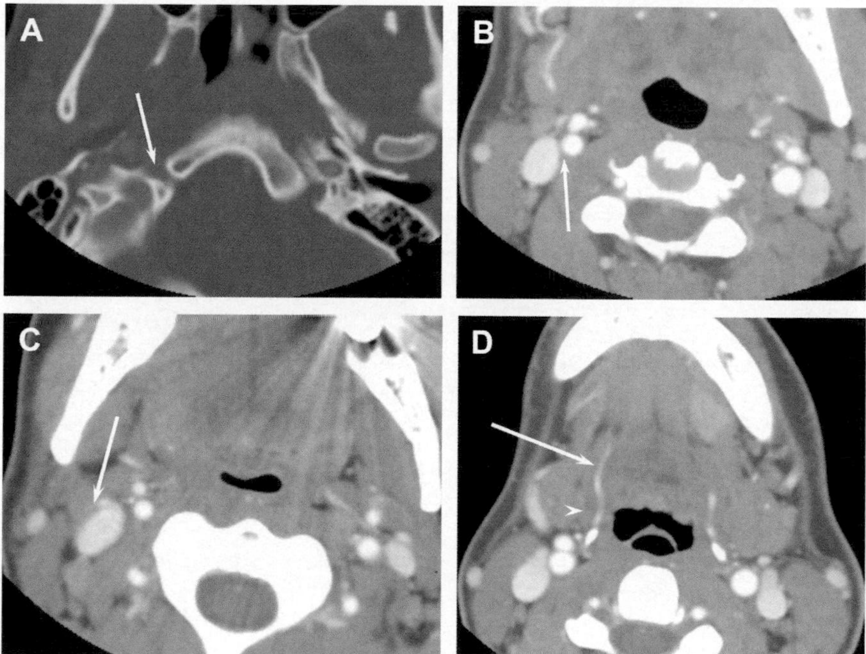

Fig. 19. Cervical course of hypoglossal nerve. Axial CT images with arrows showing the expected course of CN XII through (*A*) hypoglossal canal; (*B*) carotid space posterior to the vessels; and (*C*) medial aspect of posterior belly of digastric muscles, along with the occipital artery and (*D*) crossing the lingual artery and curving anteriorly along the surface of the hyoglossus muscle (*arrowhead*), lateral to the lingual artery within the sublingual space.

Fasciculation and tongue atrophy are absent in these cases.

When pathology affects the hypoglossal nerve at the nuclear or infranuclear level, the clinical symptoms are ipsilateral. Patients present with deviation of the tongue toward the damaged side when asked to stick out their tongue as well as possible muscle wasting and twitching of muscle fibers on the affected side, with longstanding imaging findings including fatty atrophy (**Fig. 21**).

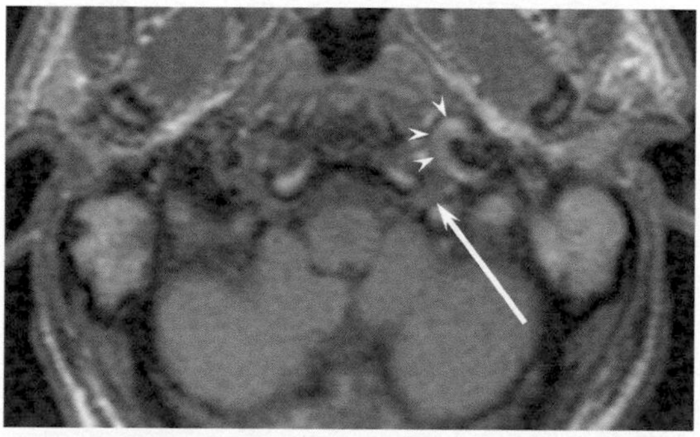

Fig. 20. Vertebral artery dissection causing hypoglossal paralysis. T1-weighted noncontrast image demonstrates crescentic region of intrinsic T1-weighted shortening (*arrowheads*) surrounding a high cervical ICA, indicating dissection. Notice its proximity to the hypoglossal nerve and canal (*arrow*).

Imaging pearl: If fatty hemiatrophy of tongue is noted on a neck CT, carefully scrutinize the posterior skull base and hypoglossal canal to exclude underlying pathology that would account for denervation of CN XII. Dedicated imaging of the brain should be considered if no cause is identified.

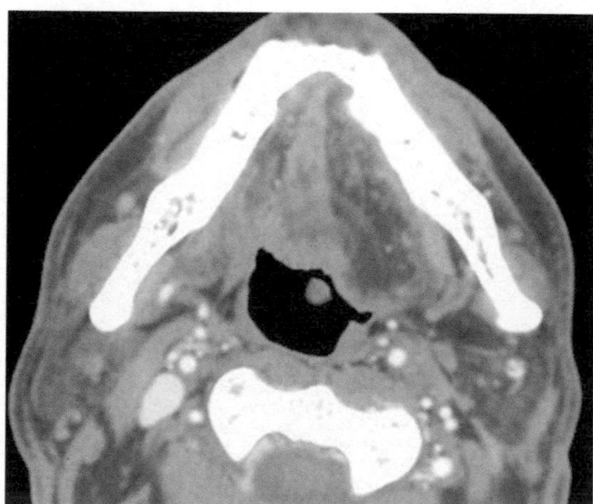

Fig. 21. Fatty atrophy of the tongue from hypoglossal denervation. CT demonstrates asymmetry of density within the tongue, with a sharp midline demarcation. The left side of the tongue musculature has atrophied from injury to CN XII.

Pathologies that involve the skull base segment of CN XII include meningiomas (**Fig. 22**); primary nerve sheath tumors; metastases; local extension of tumors, such as nasopharyngeal carcinoma, glomus tumors, or lymphoma (**Fig. 23**); and aggressive skull base infection (**Fig. 24**).

VARIANT ANATOMY AND PATHOLOGY

Bony Variants

Chamberlain line (**Fig. 25**) and Welcher basal angle (**Fig. 26**) can help quickly identify the presence of bony anomalies involving the posterior skull base and craniocervical junction.

Most anomalies of the occiput are associated with platybasia (Welcher basal angle greater 140°) and basilar invagination (cranial extension of dens and anterior arch of C1 above Chamberlain line in the setting of normal bone). These findings should prompt a search for other posterior skull base abnormalities, such as complete or partial occipital assimilation of the atlas, basioccipital hypoplasia, or condylar dysplasia.[41]

Chiari I malformations, defined as descent of the cerebellar tonsils 5 mm or more below the foramen magnum on imaging (**Fig. 27**), are also frequently associated with basilar invagination. Normal position of the cerebellar tonsils does demonstrate minor variation with age with the lowest point somewhere between 5 and 15 years of age.[42,43] Symptomatic patients demonstrate not only inferior descent of the cerebellar tonsils but also a typically a compression of the brainstem, cerebellar tonsils (which lose their normal rounded configuration and become peg like), foramen of Magendie and foramen of Luschka, and central canal of the cord (causing hydrosyringomyelia and cranial neuropathies).[44–46]

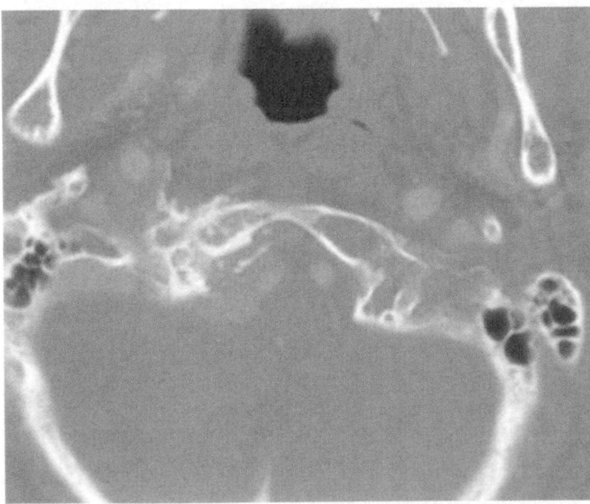

Fig. 22. Meningioma causing hypoglossal denervation. Axial-enhanced CT shows a mass surrounding the hypoglossal canal with the characteristic hyperostosis of a meningioma.

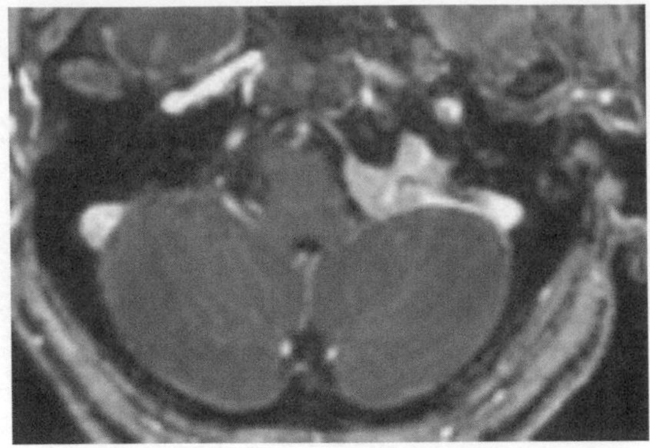

Fig. 23. Lymphoma causing hypoglossal denervation. Axial-enhanced T1-weighted image shows a broad-based dural lesion overlying and extending into the left hypoglossal canal. This could be easily mistaken for a meningioma.

Cerebrospinal fluid flow studies may be useful to assess flow surrounding the cervicomedullary junction[47] and help in selecting appropriate candidates for decompressive surgery, which include suboccipital craniectomy with or without C1/C2 laminectomy, with or without duroplasty, opening of the arachnoidal membrane, lysis of intradural adhesions, partial tonsillar resection, plugging of the obex, leaving the dura open, and/or posterior fossa reconstruction with cranioplasty.[48–51]

The variations of the arteries and veins are covered by Jindal and colleagues (See, "Imaging

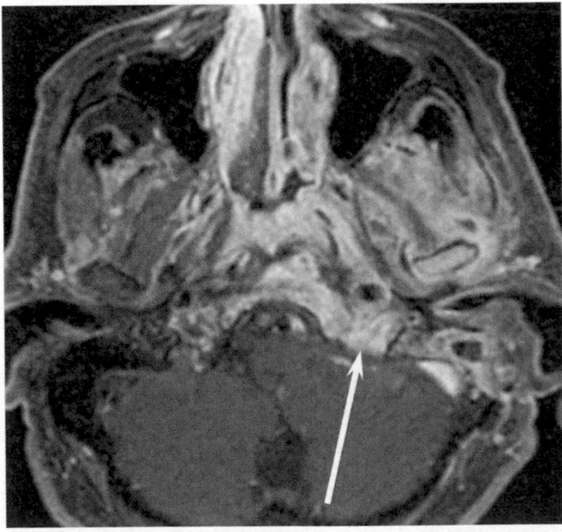

Fig. 24. Skull base osteomyelitis causing hypoglossal denervation. Axial-enhanced T1-weighted image shows extensive enhancement of the left skull base and surrounding tissues, in particular the hypoglossal canal (*arrow*).

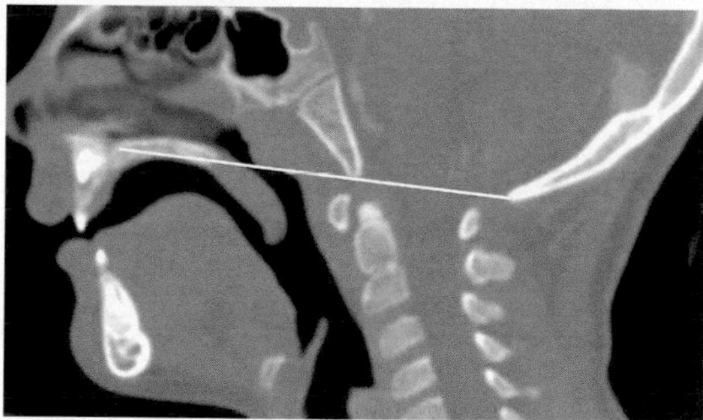

Fig. 25. Chamberlain line. This line is drawn from the hard palate to the opisthion. If the dens extends above this line, the patient has basilar invagination.

Evaluation and Treatment of Vascular Lesions at the Skull Base," in this issue.).

BONE TUMORS

Chordomas and chondrosarcomas are the most common primary bone tumors of the skull base, and there is much overlap in their clinical presentation, imaging characteristics, and management.[52–67] Both are hyperintense on T2-weighted sequences, and both are treated with wide local excision. MRI and CT play complementary roles in arriving at an accurate diagnosis.

Langerhans cell histiocytosis, although most frequently seen in children, can be seen at any age and is considered benign. Although calvarial Langerhans cell histiocytosis is most common, the preferred site of skull base involvement is the temporal bones followed by the sphenoid bone. CT is helpful in evaluation and differentiating from other pathology, by showing lack of matrix or fat within the lesion (**Fig. 28**). On MRI, although there is usually a fairly focal lesion on T1-weighted and T2-weighted sequences, associated peripheral enhancement beyond the margins of the lesion usually prompts tissue sampling to exclude a more aggressive process.

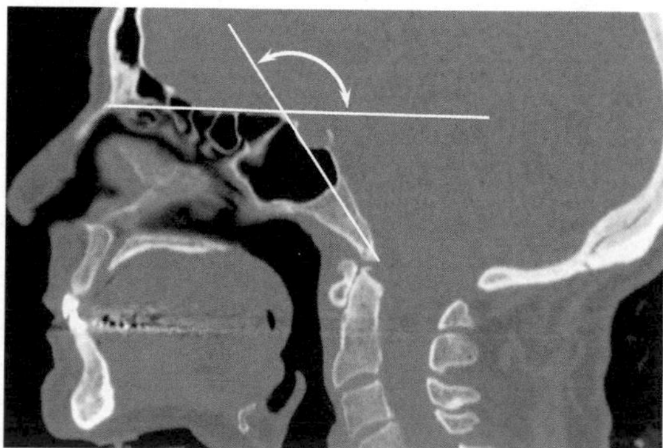

Fig. 26. Welcher basal angle. Lines are drawn between the nasion and tuberculum sella and between the basion and tuberculum sella. If the resulting angle is greater than 140°, the patient has platybasia.

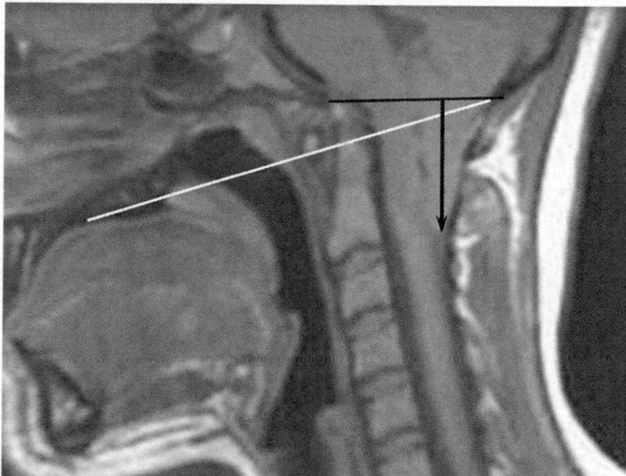

Fig. 27. Chiari I malformation. Sagittal T1-weighted image shows a black line along the foramen magnum and a black arrow depicting the severe herniation of cerebellar tonsils below the foramen magnum. Because the arrow is longer than 5 mm, and there is no posterior fossa mass or mass effect, this patient has a Chiari malformation. Note the associated basilar invagination, with the anterior arch of C1 and dens extending superior to Chamberlain line (*white line*).

Giant cell tumors, primarily occurring in the epiphyses of long bones, are rare in the skull base. Giant cell tumors are derived from differentiated mesenchymal cells of the bone marrow and should be differentiated from giant cell reparative granulomas, which are reactive bone lesions most frequently occurring in the mandible and maxilla.[68–70]

Plasmacytoma is a separate entity from multiple myeloma in that it is localized to a single site and can occur anywhere in the skull base. CT findings include an expansile, lytic slightly hyperdense lesion involving the diploic space as well as the inner and outer tables of calvarium with mass effect on the adjacent brain parenchyma. MRI characteristics of solitary plasmacytoma include T1-weighted signal isointensity and isointense or slightly hyperintense signal on T2-weighted images, with homogeneous enhancement after administration of intravenous gadolinium.[71–77]

DIFFUSE BONE ABNORMALITIES

Diffuse bony abnormalities may be secondary to metabolic disorders; chronic severe anemia from hemoglobinopathies, such as sickle cell disease; or malignancy, such as multiple myeloma.

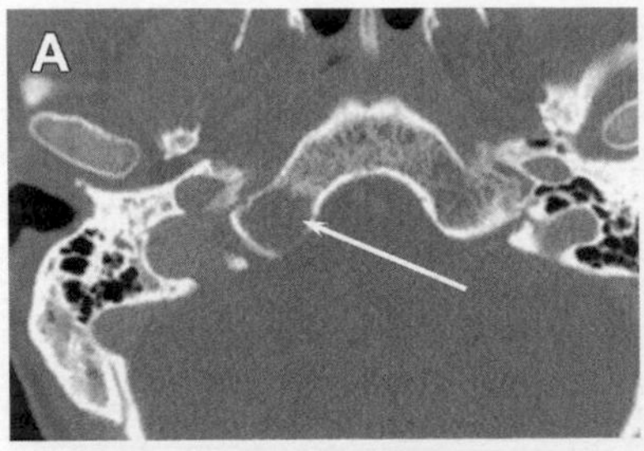

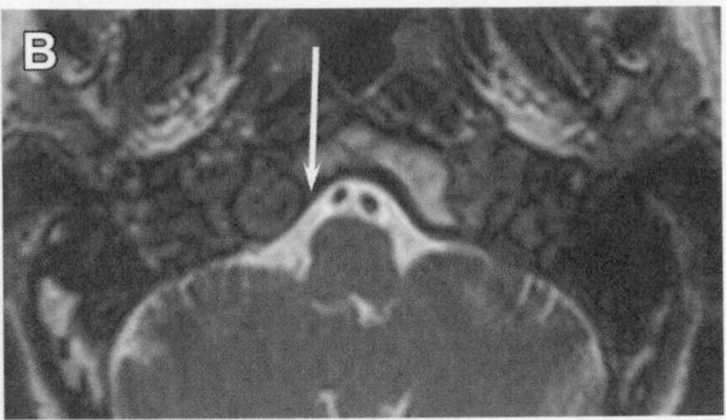

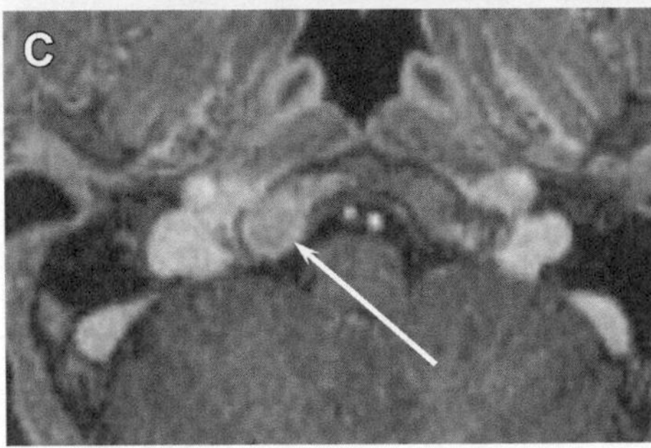

Fig. 28. Eosinophilic granuloma. (*A*) CT image shows a well-defined lytic lesion (*arrow*) in the jugular tubercle. Corresponding T2-weighted image (*B*) shows low intensity (*arrow*), which could be easily mistaken for aggressive malignancy. Enhanced T1-weighted image (*C*) shows brisk enhancement (*arrow*), also suggestive of malignancy.

The primary differential considerations for geographic areas of bony abnormality are fibrous dysplasia and Paget disease, which are discussed elsewhere in this issue (See C. Douglas Phillips and Lindsey M. Conleys' article, "Imaging of the Central Skull Base," in this issue.).

TRAUMA

There are 3 types of occipital condylar fractures:

- Type1 is a comminuted fracture of occipital bone with preservation of alar ligament and tectorial membrane (**Fig. 29**).
- Type 2 is a fracture plane extending anteriorly to involve the occipital condyle and basiocciput. The alar ligament and tectorial membrane, however, are intact by imaging.
- Type 3 is disruption of the alar ligament and tectorial membrane.

Coronal is the best plane to quickly find a small avulsion fracture off the occipital condyle (**Fig. 30**).

Clival fractures suggest a high-energy mechanism, with frequent with injury to the brainstem and posterior arterial circulation. CTA may be considered to better assess for associated vascular injury.[16]

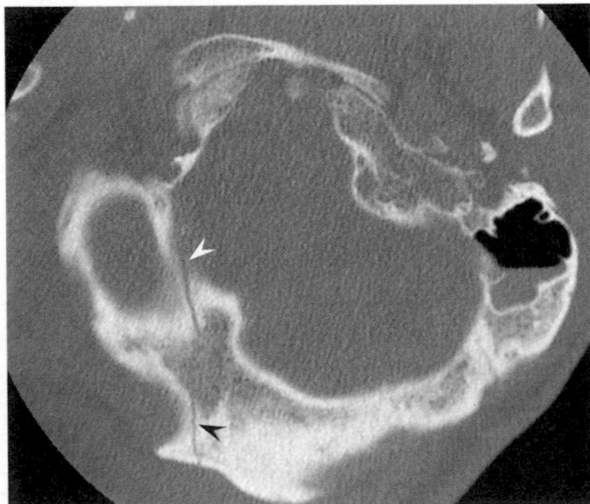

Fig. 29. Type 1 occipital bone fracture. Axial CT demonstrates a fracture line (*arrowheads*) through the lateral aspect of the condyle, where it does not affect the alar ligament or tectorial membrane.

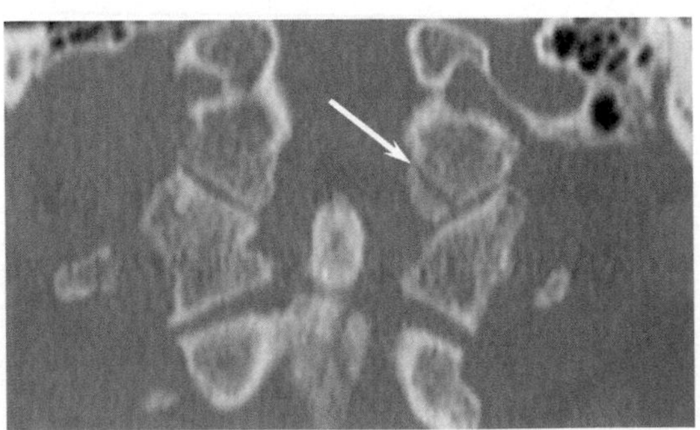

Fig. 30. Occipital avulsion. Coronal reformatted CT shows a fracture plane through the occipital condyle (*arrow*) into the atlanto-occipital junction. This is usually accompanied by an injury to the alar ligament (type 3 occipital bone fracture).

A persistent Kerckring ossicle is a small ossicle at the posterior margin of the foramen magnum, which is normally unfused in 50% of term newborns and usually fuses with the supraoccipital suture by 1 year.[3] It should not be mistaken for an avulsion fracture in this demographic.

REFERENCES

1. Kent DT, Rath TJ, Snyderman CH. Conventional and 3-dimensional computerized tomography in Eagle's syndrome, glossopharyngeal neuralgia, and asymptomatic controls. Otolaryngol Head Neck Surg 2015; 153(1):41–7.
2. Morani AC, Ramani NS, Wesolowski JR. Skull base, orbits, temporal bone, and cranial nerves: anatomy on MR imaging. Magn Reson Imaging Clin N Am 2011;19:439–56.
3. Harnsberger HR, Macdonald AJ. Diagnostic and surgical imaging anatomy. Brain, head & neck, spine. Salt Lake City (UT): Amirsys; 2006.
4. Rhoton AL Jr. Jugular foramen. Neurosurgery 2000; 47(Suppl 3):S267–85.
5. Rhoton AL Jr, Buza R. Microsurgical anatomy of the jugular foramen. J Neurosurg 1975;42:541–50.
6. Ong CK, Fook-Hin Chong V. Imaging of jugular foramen. Neuroimaging Clin N Am 2009;19:469–82.
7. Voyvodic F, Whyte A, Slavotinek J. The hypoglossal canal: normal MR enhancement pattern. AJNR Am J Neuroradiol 1995;16:1707–10.
8. Gray H, Warwick R, Williams PL. Gray's anatomy. Philadelphia: Saunders;Churchill Livingstone; 1980.
9. Murlimanju BV, Chettiar GK, Krishnamurthy A, et al. The paracondylar skull base: anatomical variants and their clinical implications. Turk Neurosurg 2015;25:844–9.
10. Drake RL, Vogl W, Mitchell AWM. Gray's basic anatomy. Edinburgh (United Kingdom): Churchill Livingstone; 2012.
11. Jo YR, Chung CW, Lee JS, et al. Vernet syndrome by varicella-zoster virus. Ann Rehabil Med 2013;37: 449–52.
12. Jackson CG. Glomus tympanicum and glomus jugulare tumors. Otolaryngol Clin North Am 2001;34: 941–70, vii.
13. Robertson JH, Gardner G, Cocke EW Jr. Glomus jugulare tumors. Clin Neurosurg 1994;41:39–61.
14. Wharton SM, Davis A. Familial paraganglioma. J Laryngol Otol 1996;110:688–90.
15. Lustrin ES, Palestro C, Vaheesan K. Radiographic evaluation and assessment of paragangliomas. Otolaryngol Clin North Am 2001;34:881–906, vi.
16. Leblanc A. Anatomy and imaging of the cranial nerves. London: Springer; 1991.
17. Mukherji S. Cranial Nerves. Neuroimaging Clin N Am 2008;18(2):xiii.
18. Hiwatashi A, Matsushima T, Yoshiura T, et al. MRI of glossopharyngeal neuralgia caused by neurovascular compression. AJR Am J Roentgenol 2008;191(2): 578–81.
19. Weissman J, Hirsch B. Beyond the promontory: the multifocal origin of glomus Tympanicum Tumors. AJNR Am J Neuroradiol 1998;19:119–22.
20. Chen RC, Khorsandi AS, Shatzkes DR, et al. The radiology of referred otalgia. AJNR Am J Neuroradiol 2009;30(10):1817–23.
21. Osborn A. Osborn's brain: imaging, pathology, and anatomy. Salt Lake City (Utah): Amirsys; 2013. p. 623–4.
22. Weissman JL. Case 21 Glomus vagale tumor. Radiology 2000;215(1):237–42.
23. Netter FH. Atlas of human anatomy. 5th edition. Philadelphia: Saunders/Elsevier; 2011. Plate 120.
24. Rubinstein D, Burton BS, Walker AL. The anatomy of the inferior petrosal sinus, glossopharyngeal nerve, vagus nerve, and accessory nervein the jugular foramen. AJNR Am J Neuroradiol 1995;16: 185–94.
25. Sreevasta MR, Srinivasarao RV. Three cases of vagal nerve shwannoma and review of the literature. Indian J Otolaryngol Head Neck Surg 2011;63(4): 310–2.
26. Abboud B, Tabchy B, Jambart S, et al. Benign disease of the thyroid gland and vocal fold paralysis. J Laryngol Otol 1999;113(5):473–4.
27. Paquette C, Manos D, Psooy BJ. Unilateral vocal cord paralysis: a review of CT findings, mediastinal causes, and the course of the recurrent laryngeal nerves. RadioGraphics 2012;32(3):721–40.
28. Gray H. Anatomy of the human body. Philadelphia: Lea & Febiger; 1918. Bartleby.com, 2000.
29. Ryan S, Blyth P, Duggan N, et al. Is the cranial accessory nerve really a portion of the accessory nerve? Anatomy of the cranial nerves in the jugular foramen. Anat Sci Int 2007;82:1–7.
30. Thompson EO, Smoker WRK. Hypoglossal nerve palsy: a segmental approach. Radiographics 1994; 14:939–58.
31. Smoker WRK. The hypoglossal nerve. Neuroimaging Clin N Am 1993;3:193–207.
32. Macedo TF, Gow PJ, Heap SW, et al. Bilateral hypoglossal nerve palsy due to vertical subluxation of the odontoid process in rheumatoid arthritis. Br J Rheumatol 1988;27:317–20.
33. Fujita N, Shimada N, Takimoto H, et al. MR appearance of the persistent hypoglossal artery. AJNR Am J Neuroradiol 1995;16:990–2.
34. Goldstein JH, Woodcock H, Phillips D. Complete duplication or extreme fenestration of the basilar artery. AJNR Am J Neuroradiol 1999;20:149–50.
35. Kodama N, Ohara H, Suzuki J. Persistent hypoglossal artery associated with aneurysms. Report of two cases. J Neurosurg 1976;45:449–51.
36. Kobanawa S, Atsuchi M, Tanaka J, et al. Jugular bulb diverticulum associated with lower cranial

nerve palsy and multiple aneurysms. Surg Neurol 2000;53:559–62.
37. Overton SB, Ritter FN. A high placed jugular bulb in the middle ear: a clinical and temporal bone study. Laryngoscope 1973;83:1986–91.
38. Weiss RL, Zahtz G, Goldofsky E, et al. High jugular bulb and conductive hearing loss. Laryngoscope 1997;107:321–7.
39. Lee M, Kim M. Image findings in bran developmental venous anomalies. J Cerebrovasc Endovasc Neurosurg 2012;14(1):37–43.
40. Alatakis S, Koulouris G, Stuckey S. CT-Demonstrated transcalvarial channels diagnostic of dural arteriovenous fistula. AJNR Am J Neuroradiol 2005; 26:2393–6.
41. Smoker W. Craniovertebral junction: normal anatomy, craniometry and congenital anomalies. Radiographics 1994;14(2):255–77.
42. Speer MC, Enterline DS, Mehltretter L, et al. Review article: chiari type i malformation with or without syringomyelia: prevalence and genetics. J Genet Couns 2003;12:297–311.
43. Kornienko VN, Pronin IN, editors. Diagnostic neuroradiology. 1st edition. Berlin: Springer Berlin; 2008. 1 online resource.
44. Sarnat HB. Disorders of segmentation of the neural tube: Chiari malformations. Handb Clin Neurol 2008;87:89–103.
45. Schijman E. History, anatomic forms, and pathogenesis of Chiari I malformations. Childs Nerv Syst 2004;20:323–8.
46. Goh S, Bottrell CL, Aiken AH, et al. Presyrinx in children with chiari malformations. Neurology 2008;71:351–6.
47. Chiapparini L, Saletti V, Solero CL, et al. Neuroradiological diagnosis of chiari malformations. Neurol Sci 2011;32(Suppl 3):S283–6.
48. Baisden J. Controversies in chiari I malformations. Surg Neurol Int 2012;3:S232–7.
49. Currarino G. Canalis basilaris medianus and related defects of the basiocciput. AJNR Am J Neuroradiol 1988;9:208–11.
50. Beltramello A. Fossa navicularis magna. AJNR Am J Neuroradiol 1998;19:1796–8.
51. Hemphill M, Freeman JM, Martinez CR, et al. A new, treatable source of recurrent meningitis: basioccipital meningocele. Pediatrics 1982;70:941–3.
52. Central Brain Tumor Registry of the United States. Statistical report: primary brain tumors in the United States, 1997–2001. Hinsdale (IL): Central Brain Tumor Registry of the United States. 2015.
53. McMaster ML, Goldstein AM, Bromley CM, et al. Chordoma: incidence and survival patterns in the United States, 1973–1995. Cancer Causes Control 2001;12:1–11.
54. Mizerny BR, Kost KM. Chordoma of the cranial base: the McGill experience. J Otolaryngol 1995; 24:14–9.
55. Dorfman HD, Czerniak B. Bone cancers. Cancer 1995;75:203–10.
56. Mindell ER. Chordoma. J Bone Joint Surg Am 1981; 63:501–5.
57. Menezes AH, Traynelis VC. Tumors of the craniocervical junction. In: Youmans JR, editor. Neurological surgery. 4th edition. Philadelphia: Saunders; 1996. p. 3041–72.
58. Lanzino G, Sekhar LN, Hirsch WL, et al. Chondromas and chondrosarcomas involving the cavernous sinus: review of surgical treatment and outcomes in 31 patients. Surg Neurol 1993;40:359–71.
59. Borba LA, Al-Mefty O, Mrak RE, et al. Cranial chordoma in children and adolescents. J Neurosurg 1996;84:584–91.
60. Erdem E, Angtuaco EC, Van Hemert R, et al. Comprehensive review of intracranial chordoma. Radiographics 2003;23:995–1009.
61. Mehnert F, Beschorner R, Kuker W, et al. Retroclival ecchordosis physaliphora: MR imaging and review of the literature. AJNR Am J Neuroradiol 2004;25:1851–5.
62. Srinivasan A. Case 133: Ecchordosis Physaliphora. Radiology 2008;247(2):585–8.
63. Heffelfinger MJ, Dahlin DC, MacCarty CS, et al. Chordomas and cartilaginous tumors of the skull base. Cancer 1973;32:410–20.
64. Korten AG, ter Berg HJ, Spincemaille GH, et al. Intracranial chondrosarcoma: review of the literature and report of 15 cases. J Neurol Neurosurg Psychiatr 1998;65:88–92.
65. Meyers SP, Hirsch WL, Curtin HD, et al. Chondrosarcomas of the skull base: MR imaging features. Radiology 1992;184(1):103–8.
66. Yeom KW, Lober RM, Mobley BC, et al. Diffusion-weighted MRI: distinction of skull base chordoma from chondrosarcoma. AJNR Am J Neuroradiol 2013;34:1056–61. s1.
67. Leonard J, Gökden M, Kyriakos M, et al. Malignant giant-cell tumor of the parietal bone: case report and review of the literature. Neurosurgery 2001; 48(2):424–9.
68. Saleh EA, Taibah AK, Naguib M, et al. Giant cell tumor of the lateral skull base: a case report. Otolaryngol Head Neck Surg 1994;111(3 Pt 1):314–8.
69. Pitkethly DT, Kempe LG. Giant cell tumor of the sphenoid. Report of two cases. J Neurosurg 1994; 80:148–51.
70. Bertoni F, Unni KK, Beabout JW, et al. Giant cell tumor of the skull. Cancer 1992;70(5):1124–32.
71. Du Preez JH, Branca EP. Plasmacytoma of the skull: case reports. Neurosurgery 1991;29:902–6.
72. Benli K, Inci S. Solitary dural plasmacytoma: case report. Neurosurgery 1995;36:1206–9.
73. Romano AJ, Shoemaker EI, Gado M, et al. Neuroradiology case of the day: plasmacytoma of the skull vault. AJR Am J Roentgenol 1989;152(6): 1335–7.

74. Provenzale JM, Schaefer P, Traweek ST, et al. Craniocerebral Plasmacytoma: MR Features. AJNR Am J Neuroradiol 1997;18:389–92.
75. Vogl TJ, Steger W, Grevers G, et al. MR characteristics of primary extramedullary plasmacytoma in the head and neck. AJNR Am J Neuroradiol 1996;17:1349–54.
76. Tabareau-Delalande F, Collin C, Gomez-Brouchet A, et al. Diagnostic value of investigating GNAS mutations in fibro-ossous lesions: a Retrospective study of 91 cases of fibrous dysplasia and 40 other fibro-osseous lesions. Mod Pathol 2013;26(7):911–21.
77. Windholz F. Osteoporosis Circumscripta Cranii: its pathogenesis and occurrence in Leontiasis Osseaand in hyperparathyroidism. Radiographics 1945;44(1):14–22.

Imaging of Vascular Compression Syndromes

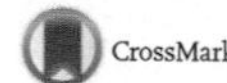

Joseph H. Donahue, MD, David A. Ornan, MD, Sugoto Mukherjee, MD*

KEYWORDS

• Neurovascular compression syndromes • Trigeminal neuralgia • Hemifacial spasm
• Vestibular paroxysmia • Glossopharyngeal and vagoglossopharyngeal neuralgia

KEY POINTS

- Neurovascular compression syndromes encompass multiple entities in which cisternal nerve segment compression by offending vessels yields symptomatic ephaptic neurotransmissions.
- Cisternal nerve segment transitional zone (TZ) between central and peripheral myelination demonstrates heightened vulnerability to pulsatile arterial mechanical irritation.
- Specialized MR imaging techniques allow identification of high-grade neurovascular conflict, which may localize to the TZ, thus adding specificity to the clinical evaluation and assisting in treatment planning purposes.

INTRODUCTION

Vascular compression syndromes are a group of disorders in which direct cranial nerve (CN) compression by blood vessels causes mechanical irritation and varying degrees of myelin injury, which facilitates symptomatic ephaptic neurotransmissions. Trigeminal neuralgia (CN V) is the most common vascular compression syndrome, followed by hemifacial spasm (HFS) (CN VII), vestibular paroxysmia (CN VIII), glossopharyngeal neuralgia (GN) (CN IX), and vagal neuralgia (CN X). The causative neurovascular conflict typically involves the cisternal segment of the CN and often localizes more specifically to the TZ between central myelination (oligodendroglial cells) and peripheral myelination (Schwann cells). Although the TZ is variable both in length and location between the CN, the heightened vulnerability of this area to chronic mechanical irritation is a commonality across the vascular compression syndromes. Thus, in this discussion of each of the vascular compression syndromes, particular attention is given to the TZ because this region is key to pathogenesis and informs accurate neuroimaging evaluation. Additionally, clinical symptoms and common differential diagnoses, imaging techniques and findings, and treatment methods are reviewed (**Box 1**, **Tables 1** and **2**).

IMAGING PROTOCOL RECOMMENDATIONS

High-resolution 3-D T2-weighted steady-state free precession sequences, represent the workhorse of evaluating the cisternal CN segments and their relationship to the adjacent vessels and, if present, characterizing the neurovascular contact. These techniques typically include variations of balanced steady-state free precession techniques, with vendor-optimized sequences. Depending on reader preferences, these sequences may obviate time-of-flight (TOF) magnetic resonance (MR) angiography, because reported sensitivities for neurovascular conflict are similar (>95%).[1,2]

Disclosure Statement: The authors have nothing to disclose.
Department of Radiology and Medical Imaging, University of Virginia Health System, PO Box 800170, Charlottesville, VA 22908, USA
* Corresponding author. Department of Radiology and Medical Imaging, University of Virginia Health System, 1215 Lee Street, PO Box 800170, Charlottesville, VA 22908-1070.
E-mail address: Sm5qd@virginia.edu

Radiol Clin N Am 55 (2017) 123–138
http://dx.doi.org/10.1016/j.rcl.2016.08.001
0033-8389/17/© 2016 Elsevier Inc. All rights reserved.

Box 1
What the referring physician wants to know

Template for radiology reporting

- Any causes of secondary disease (tumors, vascular causes, or demyelinating lesions)
- CN course, precise mapping of the proximal nerve segments, including the REZ
- Characterize the neurovascular compression
  - Identify the offending vessel (artery or vein)
  - Precise point of contact
  - Single or multiple points of contact
  - Contact ± displacement

Additional 3-D TOF MR angiography and volumetric postcontrast T1-weighted sequences help in excluding other pathologies, presurgical planning, and follow-up imaging. The 3-D imaging allows for multiplanar reconstruction at the workstation and assists in guiding neurosurgical treatment. In patients in whom MR is contraindicated, a combination of CT cisternogram and CT angiogram can help with treatment planning.

TRIGEMINAL NEURALGIA

Trigeminal neuralgia, also known as tic douloureux, is typically characterized by

- Excruciating lancinating paroxysmal facial pain
- Typically involvement of the V2 and/or V3 dermatomal distributions
- Duration of seconds to minutes and often precipitated by innocuous stimulation of the trigger zone (cold, chewing, and so forth)

Classic trigeminal neuralgia is most commonly (80%–90%) attributed to neurovascular conflict, with important secondary causes, such as multiple sclerosis and regional mass lesions, occurring less commonly.[3] When associated with multiple sclerosis, trigeminal neuralgia is more frequently bilateral and occurs at a younger age (<45). Identifying multiple sclerosis as a potential cause is important, because the underlying pathophysiology is not that of neurovascular conflict and is not appropriately treated with microvascular decompression (MVD).[4]

Anatomy

The trigeminal nerve is the largest of the CNs, with brainstem nuclei extending from the upper cervical spinal cord through the midbrain. The trigeminal nerve is a mixed sensory and motor nerve, serving facial sensation (V1, ophthalmic; V2, maxillary; and V3, mandibular) as well as the muscles of mastication via the V3 segment.

The cisternal segment of the trigeminal nerve is the most relevant nerve segment both for the evaluation of suspected trigeminal neuralgia and for treatment planning and follow-up (**Fig. 1**). The cisternal segment spans the prepontine cistern with portions, including

- Dorsal root entry zone (immediately anterior to the apparent nerve origin at the ventrolateral pons)
- TZ
- Plexus triangularis or retrogasserian segment (immediately dorsal to the porus trigeminus)

The more distal dural and foraminal nerve components are rarely the site of symptomatic neurovascular compression, although these segments should be scrutinized for perineural tumor spread or skull base mass involvement.

The TZ between central and peripheral myelination is believed particularly vulnerable to the mechanical irritation caused by neurovascular compression.[5] TZ of trigeminal sensory fibers[1,5–7]

Table 1
Diagnostic criteria for neurovascular syndromes

Cranial Neuropathy	Diagnostic Criteria
Trigeminal neuralgia	Paroxysmal lancinating facial pain commonly occurring in unilateral V2 and/or V3 dermatomal distributions of the trigeminal nerve
HFS	Involuntary synchronous spasms of one side of the face, usually beginning around the eye, only involving the muscles supplied by the facial nerve
Vestibular paroxysmia	Episodic attacks of acute vertigo with or without tinnitus and disequilibrium due to vascular compression of the vestibulocochlear nerve
GN	Intense usually unilateral paroxysmal pain referable to the sensory distribution of the glossopharyngeal nerve (CN IX)

Table 2
Differentials and mimics of neurovascular syndromes and common compressing vessels

Cranial Neuropathy	Common Differentials and Mimics	Common Compressing Vessels
Trigeminal neuralgia	Multiple sclerosis, skull base masses, herpetic neuralgia	Superior cerebellar artery (75%–88%) AICA (9.6%–25%) Venous structures (8%–10%) Multivessel conflict in as many as 38%
HFS	Facial nerve trauma, demyelinating lesions, and vascular etiologies as well as with cerebellopontine angle tumors	AICA (43%) PICA (31%) VA (23%) Venous structure (3%) Multivessel conflict in as many as 38%
Vestibular paroxysmia	Meniere disease, vestibular migraine, benign paroxysmal positional vertigo, and superior semicircular canal dehiscence	AICA (75%) Venous structure (10%)
GN	Superior laryngeal and nervus intermedius neuralgia, Eagle syndrome	PICA (68%) VA (2%) Venous structure (6%) Multivessel conflict (23%)[52]

- Measures approximately 2 mm in length
- Averages 3.6 mm from the apparent origin
- Almost never occurs within the ventral 50% of the cisternal segment

Motor fiber TZ is considerably closer to the brainstem, averaging only 0.3 mm.

Vascular Compression

Cisternal segment neurovascular conflict is the most common cause of trigeminal neuralgia, accounting for 80% to 90% of cases.[8,9] Repetitive vascular pulsation microtrauma is believed to cause focal axonal injury, leading to central oligodendroglial demyelination and variable degrees of disordered remyelination, which facilitate the symptomatic ephaptic neurotransmissions.[10]

Although neurovascular contact is incidentally identified in asymptomatic subjects (31.9%), several important observations add specificity to the evaluation of trigeminal neuralgia (**Fig. 2**)[5,11]:

- Neurovascular contact with the root entry and TZs (<3 mm from brainstem) are more likely symptomatic than contact with more ventral cisternal nerve segment.[5]
- Nerve root displacement
- Nerve root atrophy

These indicators of higher grade of neurovascular conflict are not only highly specific for symptomatic

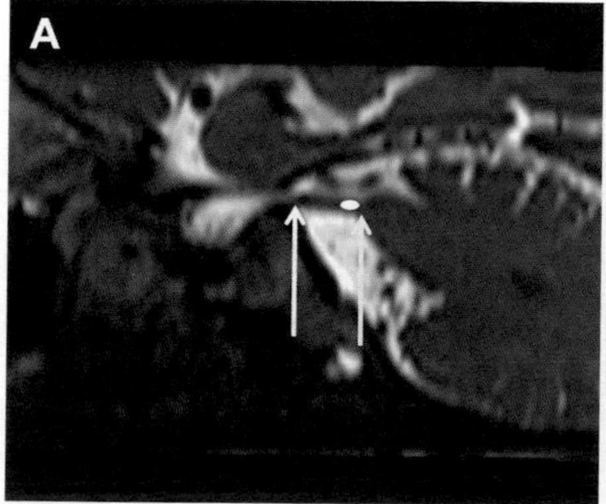

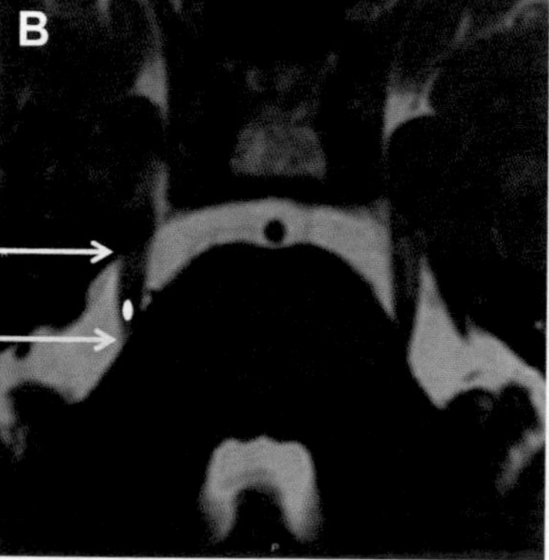

Fig. 1. Normal trigeminal nerve. (*A*) Sagittal and (*B*) axial heavily T2-weighted MR image demonstrating the normal cisternal segment of the trigeminal nerve, spanning from the apparent nerve root origin at the ventrolateral pons (*yellow arrows*) to the retrogasserian segment immediately dorsal to the porus trigeminus (*white arrows*). Approximate site of the TZ is indicated (*white ovals*).

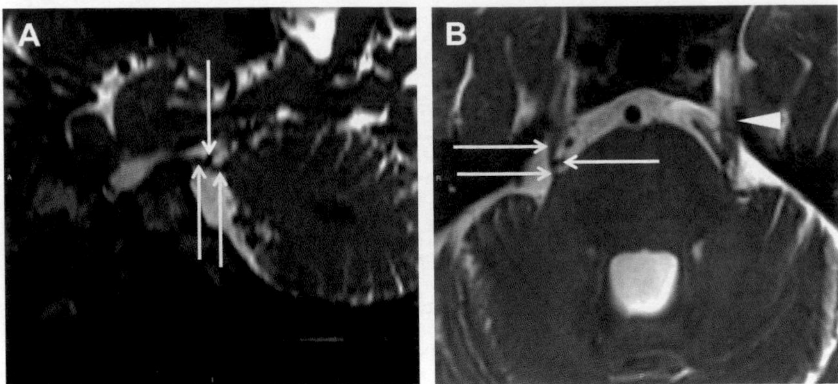

Fig. 2. High-grade trigeminal nerve neurovascular conflict. (*A*) Sagittal and (*B*) axial heavily T2-weighted MR imaging demonstrating high-grade neurovascular conflict with superior cerebellar artery (*white arrows*) compression and displacement of the cisternal segment of the right trigeminal nerve (*yellow arrows*). Subtle right trigeminal nerve volume loss is noted compared with normal left trigeminal nerve (*arrowhead*).

conflict but also prognostically important.[12] For instance, Sheehan and colleagues[13] noted improved outcomes after Gamma knife therapy when higher radiation doses were prescribed to the point of vessel impingement. Similarly, improved durability of MVD was reported in patients demonstrating preoperative nerve root atrophy.[14]

The offending vessels are most commonly arterial, with the superior cerebellar artery, 75% to 88%, and the anterior inferior cerebellar artery (AICA), 9.6% to 25%, accounting for the preponderance of cases (**Fig. 3**).[15,16]

Purely venous causes of neurovascular compression are significantly less common (8%–10%), with the transverse pontine vein and superior petrosal vein accounting for a majority of venous causes (see **Fig. 3**).[10,17] In contrast to arterial compression, venous neurovascular conflict is more commonly within the midcisternal segment and porus trigeminus.[17] Additionally, the presence of concurrent arterial and venous neurovascular conflict has been reported to be as high as 38%, emphasizing the danger of satisfaction of search after the identification of arterial neurovascular conflict.[17–19]

Less common vascular causes of trigeminal neuralgia include arteriovenous malformations, aneurysms, basilar artery dolichoectasia, and petrosal sinus engorgement secondary to carotid-cavernous fistulas (**Fig. 4**).

Tractography of Microstructural Alterations

Diffusion tensor imaging offers additional insights into the microstructural alterations within the trigeminal nerve, which occur as a result of repetitive axonal injury and subsequent disordered or reorganized remyelination.

One of the most robust measures of altered diffusivity is fractional anisotropy (FA), which quantitates the proportion of directionally constrained molecular diffusivity.[10] Intact nerve fibers demonstrate

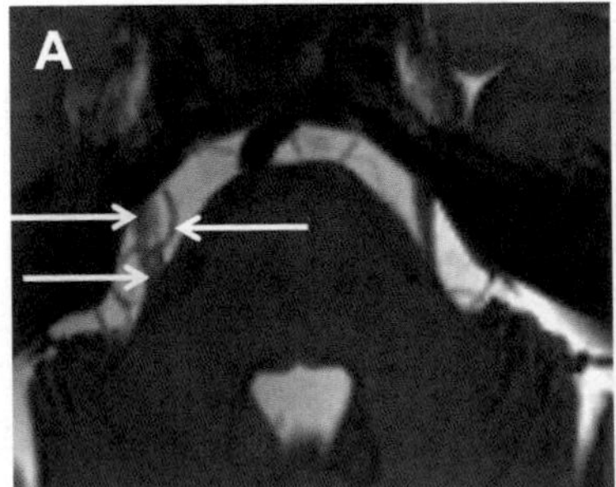

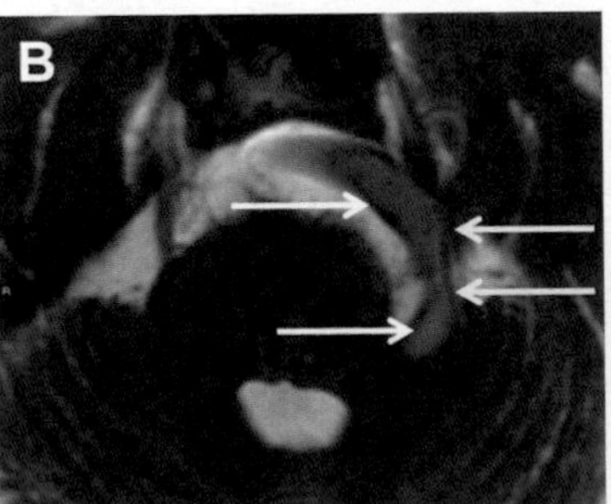

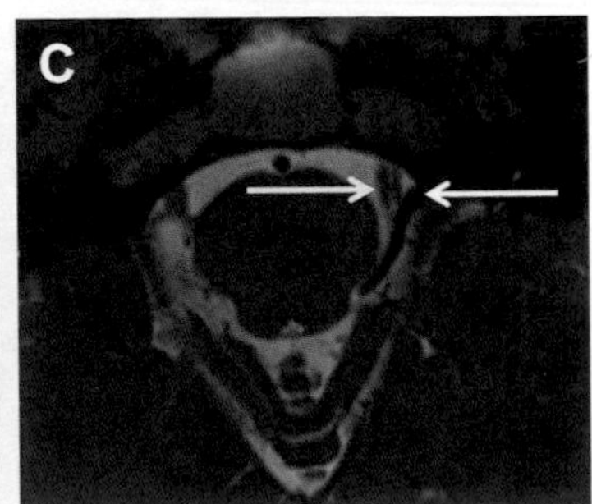

Fig. 3. Various causes of trigeminal nerve neurovascular conflict. Heavily T2-weighted MR image (*A*) axial image demonstrating superior cerebellar artery (*white arrow*) and point of contact with the cisternal segment of the right trigeminal nerve (*yellow arrows*). (*B*) Axial image demonstrating basilar artery dolichoectasia (*white arrows*) compressing and displacing the left trigeminal nerve (*yellow arrows*). (*C*) Axial image demonstrating prominent aberrant venous structure (*white arrow*) compressing and displacing the left trigeminal nerve (*yellow arrow*).

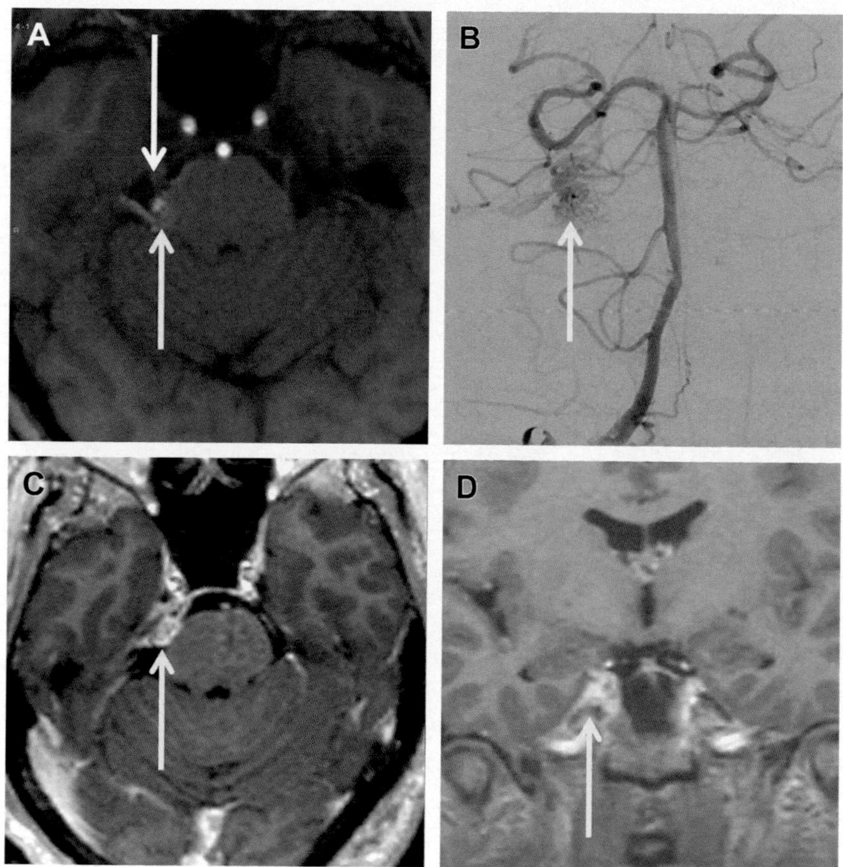

Fig. 4. Less common causes of trigeminal neuralgia. (*A*) Axial TOF MR angiogram and (*B*) corresponding right VA injection catheter angiogram demonstrating an arteriovenous malformation with the nidus (*yellow arrows*) involving the parenchymal fascicular segments and root entry zone of the right trigeminal nerve (*white arrow*). (*C*) Axial and (*D*) coronal postcontrast T1-weighted MR image demonstrating a petroclival meningioma (*C, yellow arrow*) exerting mass effect within the right prepontine cistern and Meckel cave (*D, yellow arrow*).

increased FA values compared with disordered or injured nerve fibers, which display decreased FA values (**Fig. 5**). Decreased trigeminal nerve FA values are strongly associated with atrophic changes that accompany high grade neurovascular conflict.[20]

Additionally, these microstructural alterations are evident in symptomatic neurovascular compression without appreciable atrophic changes. Furthermore, diminished FA values are evident in cases of trigeminal neuralgia without vascular compression. These 2 latter observations suggest that the changes noted in FA values may reflect early demyelination or, alternatively, dismyelination or structural myelin reorganization.[5,10]

A recent study using multitensor diffusion tractography, capable of resolving intrapontine trigeminal nerve fiber tracts, highlights the differences in pathophysiology between classic trigeminal neuralgia due to neurovascular conflict and multiple sclerosis–related trigeminal neuralgia. Cases secondary to multiple sclerosis revealed no typical cisternal segment changes; rather, the perilesion intrapontine nerve fibers displayed microstructural alterations that were unique to the multiple sclerosis cohort.[21]

Treatment Methods

Before alternative interventions are offered, trigeminal neuralgia patients typically undergo a trial of pharmacologic treatment. In cases of medically refractory disease, 2 commonly used treatment methods include surgical MVD, considered the most definitive therapy, and rhizotomy, an increasingly used minimally invasive therapy.

Microvascular decompression

MVD is considered the most durable surgical treatment option, with immediate pain relief reported in 87% to 98%, 1-year pain-free rate of 80%, and 58% to 70% pain-free at 8 to 10 years.[5]

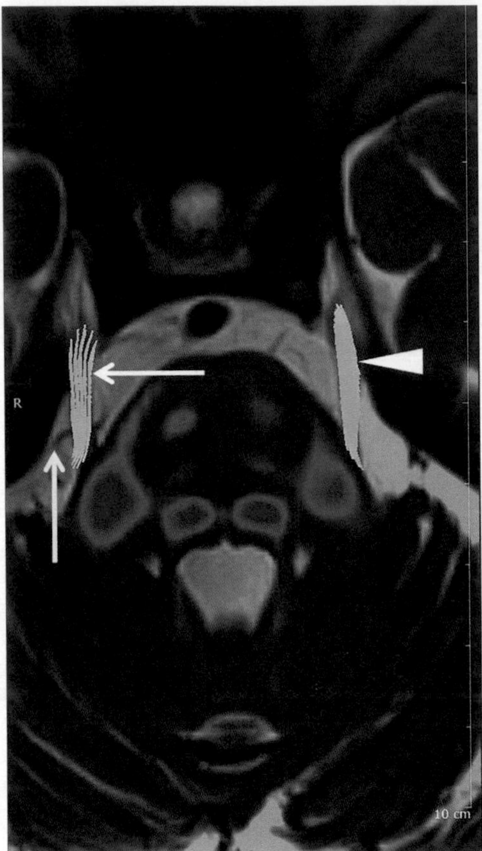

Fig. 5. Diffusion tensor tractography of right trigeminal neuralgia. Axial heavily T2-weighted MR image with diffusion tensor tractography and fractional anisotrophy color map overlay demonstrating a diminished number of right trigeminal nerve fibers (*white arrow*) compared to the contralateral normal trigeminal nerve (*arrow head*). Superior cerebellar artery approximating the cisternal segment of the right trigeminal nerve (*yellow arrow*).

The surgical approach generally entails a 2-cm triangular retrosigmoid craniotomy with mild cerebellar retraction and exposure of the cerebellopontine angle. When the offending vessel is identified, Teflon sponge or other suitable material is used to cushion the nerve and alleviate vascular compression. If the offending vessel is a vein, depending on size it can be sacrificed or decompressed in a similar fashion to the arterial culprits.[18] On cross-sectional imaging, the Teflon pledget appears as a hyperdense or hypodense prepontine structure on CT with a corresponding masslike signal void on high-resolution T2 images (**Fig. 6**).

Rhizotomy

Interruption of afferent pain fibers can be accomplished by injuring the trigeminal ganglion mechanically (percutaneous balloon compression), chemically (glycerol rhizotomy), and thermally (radiofrequency thermocoagulation). All of these procedures require general anesthesia and percutaneous placement of a needle through the foramen ovale but can be done on an outpatient basis. Although their permanent success rate is not as high as surgical microdecompression, they can be repeated to provide durable pain control and may be best suited for older patients who have surgical risk factors. An alternative noninvasive technique, radiosurgical treatment, uses stereotactic delivery of a very high dose of radiation (70–90 Gy) to a small target extending over several millimeters of the cisternal nerve segment. The midcisternal or retrogasserian segments of CN V are often targeted because these locations facilitate sharp dose falloff and limit ventral brainstem radiation exposure. Some providers also target the dorsal root entry zone at the cost of higher brainstem dose.[22] Radiosurgical treatment effects may occur via ablative mechanisms hypothesized to cause disproportionately greater nocioceptive fiber impairment or nonablative mechanisms in which radiation-related arterial wall thickening may reduce vascular pulsation transmission to the nerve root.[23]

Delayed post-treatment enhancement of the nerve root target zone is common after radiosurgery (**Fig. 7**). Although the presence of nerve root enhancement does not accurately predict symptom resolution, it does confirm treatment dose delivery to the target zone, which is pertinent in cases of poor therapeutic response. In cases requiring retreatment, enhancement of the original treatment site can inform subsequent target planning. In cases of treatment failure, the lack of expected enhancement should prompt review of the target positioning.[24] Delayed nerve root atrophy is a common postprocedural finding.[5,25] Pain relief within 3 months is reported as 70% to 75%, with 50% of patients reporting pain-free outcomes at 3 years.[26]

HEMIFACIAL SPASM

HFS is a debilitating neuromuscular disorder that causes functional, social, and cosmetic issues, typically characterized by

- Frequent involuntary contractions (spasms) of the muscles on one side (hemi) of the face (facial)
- Usually unilateral presentation, with brief clonic movements involving the orbicularis oculi
- Spreading over months to years to involve other facial muscles[27]

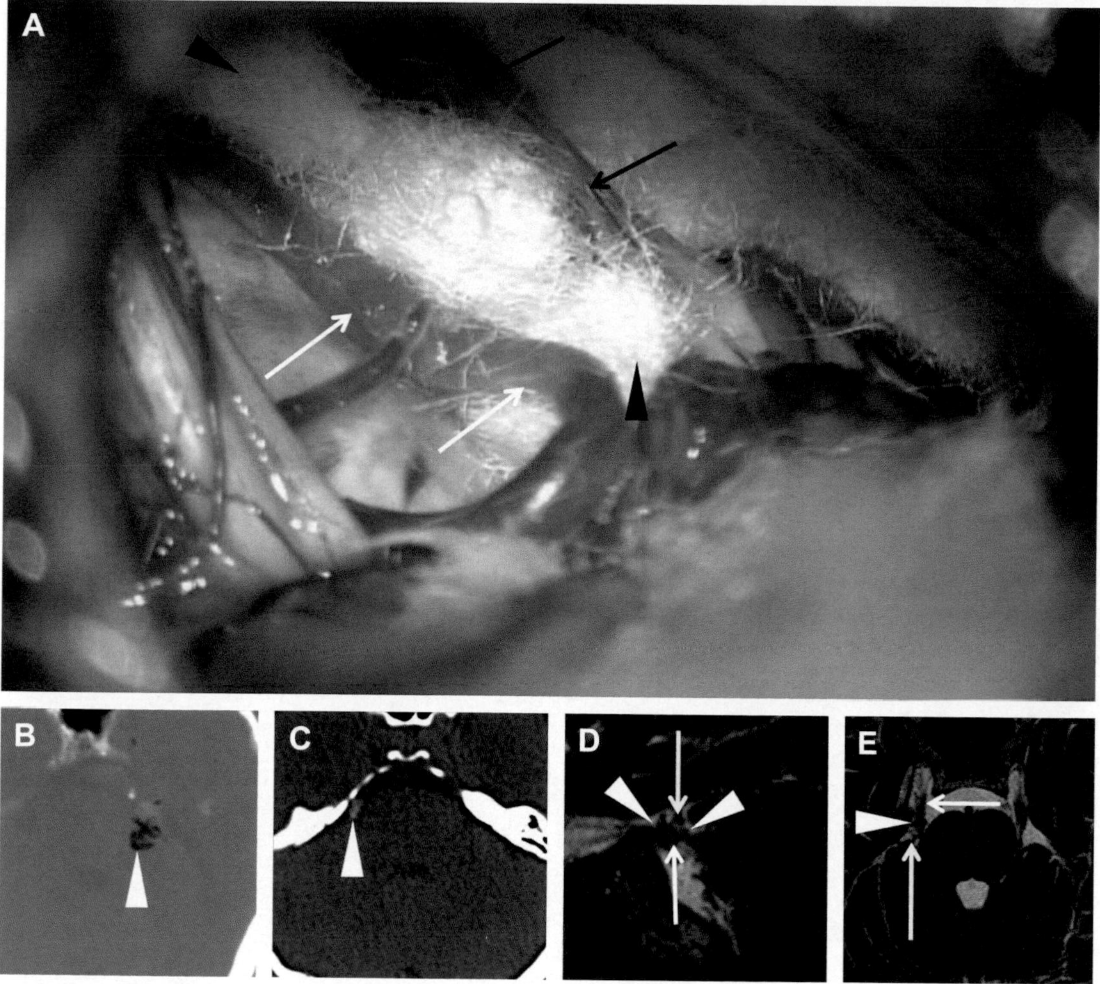

Fig. 6. MVD. (*A*) Intraoperative view demonstrating MVD pledget (*black arrowheads*) separating the superior cerebellar artery (*white arrows*) from the trigeminal nerve (*black arrows*). (*B, C*) Axial noncontrast CT demonstrating various appearances of the decompression pledget (*white arrowheads*). (*D*) Sagittal and (*E*) axial heavily T2-weighted MR image demonstrating the masslike decompression pledget (*white arrowheads*) separating the superior cerebellar artery (*yellow arrows*) from the right trigeminal nerve (*white arrows*).

- Involuntary movements that are present at rest (even in sleep) and patients unable to suppress the movements

HFS is divided into primary and secondary, based on cause. Primary HFS is defined by neurovascular compression at the nerve root entry zone of the facial nerve whereas secondary HFS is due to damage to the facial nerve along its course from the internal auditory canal to the stylomastoid foramen.[28] Secondary HFS has been rarely described with facial nerve trauma, demyelinating lesions, and vascular etiologies as well as with cerebellopontine angle tumors. An association between hypertension and primary HFS has also been described.

The work-up of HFS requires a thorough clinical history and neurologic examination; an electromyography study to distinguish it from other abnormal facial movement disorders, such as blepharospasm, tics, partial motor seizures, Meige syndrome, and neuromyotonia; and high-resolution MR imaging.

Anatomy

The facial nerve is a mixed CN with motor, sensory, and parasympathetic fibers, with the motor division the most dominant, accounting for greater than two-thirds of the total axons. The facial nerve can be broadly divided into intra-axial (within the brainstem) and the extra-axial segments (within the cistern, internal auditory canal, labyrinthine, geniculate, tympanic, mastoid, and extracranial segments).[29] The critical segment involved in HFS is the cisternal segment, which consists of the motor root and the nervus intermedius.

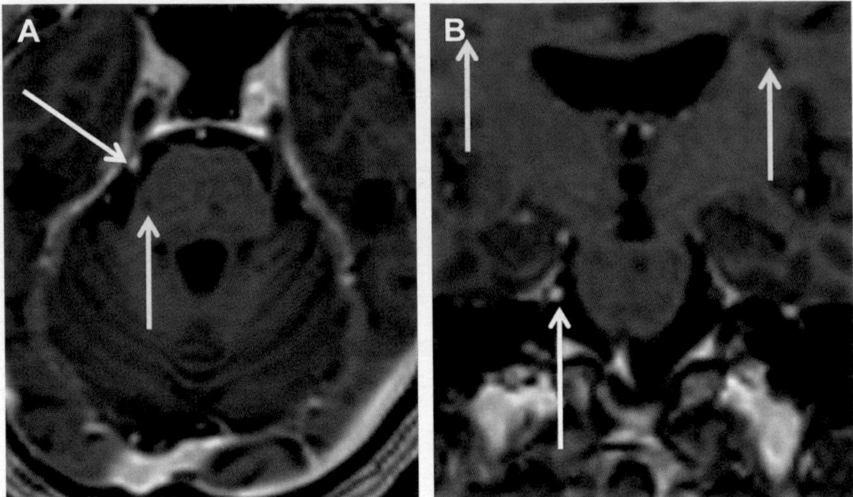

Fig. 7. Gamma knife postoperative appearance of right trigeminal neuralgia in patient with multiple sclerosis. (*A*) Axial and (*B*) coronal postcontrast T1-weighted MR image demonstrating enhancement of the retrogasserian portion of the right trigeminal nerve (*white arrows*) corresponding to and confirming appropriate treatment site targeting. Note multiple chronic demyelinating lesions within the brainstem and deep white matter (*yellow arrows*).

The facial nerve exits from the brainstem ventrolaterally from the pontomedullary sulcus near the dorsal pons and travels anterolaterally into the internal auditory canal. The cisternal segment of the facial nerve can be subdivided into 4 separate segments (**Fig. 8**), which is significant to the pathophysiology of HFS and its treatment.[30,31] High-resolution 3-D T2-weighted imaging can precisely map out the proximal cisternal anatomy of the facial nerve (**Fig. 9**).

These include

- Root exit zone (REZ) (where the facial nerve exits from the pons), the attached segment (AS) measuring 8 to 10 mm where the nerve adheres to the adjacent pons

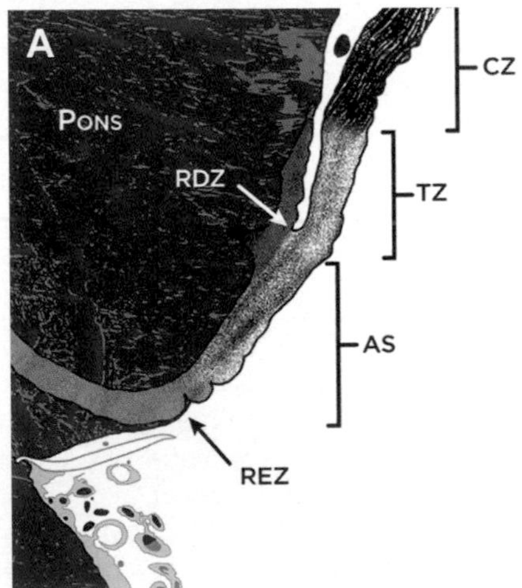

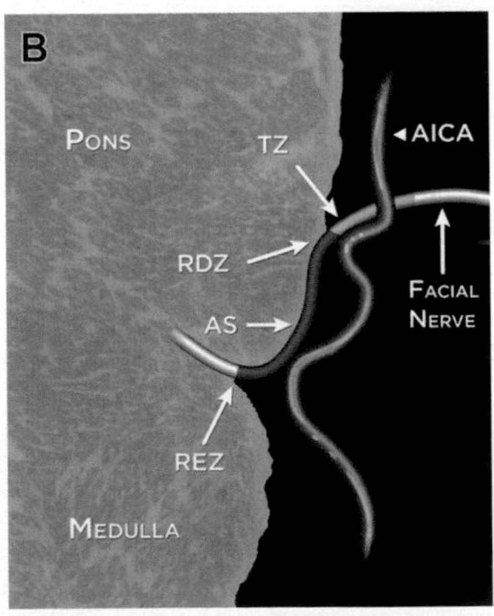

Fig. 8. Proximal facial nerve anatomy. (*A, B*) Graphic images detailing the proximal cisternal anatomy of the facial nerve as it exits from the nerve REZ at the pontomedullary sulcus. Note the REZ followed by the AS, which runs along the pons and separates at the RDZ. The TZ is the proximal 3 mm to 4 mm long segment of this nerve where the central myelin transitions to peripheral myelin followed by the true cisternal segment. (*B*) Shows a loop of AICA contacting the TZ of the left facial nerve. (*From* Campos-Benitez M, Kaufmann AM. Neurovascular compression findings in hemifacial spasm. J Neurosurg 2008;109:416–20.)

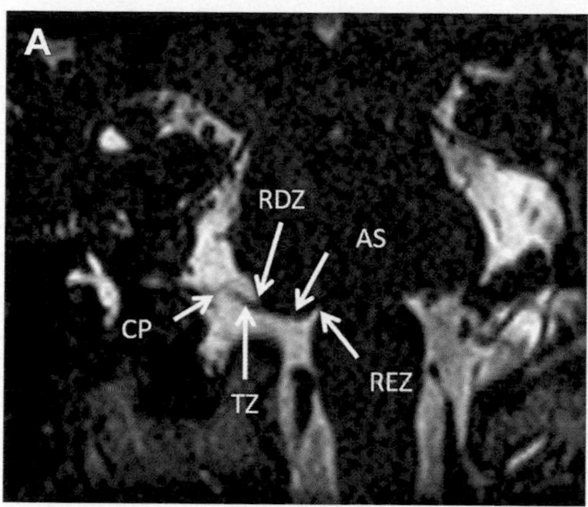

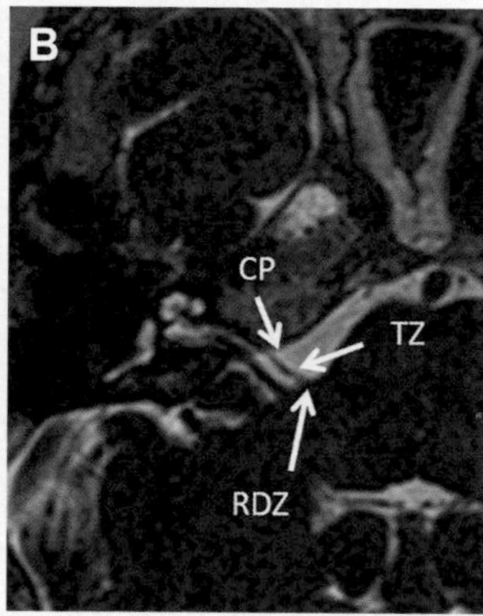

Fig. 9. MR images of facial nerve segments. (*A*) Coronal and (*B*) axial high-resolution T2-weighted MR images show the various cisternal segments of the right facial nerve. The ability of high-resolution 3-D T2-weighted imaging allows for elegant multiplanar reformations and precise mapping of neurovascular contact. CP, cisternal distal segment.

- Root detachment zone (RDZ), where the nerve separates from the pons
- TZ. The transitional myelin zone (TZ) – also known as Obersteiner-Redlich zone – where the central glial myelin transitions into peripheral Schwann cell myelin in the facial nerve is situated at the RDZ and extends further distally for approximately 3 mm to 4 mm. The myelin in the TZ is believed to be vulnerable to repeated vascular pulsation.[31]
- True cisternal zone (CZ). This final segment extends anterolateral to the porous acousticus.

The 2 current hypotheses (central and peripheral) are deficient in explaining the entire HFS pathophysiology. The central/nuclear hypothesis explains HFS on retrograde medullary changes with functional reorganization and facial nuclear hyperexcitability due to facial nerve trauma. The peripheral hyperexcitability hypothesis relies on the mechanism of fiber "crosstalk" and ectopic impulse generation due to dendritic spike generation.[32]

Vascular Compression

Neurovascular pulsatile compression is currently recognized and identified as the most common cause or HFS.[33] Although greater than 20% of normal subjects have vascular compression on imaging, the findings are significant only in patients with symptoms in the affected side.[34] Recent articles have expanded and more precisely defined the target segment of the proximal cisternal segment of the facial nerve in patients with HFS.[30,31,33] The transitional segment of the proximal facial nerve lacks both the interfascicular connective tissue and the epineurium, making these more prone to repeated axonal injury, compression, and myelin breakdown.

The vessels commonly implicated in HFS are the AICA, posterior inferior cerebellar artery (PICA), and the vertebral artery (VA) (**Fig. 10**). The incidence of veins causing HFS is rare.[33] A review of 115 patients by Campos-Benitez and Kaufman[33] identified the culprit vessel as AICA in 43%, PICA in 31%, VA in 23%, and a large vein in 3% of the cases. They also localized the precise site of compression during surgery at the root exit point in 10%, AS in 64%, root detachment/transition zone in 22%, and cisternal segment in only 3%. Moreover, 38% of patients had multiple vessels compressing the nerve (**Fig. 11**). Rarely, multiple CNs might be involved (any combination of HFS, trigeminal neuralgia and GN) due to neurovascular contact by multiple vessels (**Fig. 12**). Park and colleagues[35] have described 6 different patterns of neurovascular compression on surgery (**Fig. 13**). The pattern of compression can have implications on type of surgery and symptomatology.

Treatment Methods

Treatment of HFS includes medications, botulinum toxin injections, and MVD surgery, with surgery reserved for treatment failure and medically refractory cases.[27,30] Direct botulinum injection into the affected muscles represents the first-line treatment of HFS with a high success rate. Pharmacologic therapy (agents commonly used include carbamazepine and benzodiazepines) represent an alternative to patients who decline botulinum toxin injection.

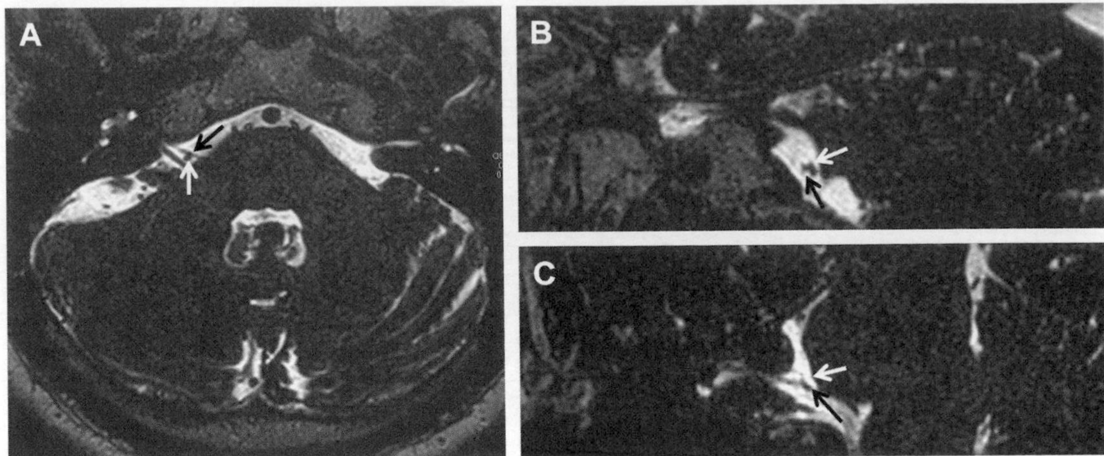

Fig. 10. Right AICA neurovascular contact. (*A*) Axial, (*B*) coronal oblique, and (*C*) sagittal oblique images in this patient with right-sided symptoms show the right AICA (*white arrows*) contacting the right facial nerve (*black arrows*) posteriorly at the transition zone, just distal to the RDZ.

MVD offers the potential for cure of HFS with success rates exceeding 90%.[36] Although MVD has its own set of risks (CN injury, cerebellar hematoma, infection, and stroke), a combination of precise presurgical imaging, patient selection, and experienced surgeons results in lower morbidity and mortality, with excellent outcomes. MVD is usually performed by a lateral retro sigmoid suboccipital craniotomy, followed by identifying and mapping the entire course of the facial nerve, the culprit neurovascular contact, and the offending vessel. The abnormal vessels causing neurovascular compression are then mobilized away from the nerve and maintained in their new positions with Teflon implants.[37] Postsurgical imaging (**Fig. 14**) allows for confirmation of the implant positioning and monitoring complications (hemorrhage, ischemia, and so forth) as well as recurrent symptoms due to persistent neurovascular contact and Teflon implant migration.

VESTIBULAR PAROXYSMIA

Vestibular paroxysmia (VP) is a debilitating disorder caused by vascular compression of the vestibulocochlear nerve (CN VIII), typically characterized by

- Episodic attacks of acute vertigo lasting seconds to minutes
- Gait or stance disturbance
- Pressure or numbness around the ear
- Unilateral tinnitus or unilateral reduced hearing[38]

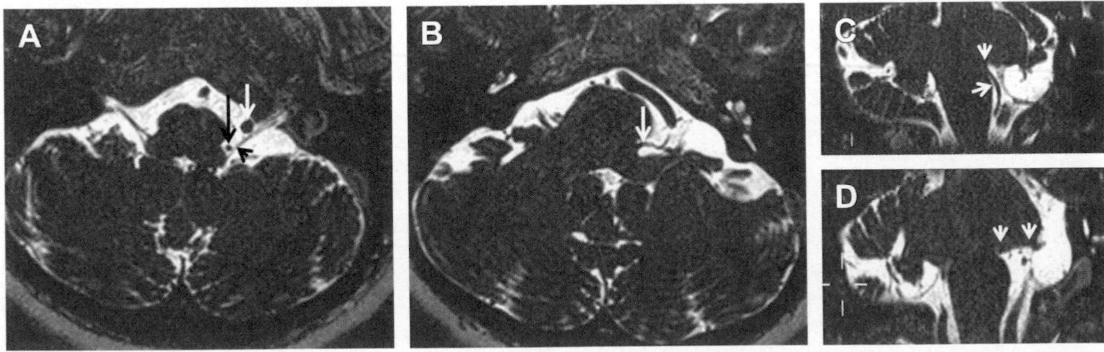

Fig. 11. Multivessel multisite neurovascular contact. (*A, B*) Axial and (*C, D*) coronal T2-weighted images with multiple sites of neurovascular contact. In this patient with left-sided HFS, imaging reveals left VA (*white arrow* [*A*]) contacting the distal cisternal segment (*short black arrow* [*A*]), left AICA (*long black arrow* [*A*]) contacting the transitional segment and also the left PICA contacting and indenting the left nerve REZ and the ASs (*long and short white arrows* [*B–D*]). Lack of careful presurgical evaluation in these patients can lead to unaddressed proximal sites of neurovascular contact and recurrence of symptoms.

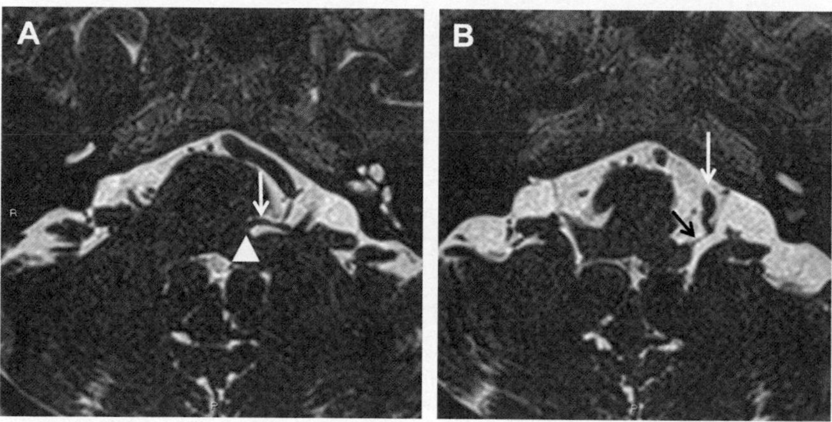

Fig. 12. Combined HFS and GN. Axial high-resolution T2-weighted MR images in a patient with combined symptoms of left HFS and GN. Careful evaluation reveals 2 distinct sites of compression involving both the left facial and glossopharyngeal nerves. (*A*) Shows superior axial slice tortuous left AICA loop (*white arrow*) indenting the REZ of the left facial nerve (*white arrowhead*). (*B*) Inferior axial slice shows an ectatic left PICA (*white arrow*) contacting and deforming the left glossopharyngeal nerve (*black arrow*).

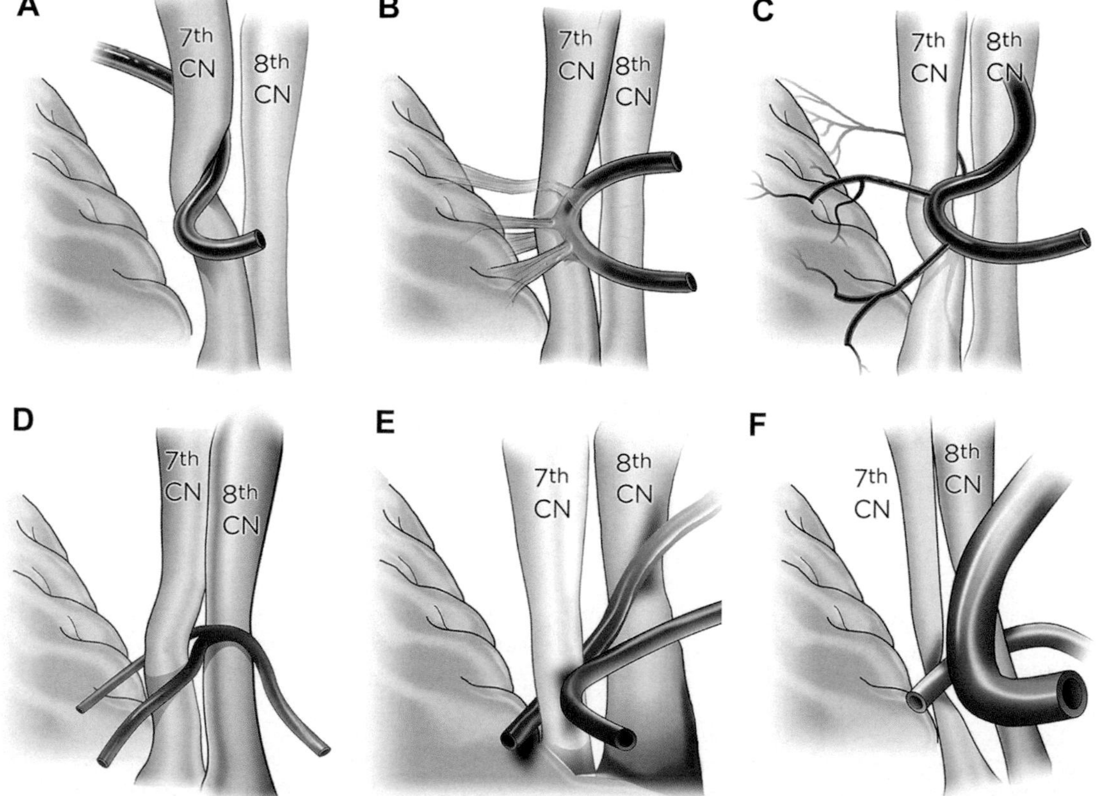

Fig. 13. Patterns of neurovascular compression, as described by Park and colleagues.[35] These include (*A*) loop-type compression where the vascular loop itself is the cause for compression, (*B*) thick arachnoid membranes causing tethering of the nerve between the brainstem and the vessel, (*C*) smaller perforating branches from the parent vessel causing tethering, (*D*) the nerve being trapped between the parent vessel and its branch, (*E*) sandwich type compression between 2 separate vessels, and (*F*) tandem type compression where one vessel compresses other vessel, which then compresses the nerve. (*Adapted from* Park JS, Kong DS, Lee JA, et al. Hemifacial spasm: neurovascular compressive patterns and surgical significance. Acta Neurochir (Wien) 2008;150(3):235–41.)

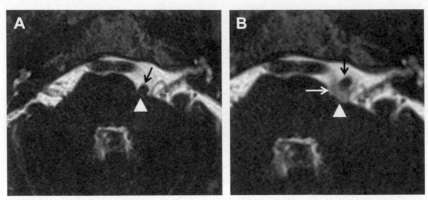

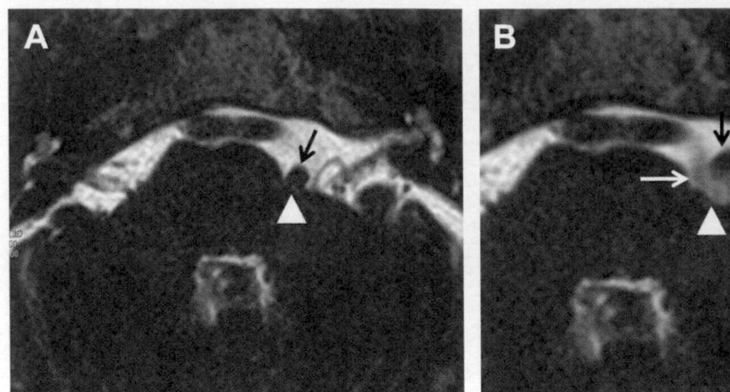

Fig. 14. Premicrovascular and post-MVD. Axial high-resolution MR images (*A*) pre-MVD and (*B*) post-MVD demonstrate the intermediate signal Teflon pledget (*white arrow*) in the left cerebellopontine angle cistern in between the left PICA (*black arrows*) and the left facial nerve exit zone (*white arrowheads*) near the left pontomedullary sulcus. The patient had left HFS, which resolved completely postsurgery.

Only in 1994 were diagnostic criteria formalized, including symptomatology, measurable neurophysiologic parameters, and response to medical treatment (eg, carbamazepine). Before then, VP was diagnosed only after exclusion of the myriad other causes of vertigo, with major differential considerations to include Meniere disease, vestibular migraine, benign paroxysmal positional vertigo, and superior semicircular canal dehiscence. The spells of vertigo associated with VP tend to be much shorter than with other entities and can be precipitated at rest or certain changes in head/body position. Hufner and colleagues[39] reported that 4% of patients seen in their dizziness clinic had symptoms attributable to VP.

Vestibulocochlear Nerve Anatomy

The vestibulocochlear nerve transmits purely sensory information from the neuroepithelial hair cells of the cochlea to mediate hearing and of the vestibular apparatus to mediate sensation of head position (gravity, linear acceleration, and rotational movement). The bipolar cochlear nerve cell bodies reside in the cochlear modiolus and connect the organ of Corti to the dorsal and ventral cochlear nuclei in the lateral pontomedullary junction, with nerve fibers traveling in the anterior-inferior quadrant of the internal auditory canal. Vestibular nerve cell bodies reside in Scarpa ganglion, located in the internal auditory canal, and link the hair cells of the utricle, saccule, and semicircular canals to the 4 vestibular nuclei in the lower pons, with nerve fibers traveling in the posterosuperior and posteroinferior quadrants of the internal auditory canal. At the level of the porus acusticus, the superior and inferior vestibular nerves merge to form a single vestibular nerve, which in turn merges with the cochlear nerve to form the CN VIII.

A unique feature of CN VIII relating to neurovascular compression is the lengthy TZ, extending 9.28 mm to 13.85 mm from the root entry zone, which leaves a much longer cisternal segment susceptible to vascular compression.[40]

Vascular Compression in Vestibular Paroxysmia

Recent studies conducted with more stringent patient selection using formalized diagnostic criteria have demonstrated the efficacy of high-resolution MR imaging in the diagnosis of VP. Best and colleagues[41] found heavily T2-weighted sequences and TOF MR angiography have a sensitivity of 100% and specificity of 65% for detecting symptomatic CN VIII neurovascular conflict compared with trigeminal neuralgia control subjects. The site of compression ranged between 0 mm and 10.2 mm from the REZ, which correlates well with the histologically defined lengthy TZ of CN VIII. AICA was the most frequent compressing vessel (75%) and venous compression accounted for 10% of cases.[41] In patients with MR imaging–detected CN VIII neurovascular conflict, symptoms included unilateral hearing loss (82%), unilateral tinnitus (80%), and dizziness (74%).[42]

These studies highlight the ability of MR to exclude VP in equivocal cases as well as the importance of including high-resolution sequences in skull base/brainstem protocols (**Fig. 15**). As with other vascular compression syndromes, medication (carbamazepine or oxcarbazepine) is the preferred first-line therapy, with surgical decompression reserved for refractory cases.

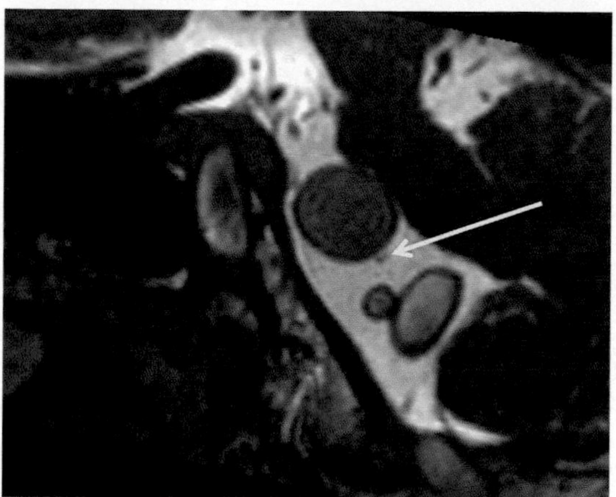

Fig. 15. Vestibular paroxysmia. A 70-year-old man with left-sided sensorineural hearing loss, tinnitus, and vertigo. Reformatted sagittal heavily T2-weighted image demonstrates dolichoectatic basilar artery compressing a markedly atrophic left CN VII/VIII complex (*yellow arrow*).

GLOSSOPHARYNGEAL AND VAGOGLOSSOPHARYNGEAL NEURALGIA

GN is a paroxysmal pain syndrome characterized by

- Typical features of intense unilateral pain localizing to the oropharynx, tonsillar fossa, and periauricular region provoked by innocuous stimulation[43]
- Atypical features of cardiac arrhythmias, syncope, and cardiac arrest, termed *vagoglossopharyngeal neuralgia* (2% of all GN cases)[44]

Ambiguous symptoms can sometimes overlap with other CN hyperactivity syndromes. The main differential considerations in this category include trigeminal neuralgia, superior laryngeal neuralgia, and nervus intermedius neuralgia.

The more common subtype of GN, the idiopathic type, is thought to result from mainly from neurovascular conflict. The less common secondary subtypes can include causative lesions, such as arterial dissection, Chiari malformation, skull base and cervical neoplasm, multiple sclerosis, infection, Paget disease, and Eagle syndrome (**Fig. 16**).

Glossopharyngeal and Vagus Nerve Anatomy

The glossopharyngeal nerve is a mixed motor, sensory, and parasympathetic nerve. It powers the stylopharyngeus muscle and receives taste information from the posterior third of the tongue and sensation from the pharynx, soft palate, tongue base, and inner surface of the tympanic membrane. It sends parasympathetic fibers to mediate salivation in the parotid gland, and it receives viscerosensory information from the carotid body and sinus. The vagus nerve (CN X) is also complex, carrying motor function to the pharynx and larynx, taste from the epiglottis, sensation

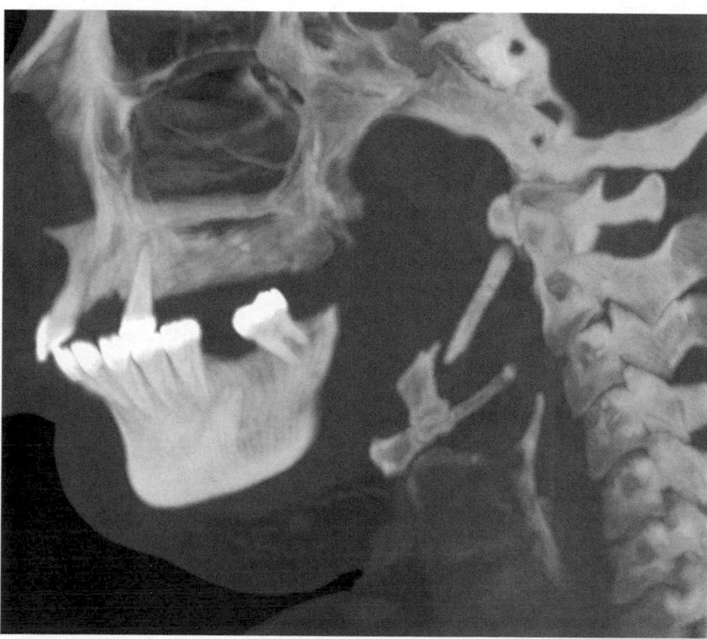

Fig. 16. Eagle syndrome. A 34-year-old woman with 3-week history of right-sided odynophagia, neck pain, and grinding sensation. Sagittal CT maximum intensity projection image demonstrates segmented, calcified stylohyoid ligament forming a pseudarthrosis with the hyoid bone, compatible with Eagle syndrome.

from the external auditory canal, central pinna, and posterior half of the tympanic membrane. It also receives viscerosensory information from the esophagus, trachea, and abdominal viscera.

The cisternal segments of these nerves exit the brainstem posterior to the medullary olive in the posterolateral sulcus, with the glossopharyngeal root entry zone slightly more rostral than the vagus. The transition zone of CN IX measures approximately 1.51 mm from the root entry zone.[45] They travel together anterolaterally through the CPA cistern in close proximity to the spinal accessory nerve (CN XI). CN IX then enters the pars nervosa of the jugular foramen and CN X and CN XI exit together through the pars vascularis. The cisternal segments of these nerves are best distinguished using very high-resolution, heavily T2-weighted sequences.[46]

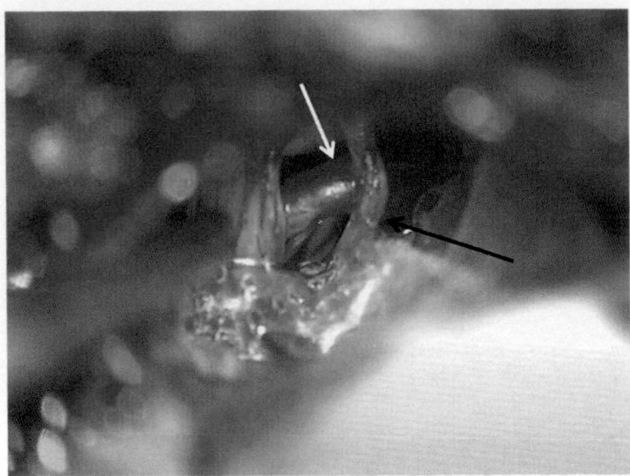

Fig. 17. Intraoperative image demonstrates left PICA (*white arrow*) compressing CN IX (*black arrow*) prior to decompression.

Vascular Compression in Glossopharyngeal Neuralgia

Laha and Jannetta[47] reported the first series of GN patients successfully treated with MVD in 1977. All compression in their series was caused by vertebral arteries, but more recently PICA has been shown the most common culprit vessel, followed by the vertebral arteries and AICA.[48,49] The proximal position of the CN IX TZ correlates nicely with MR imaging studies demonstrating very proximal neurovascular compression of the nerve at the REZ. In a series reported by Hiwatashi and colleagues,[50] all 8 cases of PICA compression occurred within the supraolivary fossette due to a vascular loop. Tanrikulu and colleagues[49] described 3 distinct patterns of neurovascular conflict at the REZ of CN IX:

- Tortuous PICA branch compression
- VA compression
- Sandwich-type compression between PICA and the VA

Although the causal relationship between neurovascular conflict and GN has been well-established, it is not entirely clear to what extent, if any, compression of CN X is responsible for the life-threatening symptoms of vagoglossopharyngeal neuralgia. Nevertheless, recent case reports have demonstrated complete remission of symptoms after MVD of the CN IX-X REZ complex.[51,52]

If medical therapy fails, MVD is considered the most effective alternative in the setting of idiopathic GN (**Fig. 17**). In the absence of neurovascular compression, surgical rhizotomy can be curative but is unfortunately associated with severe side effects, such as dysphonia and dysphagia.[53] In poor surgical candidates, less-invasive options include glossopharyngeal nerve block using either neurolytic (eg, glycerol) or non-neurolytic (eg, local anesthesia and steroids) agents, pulsed radiofrequency neurolysis, and stereotactic radiosurgery.[54]

REFERENCES

1. Hughes MA, Frederickson AM, Branstetter BF, et al. MRI of the trigeminal nerve in patients with trigeminal neuralgia secondary to vascular compression. AJR Am J Roentgenol 2016;206(3):595–600.
2. Zhou Q, Liu ZL, Qu CC, et al. Preoperative demonstration of neurovascular relationship in trigeminal neuralgia by using 3D FIESTA sequence. Magn Reson Imaging 2012;30(5):666–71.
3. Becker M, Kohler R, Vargas MI, et al. Pathology of the trigeminal nerve. Neuroimaging Clin N Am 2008;18(2):283–307, x.
4. Chan MD, Shaw EG, Tatter SB. Radiosurgical management of trigeminal neuralgia. Neurosurg Clin N Am 2013;24(4):613–21.
5. Haller S, Etienne L, Kovari E, et al. Imaging of neurovascular compression syndromes: trigeminal neuralgia, hemifacial spasm, vestibular paroxysmia, and glossopharyngeal neuralgia. AJNR Am J Neuroradiol 2016;37(8):1384–92.
6. Peker S, Kurtkaya O, Uzun I, et al. Microanatomy of the central myelin-peripheral myelin transition zone of the trigeminal nerve. Neurosurgery 2006;59(2): 354–9 [discussion: 354–9].
7. Blitz AM, Macedo LL, Chonka ZD, et al. High-resolution CISS MR imaging with and without contrast for evaluation of the upper cranial nerves: segmental anatomy and selected pathologic conditions of the cisternal through extraforaminal segments. Neuroimaging Clin N Am 2014;24(1):17–34.

8. Love S, Coakham HB. Trigeminal neuralgia: pathology and pathogenesis. Brain 2001;124(Pt 12):2347–60.
9. Bowsher D. Trigeminal neuralgia: an anatomically oriented review. Clin Anat 1997;10(6):409–15.
10. Lutz J, Thon N, Stahl R, et al. Microstructural alterations in trigeminal neuralgia determined by diffusion tensor imaging are independent of symptom duration, severity, and type of neurovascular conflict. J Neurosurg 2016;124(3):823–30.
11. Chun-Cheng Q, Qing-Shi Z, Ji-Qing Z, et al. A single-blinded pilot study assessing neurovascular contact by using high-resolution MR imaging in patients with trigeminal neuralgia. Eur J Radiol 2009;69(3):459–63.
12. Antonini G, Di Pasquale A, Cruccu G, et al. Magnetic resonance imaging contribution for diagnosing symptomatic neurovascular contact in classical trigeminal neuralgia: a blinded case-control study and meta-analysis. Pain 2014;155(8):1464–71.
13. Sheehan JP, Ray DK, Monteith S, et al. Gamma knife radiosurgery for trigeminal neuralgia: the impact of magnetic resonance imaging-detected vascular impingement of the affected nerve. J Neurosurg 2010;113(1):53–8.
14. Leal PR, Barbier C, Hermier M, et al. Atrophic changes in the trigeminal nerves of patients with trigeminal neuralgia due to neurovascular compression and their association with the severity of compression and clinical outcomes. J Neurosurg 2014;120(6):1484–95.
15. Jannetta PJ. Arterial compression of the trigeminal nerve at the pons in patients with trigeminal neuralgia. J Neurosurg 1967;26(1):Suppl:159–62.
16. Sindou M, Howeidy T, Acevedo G. Anatomical observations during microvascular decompression for idiopathic trigeminal neuralgia (with correlations between topography of pain and site of the neurovascular conflict). Prospective study in a series of 579 patients. Acta Neurochir (Wien) 2002;144(1):1–12 [discussion: 12–3].
17. Hong W, Zheng X, Wu Z, et al. Clinical features and surgical treatment of trigeminal neuralgia caused solely by venous compression. Acta Neurochir (Wien) 2011;153(5):1037–42.
18. Sade B, Lee JH. Microvascular decompression for trigeminal neuralgia. Neurosurg Clin N Am 2014; 25(4):743–9.
19. Barker FG 2nd, Jannetta PJ, Bissonette DJ, et al. The long-term outcome of microvascular decompression for trigeminal neuralgia. N Engl J Med 1996;334(17):1077–83.
20. Fujiwara S, Sasaki M, Wada T, et al. High-resolution diffusion tensor imaging for the detection of diffusion abnormalities in the trigeminal nerves of patients with trigeminal neuralgia caused by neurovascular compression. J Neuroimaging 2011; 21(2):e102–8.
21. Chen DQ, DeSouza DD, Hayes DJ, et al. Diffusivity signatures characterize trigeminal neuralgia associated with multiple sclerosis. Mult Scler 2016;22(1): 51–63.
22. Park SH, Hwang SK, Kang DH, et al. The retrogasserian zone versus dorsal root entry zone: comparison of two targeting techniques of gamma knife radiosurgery for trigeminal neuralgia. Acta Neurochir (Wien) 2010;152(7):1165–70.
23. Lettmaier S. Radiosurgery in trigeminal neuralgia. Phys Med 2014;30(5):592 5.
24. Alberico RA, Fenstermaker RA, Lobel J. Focal enhancement of cranial nerve V after radiosurgery with the Leksell gamma knife: experience in 15 patients with medically refractory trigeminal neuralgia. AJNR Am J Neuroradiol 2001;22(10):1944–8.
25. Park SH, Hwang SK, Lee SH, et al. Nerve atrophy and a small cerebellopontine angle cistern in patients with trigeminal neuralgia. J Neurosurg 2009; 110(4):633–7.
26. Gronseth G, Cruccu G, Alksne J, et al. Practice parameter: the diagnostic evaluation and treatment of trigeminal neuralgia (an evidence-based review): report of the Quality Standards Subcommittee of the American Academy of Neurology and the European Federation of Neurological Societies. Neurology 2008;71(15):1183–90.
27. Abbruzzese G, Berardelli A, Defazio G. Hemifacial spasm. Handb Clin Neurol 2011;100:675–80.
28. Colosimo C, Bologna M, Lamberti S, et al. A comparative study of primary and secondary hemifacial spasm. Arch Neurol 2006;63(3):441–4.
29. Raghavan P, Mukherjee S, Phillips CD. Imaging of the facial nerve. Neuroimaging Clin N Am 2009; 19(3):407–25.
30. Lu AY, Yeung JT, Gerrard JL, et al. Hemifacial spasm and neurovascular compression. ScientificWorldJournal 2014;2014:349319.
31. Tomii M, Onoue H, Yasue M, et al. Microscopic measurement of the facial nerve root exit zone from central glial myelin to peripheral Schwann cell myelin. J Neurosurg 2003;99(1):121–4.
32. Nielsen VK. Electrophysiology of the facial nerve in hemifacial spasm: ectopic/ephaptic excitation. Muscle Nerve 1985;8(7):545–55.
33. Campos-Benitez M, Kaufmann AM. Neurovascular compression findings in hemifacial spasm. J Neurosurg 2008;109(3):416–20.
34. Tash R, DeMerritt J, Sze G, et al. Hemifacial spasm: MR imaging features. AJNR Am J Neuroradiol 1991; 12(5):839–42.
35. Park JS, Kong DS, Lee JA, et al. Hemifacial spasm: neurovascular compressive patterns and surgical significance. Acta Neurochir (Wien) 2008;150(3): 235–41 [discussion: 241].
36. Dannenbaum M, Lega BC, Suki D, et al. Microvascular decompression for hemifacial

spasm: long-term results from 114 operations performed without neurophysiological monitoring. J Neurosurg 2008;109(3):410–5.
37. Cohen-Gadol AA. Microvascular decompression surgery for trigeminal neuralgia and hemifacial spasm: naunces of the technique based on experiences with 100 patients and review of the literature. Clin Neurol Neurosurg 2011;113(10):844–53.
38. Brandt T, Dieterich M. Vestibular paroxysmia: vascular compression of the eighth nerve? Lancet 1994;343:798–9.
39. Hufner K, Barresi D, Glaser M, et al. Vestibular paroxysmia: diagnostic features and medical treatment. Neurology 2008;71(13):1006–14.
40. Guclu B, Sindou M, Meyronet D, et al. Anatomical study of the central myelin portion and transitional zone of the vestibulocochlear nerve. Acta Neurochir (Wien) 2012;154(12):2277–83 [discussion: 2283].
41. Best C, Gawehn J, Kramer HH, et al. MRI and neurophysiology in vestibular paroxysmia: contradiction and correlation. J Neurol Neurosurg Psychiatry 2013;84(12):1349–56.
42. Markowski J, Gierek T, Kluczewska E, et al. Assessment of vestibulocochlear organ function in patients meeting radiologic criteria of vascular compression syndrome of vestibulocochlear nerve–diagnosis of disabling positional vertigo. Med Sci Monit 2011; 17(3):Cr169–73.
43. Pearce JM. Glossopharyngeal neuralgia. Eur Neurol 2006;55(1):49–52.
44. Savica R, Lagana A, Calabro RS, et al. Vagoglossopharyngeal neuralgia: a rare case of sincope responding to pregabalin. Cephalalgia 2007;27(6): 566–7.
45. Guclu B, Sindou M, Meyronet D, et al. Cranial nerve vascular compression syndromes of the trigeminal, facial and vago-glossopharyngeal nerves: comparative anatomical study of the central myelin portion and transitional zone; correlations with incidences of corresponding hyperactive dysfunctional syndromes. Acta Neurochir (Wien) 2011;153(12):2365–75.
46. Casselman J, Mermuys K, Delanote J, et al. MRI of the cranial nerves–more than meets the eye: technical considerations and advanced anatomy. Neuroimaging Clin N Am 2008;18(2):197–231. preceding x.
47. Laha RK, Jannetta PJ. Glossopharyngeal neuralgia. J Neurosurg 1977;47(3):316–20.
48. Sampson JH, Grossi PM, Asaoka K, et al. Microvascular decompression for glossopharyngeal neuralgia: long-term effectiveness and complication avoidance. Neurosurgery 2004;54(4):884–9 [discussion: 889–90].
49. Tanrikulu L, Hastreiter P, Dorfler A, et al. Classification of neurovascular compression in glossopharyngeal neuralgia: three-dimensional visualization of the glossopharyngeal nerve. Surg Neurol Int 2015; 6:189.
50. Hiwatashi A, Matsushima T, Yoshiura T, et al. MRI of glossopharyngeal neuralgia caused by neurovascular compression. AJR Am J Roentgenol 2008;191(2): 578–81.
51. Krasoudakis A, Anyfantakis D, Hadjipetrou A, et al. Glossopharyngeal neuralgia associated with cardiac syncope: two case reports and literature review. Int J Surg Case Rep 2015;12:4–6.
52. Munch TN, Rochat P, Astrup J. Vagoglossopharyngeal neuralgia treated with vascular decompression. Ugeskr Laeger 2009;171(37):2654–5 [in Danish].
53. Alafaci C, Granata F, Cutugno M, et al. Glossopharyngeal neuralgia caused by a complex neurovascular conflict: case report and review of the literature. Surg Neurol Int 2015;6:19.
54. Singh PM, Kaur M, Trikha A. An uncommonly common: glossopharyngeal neuralgia. Ann Indian Acad Neurol 2013;16(1):1–8.

Imaging of Perineural Spread in Head and Neck Cancer

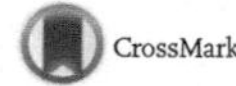

David Badger, MD, Nafi Aygun, MD*

KEYWORDS

• Perineural spread • Perineural invasion • Head and neck cancer • Skull base imaging

KEY POINTS

- Perineural spread (PNS) of tumor is a recognized pattern of metastasis occurring in the head and neck.
- Imaging plays a critical role in identifying PNS for adequate staging and treatment planning.
- Understanding the major branches and pathways of cranial nerves V and VII, key anatomic landmarks, interconnections between these nerves, and pearls and pitfalls of PNS imaging can aid in early detection, appropriate therapy, and the best possible chance for cure.

INTRODUCTION

Perineural tumor growth is a recognized pattern of malignant tumor metastasis occurring along the potential space between the nerve and the surrounding sheath. It is important to differentiate between perineural tumor spread (PNS) and perineural tumor invasion (PNI) whenever possible, as they are frequently used interchangeably in the literature and clinical practice. This interchange leads to ambiguity regarding their implications, although such differentiation may not always be feasible or accurate. We define PNS as the macroscopic tumor extension away from the primary tumor site detectable by imaging and PNI as a diagnosis made on histology, typically in a specimen including the primary tumor. Much of what is known about the prognosis and incidence of perineural tumor growth comes from pathologic studies investigating PNI, which we apply to PNS because this is done broadly in the literature and at some point they exist on the same spectrum.

The overall frequency of PNI in head and neck cancers has been reported in the range of 2.5% to 5.0%,[1] with PNS suspected to be lower. Such nerve involvement can be seen in all head and neck cancers, but certain tumors demonstrate a particular proclivity for this method of metastasis and should prompt the careful attention of the radiologist. The most commonly encountered histology is mucosal (5%) or cutaneous (5%–14%) squamous cell carcinoma (SCC), given that it is by far the most common head and neck malignancy, accounting for up to 95% of the approximately 650,000 head and neck cancers diagnosed each year worldwide.[2] The most common sites of mucosal SCC are the larynx, oral cavity, and the tonsils.[3] Adenoid cystic carcinoma (ACC) of the minor or major salivary glands is probably the most notorious offender, with reported rates of PNI in up to 50% of cases, although it comprises only 1% to 3% of all head and neck malignancies.[4] Basal cell carcinoma (BCC), melanoma, especially the desmoplastic type (1%–2%), mucoepidermoid carcinoma, and lymphoma round out the list of additional culprits.[5]

Only 30% to 40% of patients with PNI are symptomatic at presentation,[2] but the percentage is likely higher in clinical PNS, as noted in a series

The authors have nothing to disclose.
Division of Neuroradiology, Johns Hopkins University, School of Medicine, 600 North Wolfe Street Phipps B100, Baltimore, MD 21287, USA
* Corresponding author.
E-mail address: naygun1@jhmi.edu

Radiol Clin N Am 55 (2017) 139–149
http://dx.doi.org/10.1016/j.rcl.2016.08.006
0033-8389/17/© 2016 Elsevier Inc. All rights reserved.

of patients with skin cancer in which 59 of 62 patients with PNS were symptomatic.[6] Symptoms include pain, paresthesias, dysesthesias, weakness, or paralysis. Symptoms attributed to multiple nerve distributions suggest more central involvement, such as the cavernous sinus, spread from one cranial nerve (CN) to another, or leptomeningeal disease.[7,8] As in most cases, the clinical history is important to guide a careful search pattern for PNS. The clinical scenarios with which PNS presents include the following:

1. At the time of diagnosis of a primary head and neck malignancy. In this setting, PNS-specific symptoms are often absent or overshadowed by symptoms related to the primary tumor.
2. Recurrence of a previously treated tumor. In this setting, symptoms usually precede imaging diagnosis, although occasionally PNS demonstrated on imaging may be the only manifestation of recurrent disease.
3. Symptoms such as pain, paresthesia, or diplopia with no known primary tumor. Because this presentation is rare and the primary tumors are often occult, patients are frequently misdiagnosed as having, for example, trigeminal neuralgia.

The risk of developing PNI in skin cancer is higher in poorly differentiated tumors, larger primary tumor size, male gender, history of recurrence after treatment, and midface location.[9] PNI is also associated with the increased risk of local recurrence and portends a poor overall outcome with the likelihood of residual disease proportionate to the proximal extent of the tumor[6] and the diameter of the involved nerves.[10] The 5-year local control rate in one series was 25% in patients with skin carcinoma with PNI.[6] Thus, the identification of PNS has important therapeutic and prognostic implications and is critical for adequate staging and treatment planning. Changes in planned treatment may include expansion of the radiation field and/or the surgical resection; for example, the need for mastoidectomy and/or temporal bone resection in case of a parotid tumor with PNS extending into the facial canal. Failure to identify early perineural disease may delay or prevent potentially curative treatment. Knowledge of the commonly involved nerve pathways and vigilance in assessing key landmarks can allow for accurate assessment of disease extent and allow for the best chance of obtaining durable control of the disease.

GROWTH PATTERN AND PATHOPHYSIOLOGY

The pattern of growth in PNS most commonly occurs in a contiguous retrograde fashion from the primary tumor or resection site toward the intracranial cavity, although it may spread in an antegrade direction as well. Early tumor growth is described as preferentially spreading along the axis of the nerve greater than concentric growth.[1] This may explain why some patients with PNS are initially asymptomatic, as concentric growth results in compression of the nerve fibers and the previously described symptomatology. Nerve enlargement may eventually expand or erode the skull base canals and foramina. In addition, "skip" or "resurfacing" lesions with sites of tumor separated by uninvolved nerve may be present, although this pattern has been questioned in a recent study by Panizza and Warren,[11] in which they examined 50 cases of SCC and found no skip lesions. Regardless, evaluation of key landmarks distal from the tumor site remain important from an imaging standpoint.

The pathophysiology of PNS is not well understood. Previous theories suggesting spread occurring passively along paths of least resistance or via epineural lymphatics have been rejected.[12] The most recent theories describe complex interactions in the nerve environment that promote perineural tumor growth. Tumor cells have been shown to upregulate genes that increase cell proliferation and decrease rates of apoptosis in the nerve mileu.[2] Proinvasive signals, such as brain-derived neurotrophic factor, nerve growth factor, neurotrophin-3 and neurotrophin-4, glial cell line–derived neurotrophic factor, substance P, and various chemokines,[2] have been shown to facilitate tumor growth along the nerve. Neural cell adhesion molecule, which mediates cell-to-cell adhesion in neuroectodermal tissues, was found to be expressed in 93% of patients with ACC with PNS.[13] The desmoplastic type of melanoma, a variant with increased incidence of PNS, stains for high levels of p75 neurotrophin receptors mediating PNS.[14]

PNS in the head and neck most commonly involves branches of the trigeminal and facial nerves, as these are the 2 nerves responsible for most of the sensory (**Fig. 1**) and motor innervation of the face. The trigeminal nerve provides sensory information from the face and motor innervation to the muscles of mastication. Understanding the CN anatomy is critical to identifying PNS. Our goal here is to review the major branches and pathways of CNs V and VII, key anatomic landmarks, interconnections between these nerves, and pearls and pitfalls of PNS imaging.

CRANIAL NERVE V1

PNS involving the ophthalmic branch of the trigeminal nerve is uncommon compared with involvement of the maxillary and mandibular

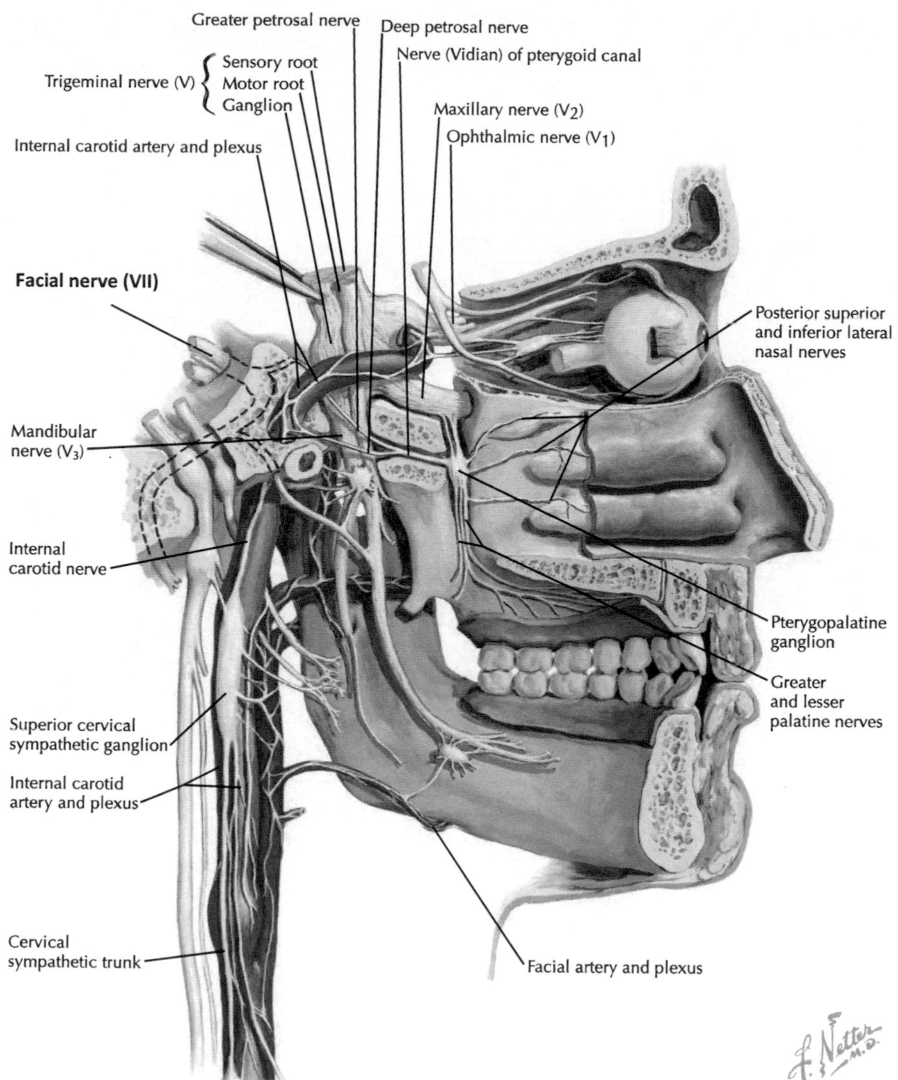

Fig. 1. Anatomic depiction of the course and major branches of the trigeminal nerve (V); ophthalmic (V1), maxillary (V2), and mandibular (V3) divisons; facial nerve (VII); and geniculate and pterygopalatine ganglia.

branches. The ophthalmic nerve branches to form the nasociliary, lacrimal, and frontal nerves. Most of the tumors are cutaneous in origin (SCC, BCC, melanoma), involving the terminal branches of the frontal nerve (supraorbital and supratrochlear nerve) which supply a large region of sun-exposed skin (forehead and eyebrow are the most common sites) (**Fig. 2**). Although less common, PNS arising from ACC of the lacrimal gland[15,16] can involve the same distribution. Shah and colleagues[17] described cases of PNS involving the nasociliary branch in medial canthus SCC and melanoma of the nasal ala. Symptoms or clinical evidence of ophthalmic branch involvement could be sinus pain or absence of the corneal blink reflex (nasociliary branch).

CRANIAL NERVE V2

The maxillary branch of the trigeminal nerve (V2) provides sensory innervation to the midfacial structures with main branches including the zygomatic, superior alveolar, and infraorbital nerves. It courses anteriorly from the cavernous sinus through the foramen rotundum and on to the pterygopalatine fossa (PPF), 3 key landmarks to assess for PNS involving V2. The PPF is located between the posterior wall of the maxillary sinus and the base of the pterygoid process with the perpendicular plate of the palatine bone at its anteromedial margin (**Fig. 3**). It serves as an important “crossroads” for PNS, connecting the masticator space laterally via the pterygomaxillary

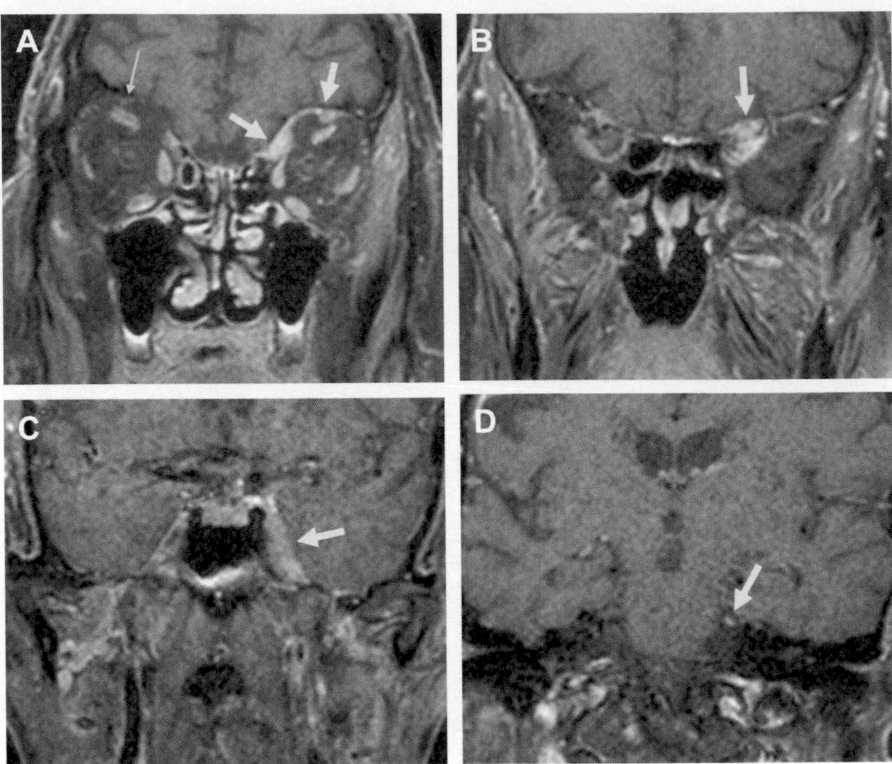

Fig. 2. A 74-year-old man with previous history of SCC of the forehead skin presents with diplopia and facial numbness. Coronal fat-suppressed contrast-enhanced image (*A*) shows enhancing tumor in the medial aspect of the orbit surrounding the superior rectus muscle compatible with PNS involving the supratrochlear nerve (ST in *A*), which extends to the frontal nerve (*F*). The normal right orbital nerve is barely visible (*thin arrow*). The orbital apex (*arrow* in *B*) and the cavernous sinus (*arrow* in *C*) are filled with tumor (presumably along the ophthalmic nerve [V1]) that reaches the cisternal segment of the trigeminal nerve (CN5) (*arrow* in *D*).

fissure, the face anteriorly via the infraorbital canal, the orbit and face superiorly via the inferior orbital fissure, the nasopharynx inferiorly via the pharyngeal (palatovaginal) canal, the palate inferiorly via the greater and lesser palatine foramina, the nasal cavity medially via the sphenopalatine foramen, and the middle cranial fossa via the foramen rotundum and vidian canal. On reaching the PPF, tumor may continue on through the foramen rotundum to the cavernous sinus and Meckel cave or anterograde along any of the previously described routes (**Fig. 4**). On reaching the Gasserian ganglion in the Meckel cave, it may spread via CN V3 through the foramen ovale. Tubular enhancement, widening of the canals, obliteration of the fat in the PPF, and denervation edema or atrophy of the masticator muscles are all characteristic imaging features of PPF involvement. PNS arising from nasopharyngeal carcinoma can involve the PPF by direct extension, via the sphenopalatine foramen or via the palatovaginal canal. Cutaneous melanoma or SCC in the V2 distribution can access the PPF via the zygomatic or infraorbital nerves (**Fig. 5**). Mucosal or minor salivary gland tumors of the palate and maxillary sinus may develop PNS via palatine, and superior alveolar branches, respectively. It bears repeating that the first sign of maxillary nerve infiltration may be discovered at a more central site such as the cavernous sinus, which should prompt careful search for a midface head or neck primary.[18]

CRANIAL NERVE V3

The mandibular branch of the trigeminal nerve (V3) carries sensory innervation from the chin, lower lip, floor of the mouth, tongue, and lateral-most side of the face. It also provides motor innervation to the muscles of mastication, tensor tympani muscle, tensor veli palatini, mylohyoid muscle, and anterior belly of the digastric muscles. The major branches are the auriculotemporal, lingual, inferior alveolar, and mental nerves. PNS of cutaneous cancers, such as melanoma or SCC of the lower lip or chin, occur along the mental nerve and follow its retrograde course through the mental

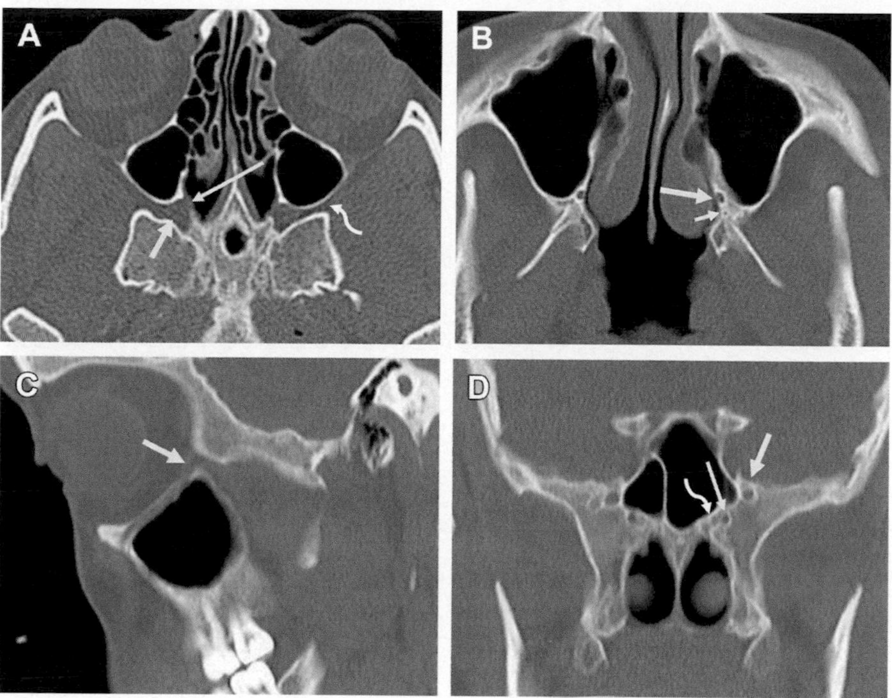

Fig. 3. Pterygopalatine fossa (PPF) (*short arrow* in *A*) is a cleft between the posterior wall of the maxillary sinus and anterior aspect of the pterygoid process containing the pterygopalatine ganglion, maxillary artery branches, and fat. Medially, it opens to the nasal cavity via the sphenopalatine foramen (*long arrow* in *A*). Laterally, PPF opens to the infratemporal fossa via the pterygomaxillary fissure, which transmits the posterior superior alveolar nerve (*curved arrow* in *A*). (*B*) Inferiorly, PPF is bound by the palatine bone and communicates with the palate through the greater (*large arrow*) and lesser palatine (*small arrow*) foramina, which house the palatine nerves. The inferior orbital fissure, which connects the PPF to the orbit, forms the superior limit of the PPF and it contains the zygomatic branch of the V2. The infraorbital nerve runs through the superior and lateral aspect of the PPF after it leaves the infraorbital nerve canal (*arrow* in *C*). Three openings are identified on the posterior wall of the PPF; from lateral to medial foramen rotundum transmitting the maxillary nerve (*thick arrow* in *D*), the vidian (pterygoid) canal (*thin arrow* in *D*), and the pharyngeal (palatovaginal) canal (*curved arrow* in *D*).

canal to involve the inferior alveolar branch along the medial aspect of the mandible to the main trunk of V3 and on to the foramen ovale. On reaching the foramen ovale, it may then involve the cavernous sinus and Meckel cave, gaining access to the trigeminal (Gasserian) ganglion (**Fig. 6**). Cancers arising from the parotid gland or skin involving the lateral-most aspect of the face that develop PNS may do so via the auriculotemporal branch of V3, which courses through the stylomandibular tunnel before arriving at the main mandibular nerve trunk (**Fig. 7**). Temporomandibular joint pain or dysfunction can occur with auriculotemporal nerve involvement. PNS may occur from any tumor arising from the masticator space or adjacent structures, such as the buccal mucosa, retromolar trigone, maxillary sinus, or nasopharynx. Denervation atrophy of the muscles of mastication may reflect perineural involvement and should be differentiated from actual muscle involvement or postradiation changes. Acute muscle denervation is T2 hyperintense without atrophy. Subacute denervation has T2 hyperintensity with some fatty replacement/loss of muscle bulk (hyperintensity may last up to a year). Chronic changes of muscle denervation show extensive fatty replacement and loss of bulk without T2 abnormality.

CRANIAL NERVE VII

The facial nerve (CN VII) provides motor innervation to the muscles of facial expression, the stylohyoid muscle, the posterior belly of the digastric muscle, and the stapedius muscles. It provides sensory innervation to the skin on and adjacent to the ear as well as taste to the anterior two-thirds of the tongue. Most cases of PNS involving CN VII occur with parotid malignancies or skin cancers invading the parotid gland. Once tumor gains access to the intraparotid segment of the facial nerve, it may spread through the

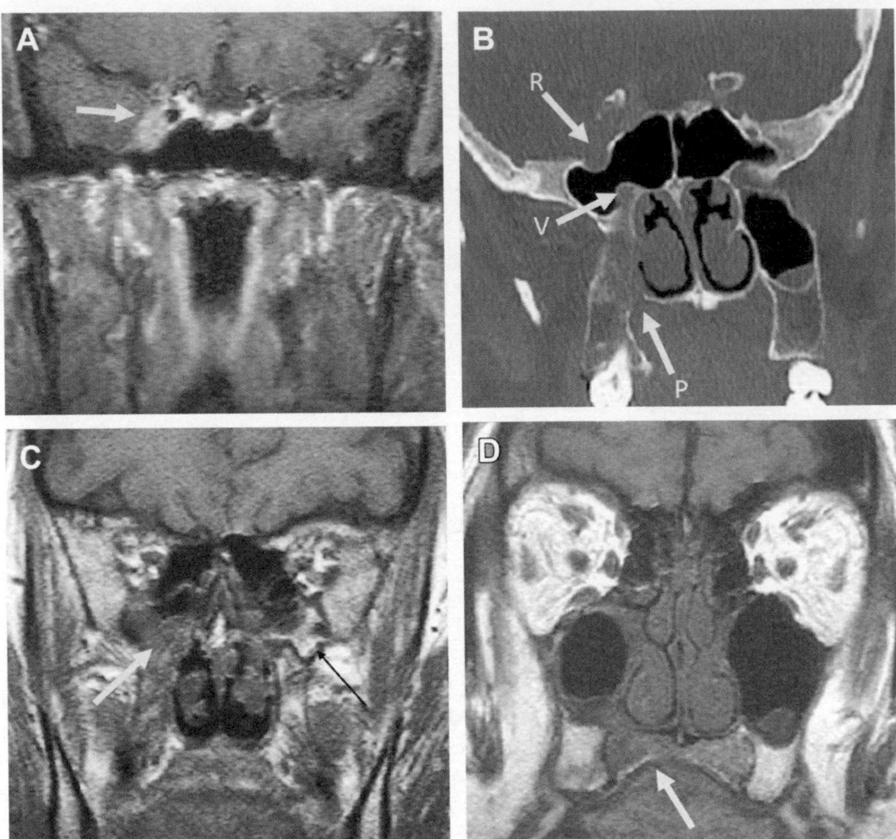

Fig. 4. A 56-year-old woman presented with diplopia. Coronal T1W image (*A*) shows a right cavernous sinus mass (*arrow*). Coronal CT (*B*) shows enlarged foramen rotundum (R), vidian canal (V), and greater palatine nerve canal (P) indicating PNS. Coronal unenhanced T1W MR image (*C*) shows effacement of the fat signal in the right PPF (*white arrow*) with preservation of fat signal in the left PPF (*black arrow*). A clinically occult tumor is seen in the right hard palate (*arrow* in *D*) which was shown to be adenocystic carcinoma arising from minor salivary gland.

stylomastoid foramen into the temporal bone, working its way through the mastoid and inner ear (**Fig. 8**).

Among salivary gland malignancies, PNS is most common in ACC (50%), followed by adenocarcinoma not otherwise specified (42%), SCC (22%), undifferentiated carcinoma (22%), mucoepidermoid carcinoma (20%), acinic cell carcinoma (11%), and carcinoma ex pleomorphic adenoma (9%).[19] Facial paralysis occurring as a result of PNS from parotid malignancy is often gradual, occurring over weeks to months, and should not be confused with the acute onset of idiopathic facial paralysis (Bell palsy).

INTERCONNECTIONS

Sites of spread that occur from one CN to another are important to be aware of when evaluating PNS, as they have clinical implications. On the most superficial level, tumors may spread between the cutaneous branches of CN V and VII, which is under the resolution of radiologic imaging. The most common route between the facial nerve and the mandibular nerve (V3) is the auriculotemporal nerve, which runs just posterior to the angle of the mandible. This allows parotid malignancies or cutaneous neoplasms access to the mandibular nerve and eventually the cavernous sinus. Less frequently, the greater superficial petrosal nerve in the vidian canal allows spread of tumor between the geniculate ganglion of the facial nerve and the pterygopalatine ganglion. The cavernous sinus (V1 and V2) and Meckel cave (V1, V2, and V3) are additional hubs for potential PNS communication involving branches of the trigeminal nerve.

IMAGING PEARLS

The most important factor in making a diagnosis of PNS is a radiologist who is aware of the clinical

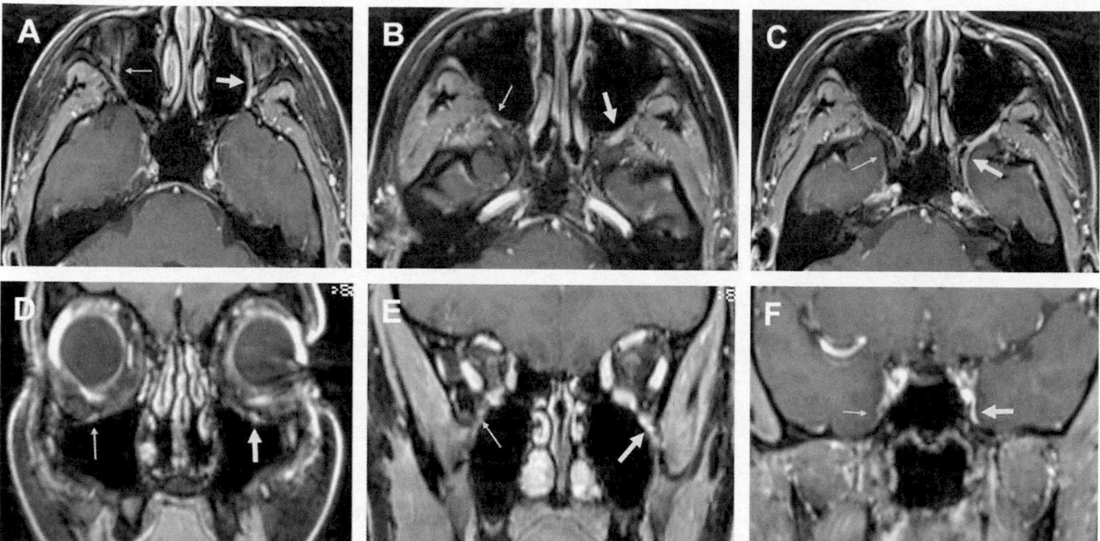

Fig. 5. A 56-year-old woman with history of facial pain refractory to medical therapy and trigeminal rhizotomy. Axial (*A–C*) and coronal (*D–F*) high-resolution postcontrast T1W images show slight thickening and abnormal enhancement of the left infraorbital nerve (*thick arrow; A, D*), extending through the infraorbital fissure into the PPF (*thick arrow; B, E*) and through the foramen rotundum and maxillary nerve into the cavernous sinus (*thick arrow; C, F*) compared with the normal nerve on the right side (*thin arrows*). The patient's remote history of a "minor dermatologic procedure" and skin SCC of the dorsum of the nose was discovered after imaging diagnosis of PNS.

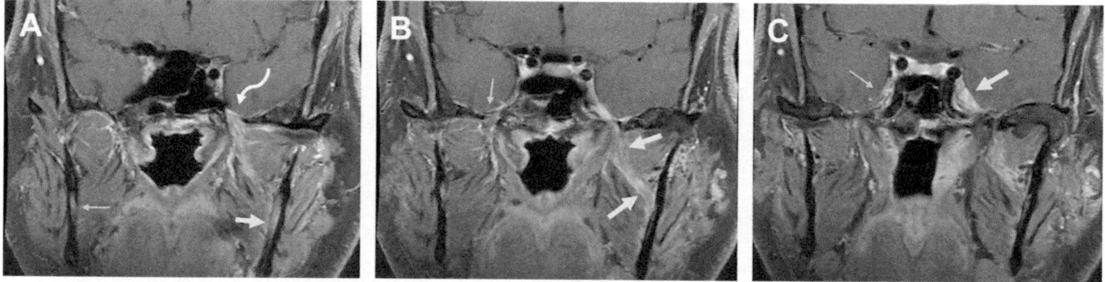

Fig. 6. Gingival SCC extending along the inferior alveolar nerve within the mandibular canal (*thick arrow* in *A*) then into the masticator (infratemporal) space (*arrows* in *B*) before reaching the foramen ovale (*curved arrow* in *A*). There is tumor extension to the Meckel cave and cavernous sinus (*thick arrow* in *C*). Thin arrows point to the normal mandibular canal (*A*), foramen ovale (*B*), and cavernous sinus (*C*).

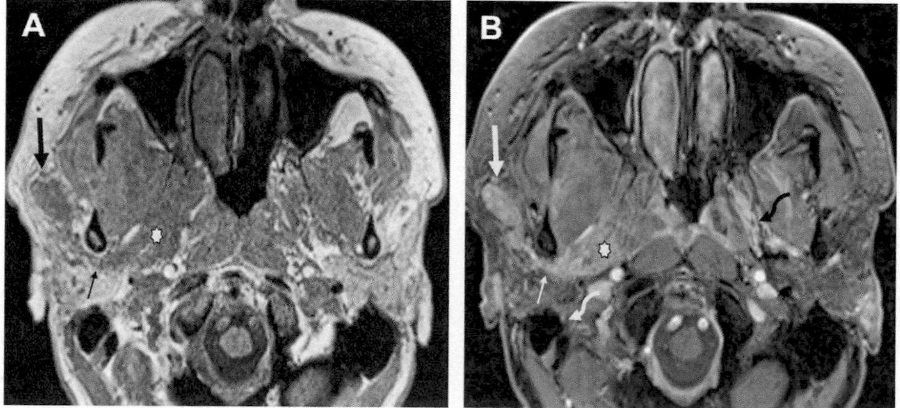

Fig. 7. PNS via the auriculotemporal nerve. Unenhanced (*A*) and contrast-enhanced fat-suppressed (*B*) T1W images show a right parotid primary malignant tumor (*thick arrows*) extending through the auriculotemporal nerve behind the mandibular angle (*thin arrows*). Bulky tumor is seen involving the mandibular nerve (V3) in the infratemporal fossa (*star*). The normal mandibular nerve (*black curved arrow* in *B*). Note that the right facial nerve (*curved white arrow*) is normal in the stylomastoid foramen.

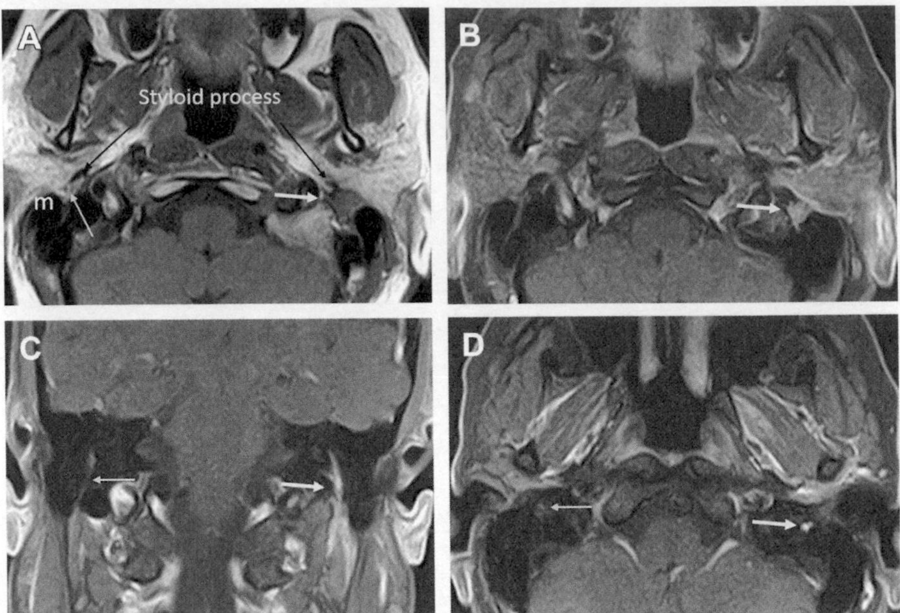

Fig. 8. PNS along the left facial nerve from high-grade parotid mucoepidermoid carcinoma. Axial T1W image through the stylomastoid foramen (*A*) shows an intermediate signal mass (*white thick arrow*). The normal right facial nerve can be seen as a tiny round structure (*white thin arrow*) surrounded by fat within the stylomastoid foramen, which is delimited by the mastoid tip (m) and the styloid process (*black arrow*). Axial fat-suppressed contrast-enhanced T1W (*B*) image shows enhancement of the mass filling the stylomastoid foramen. Coronal (*C*) and axial (*D*) fat-suppressed contrast-enhanced T1W images show extension of tumor along the mastoid segment of the facial nerve (*white thick arrows*). White thin arrows point to the normal right facial nerve.

symptoms, equipped with the anatomic knowledge, and prepared to carefully scrutinize the relevant CNs and their branches.

Knowing where the primary tumor is (or was) and the neural networks that serve that location is the most important first step to diagnosing PNS. Careful examination of the entire course of the nerve then should ensue. As a practical approach, critical examination of the PPF, stylomastoid foramen, and infratemporal fossa just below the foramen ovale would allow diagnosis of most PNS cases (**Box 1**).

A high-quality computed tomography (CT) scan, in the hands of an experienced radiologist, affords detection of most cases of PNS. Effacement of fat surrounding the CNs can readily be appreciated if proper attention to detail is given (**Fig. 9**). Findings observed on bone algorithm CT reconstructions such as foraminal destruction, erosion, or asymmetric widening, are frequently present in advanced cases and should alert radiologists to the presence of PNS (**Fig. 10**). CT is usually limited, however, in determining the extent of disease.

MR imaging is the method of choice for evaluation of PNS given its superior soft tissue contrast resolution. Many radiologists prefer high-resolution fat-saturated postcontrast images, although PNS may be identified on unenhanced T1-weighted (T1W) images as effacement of the fat pad present around each of these nerves. Some argue that non–fat-suppressed images may have better diagnostic utility because commonly present susceptibility artifacts at the skull base may obscure important foramina on fat-suppressed images.[20] Multiplanar reformations are also important in evaluation of the skull base foramina, as many are shown to better advantage in the coronal, sagittal, or oblique planes. Linear or curvilinear enhancement in a nerve distribution, infiltration of the PPF, lateral bowing of the cavernous sinus, or replacement of

Box 1
Key landmarks and contents for PNS

Key Landmarks	Nerve(s)
Pterygopalatine fossa	V2 and its branches
Stylomastoid foramen	Facial nerve
Foramen ovale	V3 and its branches
Foramen rotundum	V2 (maxillary nerve)
Cavernous sinus and Meckel cave	Cranial nerve V and its branches

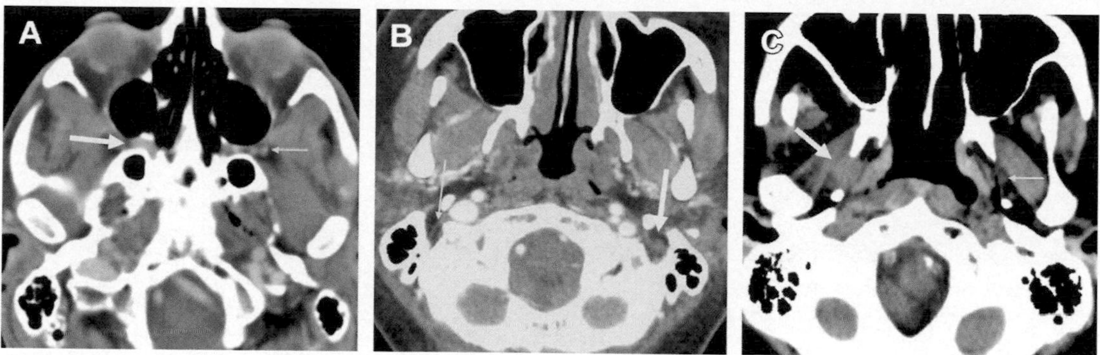

Fig. 9. Most PNS extending to the skull base will involve 1 of the 3 sites shown. Because most nerves are surrounded by fat, which can be easily identified on CT, a careful scrutiny of common locations of PNS at the skull base will allow identification of PNS in most cases. Relatively subtle nerve enlargement and effacement of surrounding fat in the right PPF (*A*), left stylomastoid foramen (*B*), and right infratemporal fossa just below the foramen ovale (*C*) indicate PNS in these patients with palate adenocystic carcinoma, parotid mucoepidermoid carcinoma and oral tongue SCC, respectively (*thick arrows*). Thin arrows point to the normal contralateral nerves.

the normally cerebrospinal fluid–filled Meckel cave can also be seen with PNS. PET CT, which is more sensitive than MR imaging and CT in detection of primary tumors and nodal metastases, is often inferior to MR imaging in diagnosis of PNS. This is related to the small volume of disease in PNS combined with limited spatial resolution of PET. Utility of diffusion-weighted imaging (DWI) is also

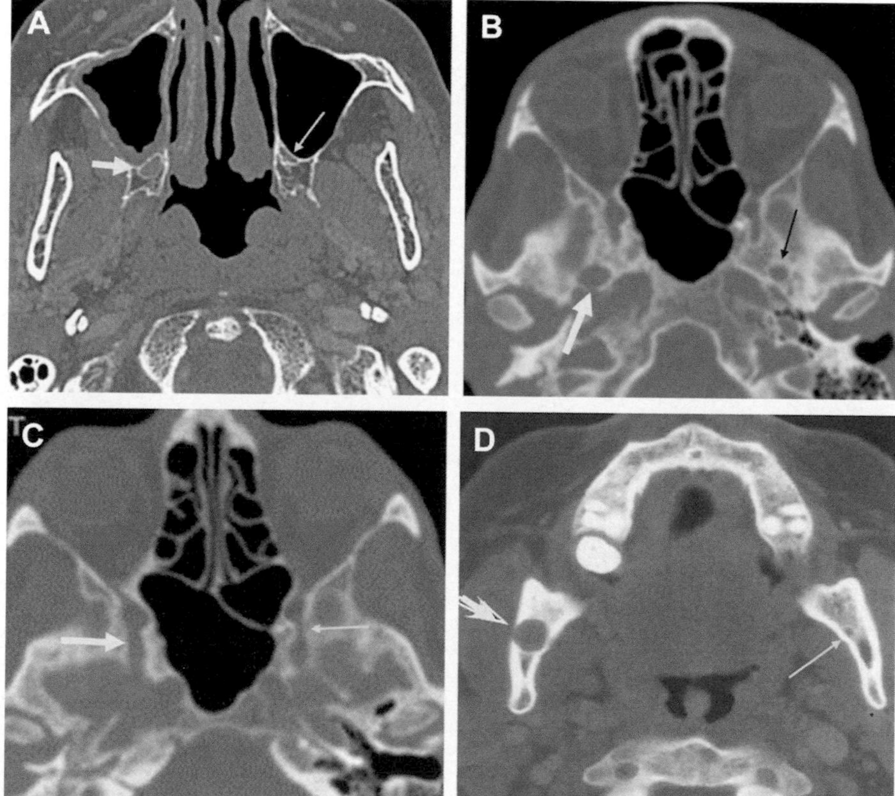

Fig. 10. Asymmetric enlargement of a nerve canal is a reliable CT finding of PNS in the proper clinical setting, although this is usually seen in advanced stages of disease. Axial CT images demonstrate enlargement of the right palatine nerve foramen (*A*), the right foramen ovale (*B*), the right foramen rotundum (*C*), and the right mandibular canal (*D*) (*thick arrows*) in separate patients with palatine nerve, mandibular nerve, maxillary nerve, inferior alveolar nerve PNS, respectively. Thin arrows point to the corresponding normal left sided nerves.

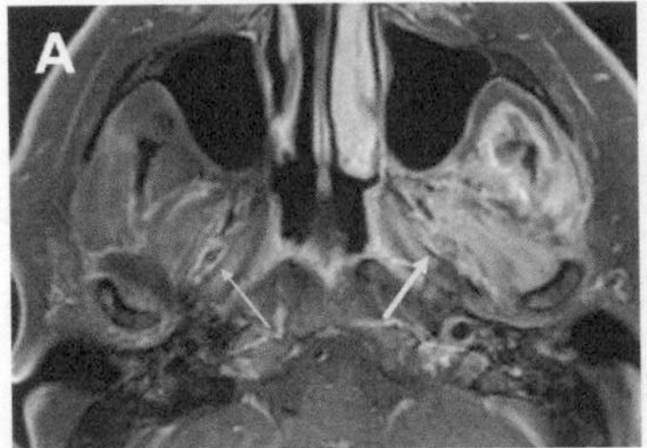

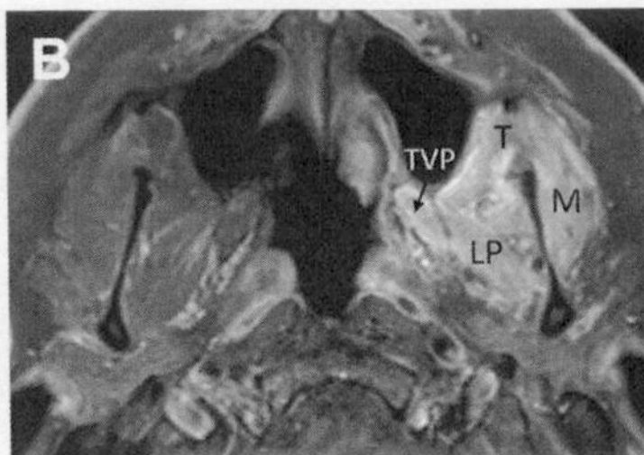

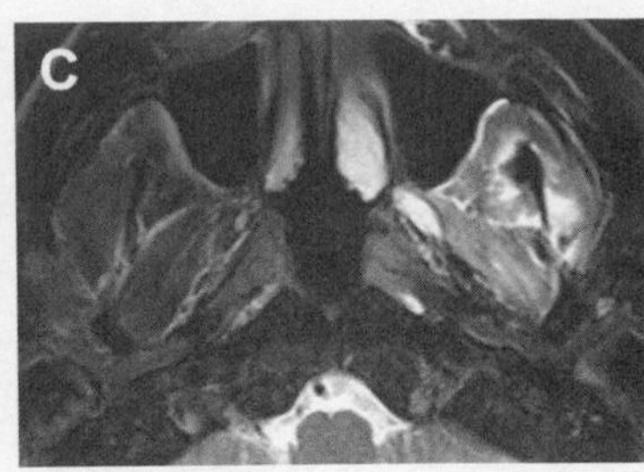

Fig. 11. Muscle denervation. Axial fat-suppressed contrast-enhanced T1W (*A, B*) and axial fat-suppressed T2W (*C*) images show enlarged and abnormally enhancing left mandibular nerve (V3) in the infratemporal fossa (*thick arrow* in *A*) compared with the normal right V3 (*thin arrow* in *A*) secondary to PNS from skin SCC. The muscles of mastication innervated by V3 show abnormal enhancement (*B*) and increased T2 signal (*C*). Other muscles innervated by the V3, not shown here, include medial pterygoid and tensor tympani muscles. LP, lateral pterygoid muscle; M, masseter muscle; T, temporalis muscle; TVP, tensor veli palatini muscle.

limited in diagnosis of PNS due to the common susceptibility artifacts at the skull base that create marked image distortion on DWI.

PITFALLS

Contrast enhancement is often seen in the perineural venous plexus surrounding the normal CNs and may mimic abnormal nerve enhancement, hence PNS. This is particularly problematic for small nerves and low-quality MR image studies that do not allow resolution of nerves from veins. The proximal greater superficial petrosal nerve, the geniculate ganglion, and the tympanic and mastoid segments of the facial nerve are common sites that may pose this problem. Comparison to the opposite site may be helpful, although venous plexus enhancement is often asymmetric as well. The perineural venous plexus may contribute to the enhancement seen involving the trigeminal ganglion and proximal portions of V1, V2, and V3. Crescent-shaped enhancement along the inferior aspect of the Meckel cave is routinely seen in the normal Gasserian ganglion on high-resolution MR imaging and should not be mistaken for PNS, which is usually larger and more rounded. Disruption of the blood-brain barrier secondary to ischemia, infarction, inflammation, trauma, or demyelination may result in segmental intracranial nerve enhancement, which should not be confused with PNS.[21] Last, as was mentioned before, understanding the imaging appearance of denervated muscles is important to avoid misinterpreting muscle enhancement seen in subacute denervation for tumor infiltration (**Fig. 11**). Other enhancing lesions besides PNS may involve the skull base foramina, such as meningiomas, schwannomas, or granulomatous diseases. Enlargement and enhancement of CNs also can be seen in rare demyelinating conditions and fungal or viral infections. Consideration of the clinical context is always key to the correct diagnosis.

SUMMARY

Identification of PNS has important therapeutic and prognostic implications and is critical for adequate staging and treatment planning. Careful attention to the neural pathways of the head and neck with routine evaluation of key landmarks can aid in early detection, appropriate therapy, and the best possible chance for cure.

REFERENCES

1. Fowler BZ, Crocker IR, Johnstone PA. Perineural spread of cutaneous malignancy to the brain: a review of the literature and five patients treated with stereotactic radiotherapy. Cancer 2005;103(10):2143–53.
2. Roh J, Muelleman T, Tawfik O, et al. Perineural growth in head and neck squamous cell carcinoma: a review. Oral Oncol 2015;51(1):16–23.
3. Hayat MJ, Howlader N, Reichman ME, et al. Cancer statistics, trends, and multiple primary cancer analyses from the Surveillance, Epidemiology, and End Results (SEER) Program. Oncologist 2007;12(1):20–37.
4. Barrett AW, Speight PM. Perineural invasion in adenoid cystic carcinoma of the salivary glands: a valid prognostic indicator? Oral Oncol 2009;45(11):936–40.
5. Kalina P, Bevilacqua P. Perineural extension of facial melanoma. Neuroradiology 2005;47(5):372–4.
6. Galloway TJ, Morris CG, Mancuso AA, et al. Impact of radiographic findings on prognosis for skin carcinoma with clinical perineural invasion. Cancer 2005;103(6):1254–7.
7. Woddruff WW, Yeates AE, McLendon RE. Perineural tumor extension to the cavernous sinus from superficial facial carcinoma: CT manifestations. Radiology 1986;161:395–9.

8. Banerjee TK, Gottschalk PG. Unusual manifestations of multiple cranial nerve palsies and mandibular metastasis in a patient with squamous cell carcinoma of the lip. Cancer 1984;53:346–8.
9. Cernea CR, Ferraz AR, de Castro IV, et al. Perineural invasion in aggressive skin carcinomas of the head and neck. ORL J Otorhinolaryngol Relat Spec 2009;71:21–6.
10. Ross AS, Whalen FM, Elenitsas R, et al. Diameter of involved nerves predicts outcomes in cutaneous squamous cell carcinoma with perineural invasion: an investigator-blinded retrospective cohort study. Dermatol Surg 2009;35(12):1859–66.
11. Panizza B, Warren T. Perineural invasion of head and neck skin cancer: diagnostic and therapeutic implications. Curr Oncol Rep 2013;15(2):128–33.
12. Binmadi NO, Basile JR. Perineural invasion in oral squamous cell carcinoma: a discussion of significance and review of the literature. Oral Oncol 2011;47(11):1005–10.
13. Gandour-Edwards R, Kapadia SB, Barnes L, et al. Neural cell adhesion molecule in adenoid cystic carcinoma invading the skull base. Otolaryngol Head Neck Surg 1997;117(5):453–8.
14. Iwamoto S, Odland PB, Piepkorn M, et al. Evidence that the p75 neurotrophin receptor mediates perineural spread of desmoplastic melanoma. J Am Acad Dermatol 1996;35:725–31.
15. Eneh A, Parsa K, Wright KW, et al. Pediatric adenoid cystic carcinoma of the lacrimal gland treated with intra-arterial cytoreductive chemotherapy. J AAPOS 2015;19(3):272–4.
16. Mardi K, Kaushal V, Uppal H. Cytodiagnosis of intracranial metastatic adenoid cystic carcinoma: spread from a primary tumor in the lacrimal gland. J Cytol 2011;28(4):200–2.
17. Shah K, Esmaeli B, Ginsberg LE. Perineural tumor spread along the nasociliary branch of the ophthalmic nerve: imaging findings. J Comput Assist Tomogr 2013;37(2):282–5.
18. Ginsberg LE, Demonte F. Palatal adenoid cystic carcinoma presenting as perineural spread to the cavernous sinus. Skull Base Surg 1998;8(1):39–43.
19. Carlson ML, Patel NS, Modest MC, et al. Occult temporal bone facial nerve involvement by parotid malignancies with perineural spread. Otolaryngol Head Neck Surg 2015;153(3):385–91.
20. Curtin H. Detection of perineural spread: fat suppression vs no fat suppression. AJNR Am J Neuroradiol 2004;25:1–3.
21. Maroldi R, Farina D, Borghesi A, et al. Perineural tumor spread. Neuroimaging Clin N Am 2008;18:413–29.

Imaging Evaluation and Treatment of Vascular Lesions at the Skull Base

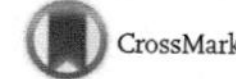

Gaurav Jindal, MD*, Timothy Miller, MD, Prashant Raghavan, MD, Dheeraj Gandhi, MD

KEYWORDS

- Paraganglioma • Juvenile nasopharyngeal angiofibroma • Cavernous carotid fistula
- Dural arteriovenous fistula • Preoperative embolization • Dissection

KEY POINTS

- Arterial and venous anomalies at the skull base tend to be asymptomatic; however, failure to recognize them can also have major clinical implications.
- Vascular tumors at the skull base may arise de novo in the skull base or originate in the orbits or sinonasal cavities and involve the skull base by extension.
- Preoperative embolization can be a useful and cost-effective adjunctive tool before surgical resection of hypervascular skull base tumors.
- Intracranial dural arteriovenous fistulas account for 10% to 15% of intracranial arteriovenous malformations, and they most commonly involve the wall of a major dural venous sinus.
- At the skull base, these lesions can involve the cavernous sinus and posterior fossa skull base veins.

INTRODUCTION

The skull base, which is composed of osseous, vascular, and cartilaginous elements, represents the interface between the cranial cavity and the face and neck. Major vascular and neural structures traverse the skull base through paired and unpaired foramina. Vascular skull base abnormalities generally arise owing to congenital abnormalities, consequent to dural arteriovenous shunts, trauma, or as a result of neoplastic transformation of vascular and nonvascular cellular elements.

A detailed discussion of all such abnormalities being beyond the scope of this review, we confine ourselves to a discussion of the more common, clinically relevant entities (**Box 1**), with an emphasis on those for which surgical and/or image-guided treatment options are available. A brief overview of the principles and practice of endovascular treatment strategies for some of these vascular lesions is also provided.

CONGENITAL VASCULAR VARIANTS OF THE SKULL BASE

The major vessels that traverse the skull base include the internal carotid and vertebral arteries and the internal jugular veins. In addition to these, meningeal branches of the external carotid artery (ECA) and emissary veins pass through the skull

Authors Disclosures: Dr G. Jindal has research grants from Stryker Neurovascular, Medtronic, Microvention, and Codman Neurovascular; Dr T. Miller has research grants from Stryker Neurovascular and Medtronic; Dr P. Raghavan has no relevant disclosures; Dr D. Gandhi has research grants from Stryker Neurovascular and Medtronic.

Department of Radiology, University of Maryland Medical Center, 22 South Greene Street, Baltimore, MD 21201, USA

* Corresponding author.

E-mail address: drjindal@gmail.com

Radiol Clin N Am 55 (2017) 151–166

http://dx.doi.org/10.1016/j.rcl.2016.08.003

0033-8389/17/© 2016 Elsevier Inc. All rights reserved.

Box 1
Vascular abnormalities at the skull base

- Congenital vascular variants of skull base
  - Aberrant internal carotid artery
  - Dehiscence of the internal carotid artery
  - Persistent carotid basilar anastomoses
  - Persistent stapedial artery
  - High riding jugular bulb, jugular bulb dehiscence, jugular bub diverticulum
  - Sigmoid sinus wall anomalies
  - Posterior fossa emissary veins
- Hypervascular tumors of the skull base
  - Paraganglioma
  - Metastases
  - Juvenile nasopharyngeal angiofibroma
  - Intratemporal benign vascular tumors
- Dural arteriovenous and carotid cavernous fistulae
- Arterial dissection and aneurysms

base. Congenital variants are more common in the venous circulation and rarely tend to be of clinical significance. Although arterial variations are less commonly encountered in routine practice, failure to recognize them can have major clinical implications.

Aberrant Internal Carotid Artery

The most common congenital arterial variant at the skull base is the aberrant internal carotid artery (ICA).[1] Here, the ICA deviates from its normal anteromedial course through the petrous carotid canal to extend laterally into the middle ear. This variant is thought to arise when the cervical portion of the ICA fails to develop normally, or regresses. Consequently, 2 embryonic vessels, the inferior tympanic and caroticotympanic arteries, enlarge to reconstitute the ICA at the level of the missing segment. Because the inferior tympanic artery normally extends laterally through the temporal bone and into the middle ear via the inferior tympanic canaliculus, the aberrant ICA follows a similar course.[1] On otologic examination, an aberrant ICA appears as a vascular, pulsatile, retrotympanic structure. On imaging, the aberrant ICA is evident as an absent or hypoplastic vertical segment of the carotid canal with a corresponding enlarged inferior tympanic canaliculus and canal and a reduced caliber aberrant ICA traversing through it.[2] On angiography, there is an enlarged tympanic branch of ascending pharyngeal artery and a more lateral and posterior route of the petrous part of ICA than usual with a focal pinched contour of the vessel.[3] Failure to recognize this entity may lead to inadvertent biopsy, because these lesions can be mistaken for a vascular tumor, with catastrophic consequences.

Dehiscence of the Internal Carotid Artery

Dehiscence of the ICA canal is an anatomic variant that generally does not merit treatment consideration. Dehiscence of the carotid canal may cause pulsatile tinnitus and can present as a vascular retrotympanic mass. On imaging, thinning or absence of the normal bony covering of the ICA will be present, typically near the basal turn of the cochlea.[4]

Persistent Carotid–Vertebrobasilar Anastomoses

Failure of vessels to regress during embryonic development results in various persistent carotid–vertebrobasilar anastomoses. The persistent trigeminal artery is the most common and most cephalic of these[5] with a reported prevalence of 0.1% to 0.6%.[6] This artery originates from the ICA after its exit from the carotid canal and anastomoses with the midbasilar artery. The part of the basilar artery that is caudal to the anastomosis with the trigeminal artery is usually hypoplastic. Associated anomalies include intracranial aneurysms, which are seen in approximately 14% of patients.[7] Additional variants of the persistent trigeminal artery are not discussed here. The persistent hypoglossal artery is the second most common carotid–vertebrobasilar artery anastomosis, with a prevalence of 0.02% to 0.10%.[8] The persistent hypoglossal artery originates from the ICA at the levels of the C1 through C3 vertebral bodies and courses through the hypoglossal canal to anastomose with the basilar artery; this artery does not pass through the foramen magnum. A persistent proatlantal intersegmental artery has been reported in the medical literature to originate from the common carotid artery bifurcation, ECA, or ICA at the levels of the C2 through C4 vertebral bodies; it joins the horizontal part of the vertebral artery in the suboccipital region.[9] The medical literature contains a few descriptions of a persistent otic artery arising from the petrous ICA within the carotid canal, coursing laterally through the internal auditory canal, and anastomosing with the proximal basilar artery.[9]

Persistent Stapedial Artery

Occasionally, a persistent stapedial artery (PSA) may be a cause of pulsatile tinnitus and a vascular retrotympanic mass.[4,10] This vessel can be identified as a small artery arising from the petrous ICA, which courses into the hypotypanum and through the obturator foramen, located between the crura of the stapes, to exit via the tympanic segment of the facial nerve canal and geniculate fossa.[4] In these instances, the PSA will supply the normal vascular territory of the middle meningeal artery, with the more proximal portion of the middle meningeal artery, as well as the foramen spinosum, being absent. A PSA may occur as an isolated anomaly or in conjunction with an aberrant ICA. On computed tomography (CT) scans, the combination of a soft tissue density overlying the cochlear promontory and traversing the oval window niche, a widened tympanic facial canal, and an absent foramen spinosum is typical of a PSA.[11,12]

High Riding Jugular Bulb, Jugular Bulb Dehiscence, and Jugular Bulb Diverticulum

A high riding jugular bulb is distinguished from an asymmetrically large jugular bulb by its dome reaching a plane superior to the internal acoustic meatus.[11,12] A high riding jugular bulb has an intact thin bone, the sigmoid plate, separating it from the middle ear cavity. This is evident on high-resolution CT scans.[11,12] If the bony plate is thin or deficient, the anomaly is termed a dehiscent jugular bulb. When the bulb protrudes into the middle ear cavity, it may be evident as a retrotympanic vascular mass.[11,12] As opposed to aggressive hypervascular tumors in the region of the jugular bulb discussed below, the high-resolution CT hallmark of these anomalies is the smooth, intact osseous margin of the jugular foramen.[13]

Sigmoid Sinus Wall Anomalies

Although perhaps not entirely congenital in origin, these are an increasingly recognized diagnosis in the workup of pulse synchronous tinnitus. The spectrum of sigmoid sinus wall anomalies includes thinning/dehiscence of the sigmoid plate mentioned, sigmoid sinus diverticulum formation with a focal protrusion of vascular elements into the mastoid air cells, and ectasia with smooth bulging of the sigmoid sinus into the mastoid air cells without a focal diverticulum. There seems to be a strong association between high body mass index, female gender, and features of idiopathic intracranial hypertension and the incidence of these anomalies.

VASCULAR TUMORS OF THE SKULL BASE

Vascular tumors may arise de novo in the skull base or originate in the orbits or sinonasal cavities and involve the skull base by extension. Of the former, paragangliomas are the most frequent. In the latter category, juvenile nasopharyngeal angiofibromas (JNAs) are perhaps the most common. Other tumors that may manifest significant vascularity include benign vascular tumors such as meningiomas and hemangiomas of the temporal bone and more aggressive processes such as endolymphatic sac tumors and hypervascular metastases from renal or thyroid primary malignancies, among others.

Paraganglioma

Paragangliomas, also known as glomus tumors, are slow-growing neuroendocrine tumors that can be located in the head and neck, adrenal gland (pheochromocytoma), spinal regions, and other locations.[14] They account for 0.6% head and neck neoplasms[14,15] and are located at the common carotid bifurcation (glomus caroticum), along the vagus nerve (glomus vagale), the jugular foramen (glomus jugulare), and in the middle ear (glomus tympanicum). About 80% of all paragangliomas are either carotid body tumors or glomus jugulare tumors.[16] Women are affected more often than men, usually between 40 and 60 years of age.[14,17] They may be familial and multicentric, and may manifest as unilateral or bilateral lesions, either synchronously or metachronously.[18,19] Malignant behavior, that is, metastasis to different sites, is seen in 2% to 10% of cases.[20,21]

Glomus jugulare tumors arise within the jugular foramen along the jugular bulb, from paraganglia located along Jacobson's nerve, a branch of the glossopharyngeal nerve, or along Arnold's nerve, a branch of the vagus nerve. Glomus tympanicum tumors often manifest as a small, discrete mass arising along Jacobson nerve in the mucosa covering the cochlear promontory.[11,12,22] Clinical manifestations of skull base paragangliomas include pulsatile tinnitus, conductive hearing loss, vertigo, hoarseness, and aural pain or discharge. A retrotympanic vascular mass may be visible on otoscopic examination. Local soft tissue and bony invasion is common for skull base, jugulotympanic lesions. Regional lymph node involvement and distant metastases are rare.

Contrast-enhanced MR imaging and CT scans depict these highly vascular, soft tissue masses well.[23–25] Angiography is also very sensitive in the detection of these lesions (**Fig. 1**).[26] CT imaging is excellent for evaluating the integrity of the temporal bone and aids in defining regional surgical anatomy. A moth-eaten, permeative pattern of osteolysis of the margins of the jugular foramen is the hallmark of glomus jugulare tumors. Destruction of the adjacent carotid crest, osseous jugular

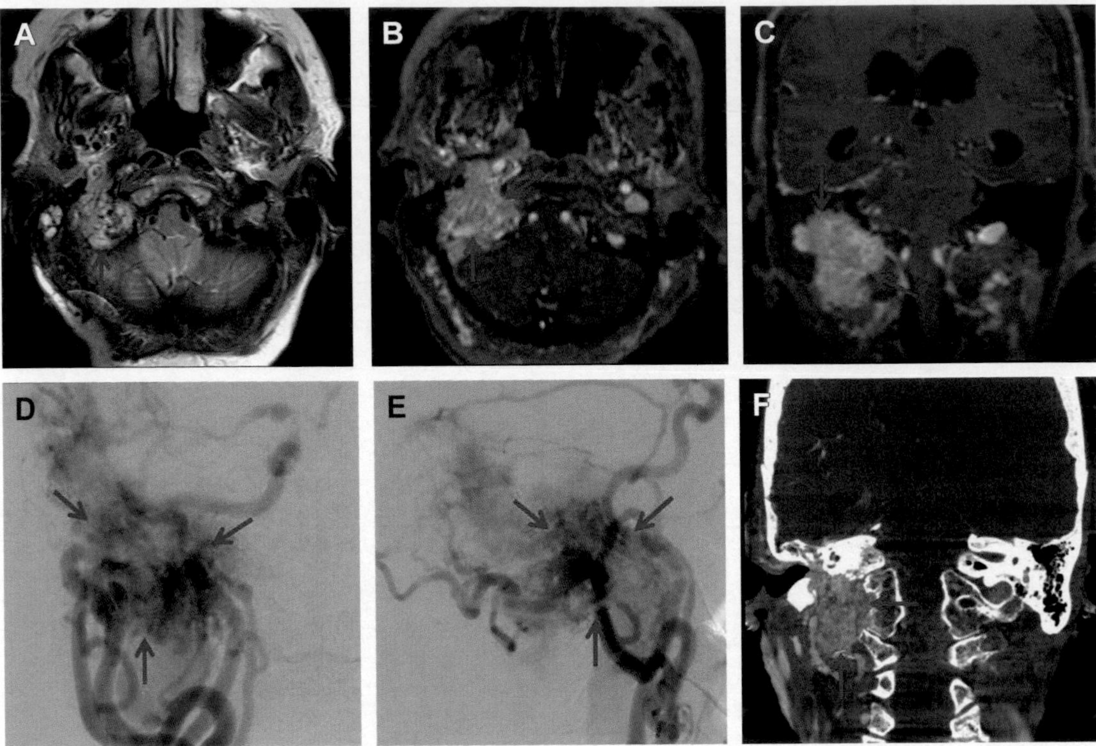

Fig. 1. A 90-year-old woman presented with chronic, progressive headaches. T2-Weighted axial MR imaging (*A*) demonstrates a heterogeneous right skull base mass with a "salt and pepper" appearance centered at the right jugular foramen (*red arrows*). The mass demonstrates marked enhancement (*red arrows*) after gadolinium administration on axial (*B*) and coronal (*C*) T1-weighted MR images, with involvement of a large portion of the right temporal bone. Catheter angiography demonstrates prominent tumor blush (*red arrows*) with arterial supply from multiple enlarged right external carotid artery branches (*D, E*). Flat panel rotational computed tomography scans performed at the same time (*F*) demonstrates the associated bony destruction with extension of the lesion into the right middle ear cavity (*red arrows*). Findings are consistent with a glomus jugulare tumor.

spine, and surrounding bony labyrinth can be seen.[27,28] These tumors initially spread superiorly. Invasion of the hypotympanum, mesotympanum, ossicles, and sinus tympani is common. Inferior spread of the tumor results in infiltration of the internal jugular vein and infratemporal fossa. Laterally, the tumor may destroy and infiltrate the facial nerve and its canal.[11,12] The tumor may extend posteriorly directly through the petrous bone,[11,12,22] medially via the inframeatal route directly into the cerebellopontine angle, or via the infralabyrinthine–inframeatal route into the cerebellomedullary angle.[22] Intracranial extension occurs in 15% to 20%[29,30] of cases, although many remain extradural. Glomus tympanicum tumors generally present as small sessile enhancing lesions located on the promotory. Ossicular encasement, spread into the bony labyrinth, and, rarely, invasion of the mastoid air cells and Eustachian canal with subsequent spread into the nasopharynx may occur.[11,12,27,31–33] The radiologist must be aware that what seems to be a "glomus tympanicum" clinically may actually represent the cranial extent of a glomus jugulare. The latter may invade the middle ear cavity using the canaliculi of Arnold's and Jacobson's nerves or via hypotympanic air cells. The jugular foramen must always be carefully inspected when the inferior margin of a glomus tympanicum is not well-delineated.

Paragangliomas typically exhibit low signal intensity on T1-weighted images and high signal intensity on T2-weighted sequences. Intense enhancement is typically seen.[34,35] Multiple foci of signal loss, owing to intratumoral vessels may be present and evident on all MR imaging sequences.[34–36] The classic "salt-and-pepper" appearance is owing to multiple signal voids (pepper) and hyperintense foci (salt) from slow flow and/or hemorrhage.[34,36] In addition to providing superior definition of location, extent, and characterization of paragangliomas, MR imaging also better demonstrates tumor involvement of the ICA and internal jugular vein compared with that seen with CT imaging.[36]

Digital subtraction angiography remains the most reliable preoperative imaging study for assessing vascular invasion. The typical angiographic appearance of a paraganglioma is that of a hypervascular mass[37] with enlarged feeding arteries, intense tumor blush, and early draining veins[13] supplied predominantly, in the case of glomus jugulare tumors, by the ascending pharyngeal artery. This artery supplies the inferomedial portions of the tumor at the jugular foramen and the cochlear promontory, whereas supply to the posterolateral compartment arises from the stylomastoid artery a branch of the posterior auricular artery or occipital artery, or from other branches of these arteries. The anterior compartment is often supplied by the anterior tympanic artery, whereas the superior compartment receives supply from middle meningeal and accessory meningeal arteries.[26] Arterial supply may also be recruited from other ECA branches or from the ICA or vertebral arteries.[22,38] Parenchymal branches from the cerebellar arteries may supply an intradural component of a glomus jugulare tumor.[22,26] In discrete glomus tympanicum tumors, the inferior tympanic artery is the most common vascular supply.[39]

Indium-111 octreotide is the agent of choice for nuclear medicine imaging of paragangliomas. Octreotide is a somatostatin analog that binds to receptors on paraganliomas and is tagged with indium-111. Single photon emission computed tomographic images are obtained at 4 hours after intravenous injection of this tracer. Imaging can be repeated at 24 hours if needed. A focal area of intense early radiotracer uptake corresponds to the location of the paraganglioma on the 4-hour study. Indium-111 octreotide scanning is useful in the early detection of lesions in patients at high risk (e.g., those with a history of familial paragangliomas), differentiation of a paraganglioma from a nerve sheath tumor (which is not octreotide avid), detection of multicentric or metastatic paragangliomas, and distinguishing scar from recurrent or residual tumor after surgery.[40]

The differential diagnosis of masses in the jugular foramen includes jugular schwannomas and meningiomas. Nerve sheath tumors of the jugular foramen arise either from the lower cranial nerves or the spinal nerves. Unlike paragangliomas, these lesions are sharply demarcated and surrounded by smooth osseous margins. They may demonstrate a dumbbell shape with intracranial and extracranial components.[41] Larger lesions are heterogeneous and contain areas of cystic degeneration. These lesions are not as highly vascular and, as a result, do not characteristically have internal flow voids.[41] The jugular foramen meningioma is a dural-based, well-circumscribed mass with areas of calcification. On high-resolution CT scans, the adjacent cortex demonstrates sclerosis, remodeling, or erosion in rare cases.[42] Digital subtraction angiography usually reveals that jugular foramen meningiomas are hypovascular or mildly vascular.[42]

Surgery is the treatment of choice for skull base paragangliomas, although resection can be challenging owing to the complexity of the tumor location and anatomy as well as robust tumor vascularity.[43,44] Complications are not uncommon owing to the large number of sensitive structures in the region and include, in addition to blood loss, cranial nerve deficits and cerebrospinal fluid/endolymphatic fluid leak. Recurrence and local invasion are common, occurring in 40% to 50% of cases.[14] Although most cervical paragangliomas (e.g., carotid body tumors) are considered relatively radioresistant, base of skull paragangliomas are radiosensitive, and, thus, large inoperable tumors or tumors in poor surgical candidates are often treated with radiotherapy.[30,45]

Metastatic Tumors

Vascular bony metastases, such as from renal cell carcinoma or thyroid cancer, can appear very similar to paragangliomas, although metastases may not have internal flow voids or a "salt-and-pepper" appearance and do not follow the usual routes of spread seen in paragangliomas.[13] Other neoplastic lesions in this region include primary bone lesions such as multiple myeloma, lymphoma, and Langerhans cell histiocytosis.[7] The differential diagnostic considerations for a middle ear mass include neoplasms such cholesteatoma, cholesterol granulomas, squamous cell carcinoma, endolymphatic sac tumor, choristoma, adenocarcinoma, and sarcomas.[46]

Juvenile Nasopharyngeal Angiofibroma

JNAs are rare, benign but locally aggressive vascular tumors. They occur almost exclusively in males and usually in adolescence. JNAs are thought to arise from the lateral margin of the posterior nasal cavity, adjacent the sphenopalatine foramen. The presentation is typically with obstructive symptoms such as sinusitis and chronic otomastoiditis and/or epistaxis,[47] which can lead to severe blood loss. Anosmia, proptosis, facial/temporal swelling, and extraocular muscle palsies may be seen. On endoscopic examination, the mass may be seen as a reddish-blue, gray mass; biopsy can be catastrophic owing to intense tumor vascularity.[48]

These masses usually present when they have reached considerable size, frequently with extension medially into the nasopharynx and paranasal sinuses and laterally into the pterygopalatine fossa and infratemporal fossa.[49] JNA can spread superiorly into the sphenoid sinus, orbit, cavernous sinus, sella, and middle cranial fossa. Occasionally, the greater wing of the sphenoid bone may be eroded, which can expose the dura mater. A classification scheme for these tumors was devised by Fisch[50] and is summarized in **Table 1**.

On imaging, typically a lobulated, nonencapsulated soft tissue mass is seen centered in a widened sphenopalatine foramen. The pterygomaxillary fissure may be widened. There may be bowing the posterior wall of the maxillary antrum anteriorly. CT scanning is particularly useful at delineating local bony changes related to JNA. The tumor generally does not invade bone, but does cause bony erosion and remodeling.[51] This feature may be helpful in differentiating JNA from other more aggressive lesions such as nasopharyngeal carcinoma or other malignant tumors in this region. Avid contrast enhancement is seen, reflecting prominent tumor vascularity.[51]

MR imaging best demonstrates the soft tissue extent of tumor, including intracranial and/or intraorbital extension of disease, and is useful for differentiation of obstructed sphenoid sinus secretions versus soft tissue mass.[34,52] The mass is often of intermediate signal intensity on T1-weighted images and heterogeneous signal intensity on T2-weighted images. There can be flow voids from vascular channels within the mass and a "salt-and-pepper" appearance, as a result of flow voids and intrinsic hyperintensities, similar to paragangliomas described.[34] There is prominent enhancement after contrast administration (**Fig. 2**). Differential diagnostic considerations on imaging include angiomatous polyp, a variant of the sinonasal polyp, rhabdomyosarcoma, nasopharyngeal carcinoma, nasopharyngeal teratoma, in addition to other tumors.

Angiography is useful in defining the feeding vessels as well as in preoperative embolization planning.[53] An early appearing, intense vascular blush is seen that persists until the late venous phase. Arteriovenous shunting can be seen. The arterial supply is often from internal maxillary artery branches, such as the palatine and sphenoidal arteries, anterior ascending pharyngeal artery branches, and accessory meningeal artery.[53] As the tumor grows, there can be supply from facial artery branches such as the ascending palatine artery, ethmoidal branches of the ophthalmic artery, and ICA branches such as the mandibulovidian/pterygovaginal artery, inferolateral trunk, meningohypophyseal trunk, and other petrous ICA segment branches.[54] Tumors that cross the midline may have a bilateral arterial supply.[54]

Surgical resection is the treatment of choice and is usually performed with preoperative embolization to aid in hemostasis during surgery. Irradiation may be an option if surgery is not possible or only incomplete resection is expected, such as with extensive intracranial spread of disease.[52,53,55]

Table 1
Fisch classification for juvenile nasopharyngeal angiofibromas

Type	Characteristics
I	Tumor limited to the nasopharynx and nasal cavity without significant bone destruction.
II	Tumor invades the pterygopalatine fossa or sinuses with bone destruction.
IIIa	Tumor invades the infratemporal fossa or orbit without intracranial spread.
IIIb	Tumor invades the infratemporal fossa or orbit without intracranial extradural (parasellar) involvement.
IVa	Intracranial intradural tumor without infiltration of cavernous sinus, pituitary fossa, or optic chiasm.
IVb	Intracranial intradural tumor with infiltration of cavernous sinus, pituitary fossa, or optic chiasm.

Image-guided treatment of vascular skull base tumors

As early as 1975, preoperative embolization has been advocated as a useful and cost-effective adjunctive tool before surgical resection of hypervascular skull base tumors for reduction of intraoperative blood loss, intraoperative time, and recovery time, in addition to affording better visualization of surgical planes.[22,43,56–64] This is especially true for skull base paragangliomas and JNAs.[59,60,62] Murphy and Brackmann[59] described a reduction in intraoperative blood loss from 2769 mL to 1122 mL using preoperative embolization in skull base glomus jugulare tumors. In another series, the mean blood loss for glomus jugulare and glomus vagale tumors with skull base extension was between 450 mL and 494 mL after preoperative embolization.[60] Moulin and colleagues[62] demonstrated a significant difference in blood loss between embolized and

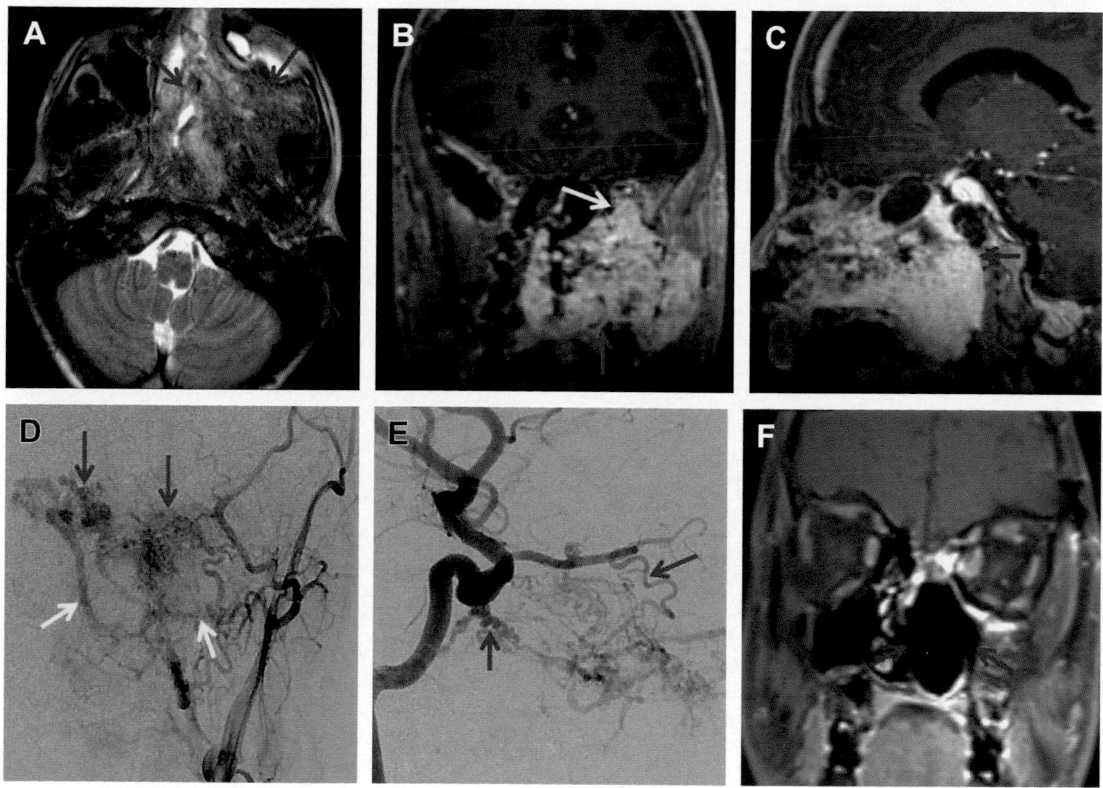

Fig. 2. A 15 year-old boy presented with a reported history of epistaxis and nasal discharge. The patient reportedly underwent biopsy at an outside hospital for a nasal mass. T2-Weighted axial MR imaging (*A*) demonstrates a heterogeneous right skull base mass (*red arrows*) centered in the left nasal cavity and infratemporal fossa. The lesion demonstrates avid enhancement after gadolinium administration on coronal (*B*) and sagittal (*C*) T1-weighted MR images, with extension into the left orbital apex (*yellow arrow* in *B*), as well as the oropharynx and nasopharynx (*arrows* in *C*). On left external carotid (*D*) and left internal carotid (*E*) catheter angiography, the lesion demonstrates prominent vascular blush (*red arrows* in *D*) with arterial supply from enlarged branches of the left external carotid artery branches (*yellow arrows* in *D*). Additional arterial supply arises from branches of the left inferolateral trunk and ophthalmic artery (*arrows* in *E*). Findings are consistent with juvenile angiofibroma. The patient subsequently underwent transarterial polyvinyl alcohol particle embolization followed by surgical resection, with no significant residual tumor on postoperative gadolinium enhanced MR imaging (*arrows* in *F*).

nonembolized surgical groups for JNA. Oka and colleagues[63] demonstrated that preoperative embolization improved clinical outcomes in skull base meningiomas. Although not a report on skull base lesions, a recent metaanalysis on cervical carotid body tumors demonstrated significant improvement in blood loss and surgical time after preoperative embolization.[45] Tumors larger than 3 cm may be ideally suited for embolization,[65] and the benefit is less clear for embolization of small lesions. However, very large tumors can have collateral blood supply and/or supply from pial branch arteries, which may render embolization relatively less useful.[63,66] Other skull base tumors that may require preoperative embolization include hypervascular metastases, esthesioneuroblastomas, schwannomas, rhabdomyosarcomas, plasmacytomas, chordomas, and hemangiopericytomas.[61]

The goal of tumor embolization is to selectively occlude ECA feeders through intratumoral deposition of embolic material. Embolization is ideally performed 24 to 72 hours before surgical resection to allow maximal thrombosis of the occluded vessels and prevent recanalization of the occluded arteries or formation of collateral arterial channels.[53,61] Since modern techniques have been adopted, these tumors have been more readily embolized with embolic agents such as polyvinyl alcohol particles, liquid embolic agents such as *N*-butyl cyanoacrylate (n-BCA), or "glue," and ethylene vinyl alcohol copolymer, gelatin sponge, and coils.[67–69] Most arteries can be embolized by using polyvinyl alcohol particles, typically varying in size from 150 to 550 μm.[57] Endovascular treatment consists of performing detailed cerebral angiography, including selective injections of the ICA and the ECA to assess for dangerous anastomoses between the ECA and ICA and/or vertebral artery branches. If critical anastomoses are present, the anastomotic connection can first be occluded with coils followed by particulate and/or liquid embolization. Notably, anastomotic pathways may not be evident on initial angiography but may reveal themselves only as changes in regional blood flow occur during embolization.[61] One should also be aware of the risk of injury to the cranial nerves and the skin.[61] The stylomastoid branch of the occipital artery and proximal posterior middle meningeal artery branches, for example, supply cranial nerve VII. The neuromeningeal trunk of the ascending pharyngeal artery supplies cranial nerves IX through XII. The ophthalmic artery can have anastomotic connections to the internal maxillary artery, middle meningeal artery, superficial temporal artery, and facial artery.[56,70] During embolization of a JNA, for example, one must take great care to avoid central retinal artery occlusion attributable to potential communication with the ophthalmic artery from ethmoidal arterial or other collaterals.[61]

Direct percutaneous puncture under fluoroscopic guidance, CT, or sonography has also been described to embolize many different types of tumors. Advantages of this technique include direct and easy access to the vascular tumor bed that is not hindered by arterial tortuosity, the small size of arterial feeders, atherosclerotic disease, or catheter induced vasospasm.[61] This method was initially reported for tumors in which transarterial embolization was technically impossible owing to the small size of the arterial feeders or in cases in which the risks of such an approach were considered too high.[71] Excellent results obtained by this technique have extended its application to smaller and less complex tumors.[72] Complete devascularization of the tumor can be obtained with decreased risk to the patient by direct tumoral injection of ethylene vinyl alcohol copolymer or n-BCA.[71,72]

Minor complications of preoperative embolization include postembolization fever and ear pain. They are attributed to tumor ischemia, are transient, and suggest successful treatment.[56,73] Embolization-related local edema may be present immediately after the procedure, although this is generally not severe enough to hinder surgical management.[37,65] Serious complications occur in less than 2% of patients.[71,74] These are usually related to particle reflux, poor technique, and/or nonvisualization of dangerous anastomoses resulting in transient or permanent neurologic deficits, including cranial nerve palsies and blindness in the setting of central retinal artery occlusion. Stroke may occur if embolic material travels into the vertebrobasilar system or ICA via existing anastomoses between the ECA and ICA or vertebral artery.[75] Complications can be minimized by meticulous evaluation of the preembolization angiogram and/or provocative testing, such as with lidocaine for facial nerve supply or with amytal if concerned about the possibility of nontarget embolization.[56,76]

SKULL BASE ARTERIOVENOUS FISTULAE

Intracranial dural arteriovenous fistulas (dAVFs) are sporadic pathologic communications between dural arteries and dural venous sinuses, meningeal veins, cortical veins, or a combination of veins. They account for 10% to 15% of intracranial arteriovenous malformations.[77–79] The pathogenesis of dural arteriovenous fistulas is not yet well-understood, but they are considered by most authors to be acquired lesions, after thrombophlebitis or head trauma.[78,80,81] They most commonly involve the wall of a major dural venous sinus such as the transverse, sigmoid, cavernous, or superior sagittal sinus.[82,83] We confine our discussion in this report to dAVFs that occur at the skull base, including cavernous carotid and posterior fossa skull base fistulae.

Patients with dAVF may be asymptomatic or experience symptoms ranging from mild, nonaggressive symptoms such as tinnitus to aggressive symptoms such as neurologic deficits from intracranial hemorrhage.[84–86] The venous drainage pattern of dAVFs is the most predictive factor of aggressive symptoms.[82] dAVFs that drain in a retrograde fashion via leptomeningeal cortical venous channels show a relatively high rate of aggressive symptoms.[87–89] Although several classification systems have been developed to grade the risks of dural AVFs, those devised by Cognard and colleagues[86] and Borden and colleagues[90] are the most widely used. Grading dAVFs is based on the direction of venous flow within the dural venous sinus (anterograde vs retrograde) and/or the presence of cortical venous reflux.[90] Regardless of symptomatology, the natural history of dAVFs can be progressive, and intervention aimed at closure of the fistula should be considered in many cases—either endovascularly, surgically, or radiosurgically.[82]

Cavernous Carotid Fistula

Cavernous carotid fistulas (CCF) are abnormal communications between the carotid circulation and the cavernous sinus. The most common symptoms of CCF are ocular symptoms such as conjunctival injection, chemosis, proptosis, and extraocular muscle palsies caused by cranial neuropathy and/or anterior venous drainage.[91] Aggressive neurologic symptoms such as intracranial hemorrhage are extremely rare because of the often benign venous drainage pattern, but can occur in association with cortical venous reflux or drainage deep venous.[92,93]

CCFs can be classified as direct or indirect, which are distinct conditions with different etiologies. Direct CCFs are often secondary to trauma and, as such, are seen most commonly in young, male patients. The presentation is acute, and symptoms develop rapidly. Indirect CCFs have a predilection for the postmenopausal female patient, and the onset of symptoms is often insidious. Indirect CCFs are supplied by branches of the ECA and/or ICA branches, and are thought to occur secondary to cavernous sinus thrombosis with revascularization. Other predisposing factors seem to be pregnancy, changes from surgery in the region, and invasive sinusitis.[94] A method of classification is outlined in **Table 2**.[94]

Cross-sectional imaging findings include proptosis and enlarged superior ophthalmic veins; extraocular muscle enlargement and orbital edema are possible. Intracranial hemorrhage may be seen rarely from rupture of an arterialized or aneurysmal cortical vein.[95] Digital subtraction angiography often demonstrates rapid shunting from the ICA to the cavernous sinus in direct lesions and similar but less rapid shunting in indirect lesions. The draining veins are often enlarged; drainage is often into the superior ophthalmic vein, other ophthalmic veins, facial vein, inferior petrosal sinus, superior petrosal sinus, ptyergoid venous plexus, the contralateral cavernous sinus and contralateral veins, and occasionally the sphenoparietal sinus and cortical veins (**Fig. 3**).[96]

Table 2
Classification scheme of cavernous carotid fistula

Type	Characteristics
A	Direct connection between ICA and CS
B	Dural shunts between ICA branches and CS
C	Dural shunts between meningeal branches of the ECA and CS
D	Combination of types B and C

Abbreviations: CS, cavernous sinus; ECA, external carotid artery; ICA, internal carotid artery.

Posterior Skull Base Arteriovenous Fistula

Fifty percent of intracranial dAVFs occur in the posterior fossa and usually involve the transverse or sigmoid sinus,[79] although they may also be located along the tentorium and in the region of the hypoglossal canal and foramen magnum.

Dural AVFs in the region of the hypoglossal canal (HCDAVFs) represent a rare subtype of dAVFs involving the anterior condylar confluence and/or the anterior condylar vein.[97,98] They have been previously referred to as dAVFs of the inferior petrosal sinus, jugular bulb, marginal sinus, skull base, or foramen magnum.[97,99] Distinguishing HCDAVF from other skull base dAVFs, such as these or such as posterior condylar canal or inferior petroclival vein fistulas may be challenging and requires a thorough knowledge of the complex venous here anatomy.[100,101]

The anterior condylar confluence is located at the extracranial aperture of the hypoglossal canal at the skull base and, because of its connection to a rich venous network, represents a major venous cross-road. It originates at the junction of the jugular bulb and inferior petrosal sinus and extends into the hypoglossal canal. The anterior condylar vein traverses the hypoglossal canal and, along with other emissary veins, joins the inferior petrosal sinus and internal jugular vein to the intradural sinuses, suboccipital venous plexus, vertebral or paravertebral veins, marginal sinus, basilar/clival venous plexus, and the internal and external vertebral venous plexus.[100] Notably, the venous networks here can communicate with intracranial pial and perimedullary veins of the posterior fossa. This is particularly relevant in this region, because craniocervical junction dAVFs with subarachnoid venous drainage have a higher risk of intracranial hemorrhage in comparison with similar lesions elsewhere.[102]

Owing to the complexity of venous networks here, HCDAVFs may present with a variety of clinical presentations that may mimic fistulas in other locations such as the cavernous sinus. These dAVFs most often present with pulse synchronous tinnitus,[100] but can also present with orbital symptoms, dizziness, hypoglossal nerve palsy, myelopathy, and intracranial hemorrhage.[103,104] As with other cranial dAVFs, the anatomy of the venous outflow is the critical factor in patient presentation and treatment planning.

Cross-sectional imaging with CT or MR angiography demonstrates an arterialized venous pouch corresponding to a dilated anterior condylar confluence and/or anterior condylar vein; dilated and tortuous pial or perimedullary veins and intraosseous fistula components may exist. Standard

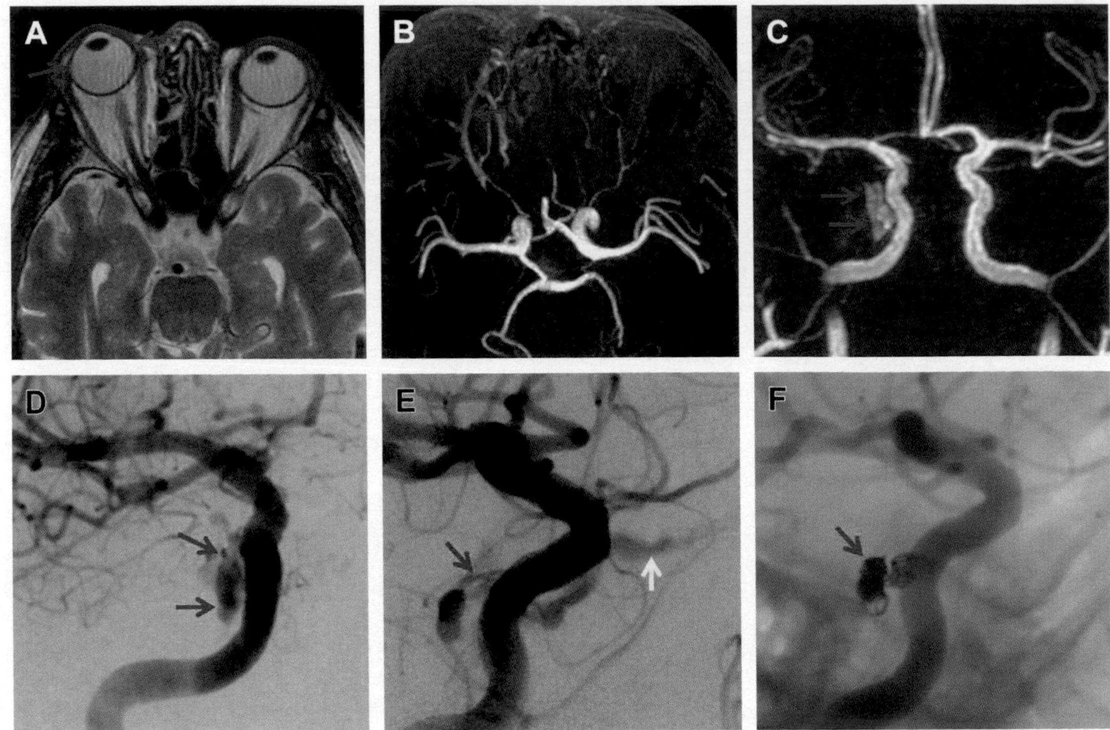

Fig. 3. A 70-year-old man presented with right-sided proptosis, chemosis, and ophthalmoplegia. High resolution T2-weighted axial MR imaging (*A*) demonstrates the right-sided proptosis (*red arrows*). On 3-dimensional time of flight MR angiography (*B*), there is abnormal flow-related enhancement in the right superior ophthalmic vein (*red arrows*), and reconstructed maximum intensity projection images from gadolinium bolus MR angiography (*C*) shows abnormal early filling of the right cavernous sinus (*red arrows*). Catheter angiography (*D, E*) confirms the presence of an indirect dural arteriovenous fistula involving the right cavernous sinus (*red arrows D*). Arterial supply is via small meningeal branches arising from the right internal carotid artery (*red arrow* in *E*), with retrograde opacification of the right superior ophthalmic vein (*yellow arrow* in *E*). The patient subsequently underwent successful transvenous coil embolization of the lesion (*F*).

MR imaging is not sensitive in detecting dAVFs and may fail to demonstrate an HCDAVF entirely.[105,106] Conventional digital subtraction angiography, especially if coupled with 3-dimensional rotational angiography and C-arm cone-beam CT imaging, remains the gold standard for characterizing the fistulous location, arterial supply, and venous drainage routes. Angiography additionally allows for the assessment of arterial and venous access to the site of fistula, which is important for treatment planning.

Endovascular treatment of skull base arteriovenous fistula

Cavernous sinus dAVFs that do not regress or those with progressive symptoms and dangerous drainage patterns require treatment. Treatment options include irradiation, transarterial embolization and transvenous embolization (TVE). TVE is considered the first-line curative therapy in cavernous sinus dAVF as well as direct CCF.[107] Transarterial embolization may be used in combination with TVE for direct CCF to access and embolize the venous outflow if the communication between the artery and vein allows for catheterization. The embolic material of choice varies depending on lesion anatomy and operator preference. Detachable coils for embolization of the cavernous sinus and relevant venous outflow tracts have the advantage of precise, controlled delivery. The approach in most cases of TVE is via the inferior petrosal sinus into the cavernous sinus. Other common approaches involve facial venous or superficial temporal venous access, as well as surgical superior ophthalmic venous access.[108–110] A transcontralateral cavernous sinus approach may also be considered. Outlets of cavernous sinus reflux to dangerous venous drainage systems, such as cortical and deep cerebral veins, and ophthalmic veins, should be occluded. Incomplete or inadequate embolization of such venous outlets could increase venous hypertension. Moreover, the low-risk drainage patterns of dAVFs may develop into high-risk patterns with progressive thrombosis and/or iatrogenic restriction of venous outlets.[111]

The treatment strategy for HCDAVFs is also determined by the risk of aggressive symptoms and the efficacy of each technique, which depends on lesion accessibility and the skill of the endovascular specialist and neurosurgeon. TVE is an effective treatment of HCDAVFs,[97,101] although the complex drainage patterns and connections can prove challenging in some cases. A fistula located along the posterior rim of the foramen magnum may be accessed surgically as well.[100] Most of these lesions are supplied by the ascending pharyngeal artery, and although transarterial embolization is feasible in select cases, great care must be taken during embolizing this

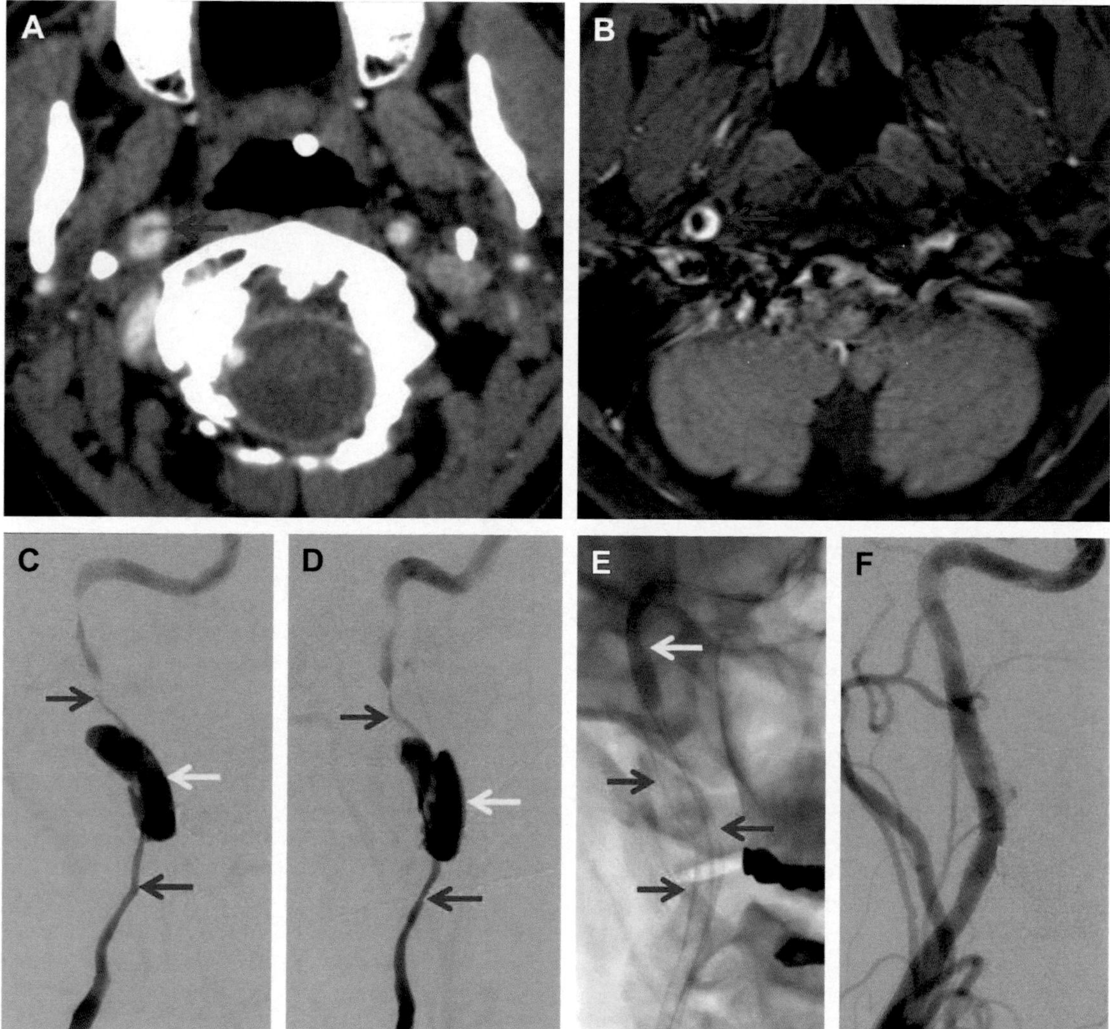

Fig. 4. A 60-year-old man presented after severe blunt trauma with dissection of the cervical right internal carotid artery extending into the petrous segment/skull base. Source imaging from computed tomography angiography of the head and neck (*A*) demonstrates a dissection flap in the distal cervical right internal carotid artery (*red arrows*). (*B*) A mural hematoma (*red arrows*) was demonstrated in the same region on fat saturated T1-weighted axial imaging performed a few days later. The patient was initially treated conservatively with anticoagulation, but follow-up right internal catheter angiography (*C, D*) performed 1 week after presentation demonstrated marked worsening stenosis of the dissected vessel (*red arrows*) as well as a large pseudoaneurysm formation (*yellow arrows*). Consequently, the patient underwent endovascular stent reconstruction (*E*) of the dissected right internal carotid artery, with the stent construct extending from the proximal cervical to petrous segments (*red arrows* in *E*). An angioplasty balloon is noted in the distal aspect of the stent construct (*yellow arrow* in *E*). A follow-up catheter angiogram performed approximately 1 year later (*F*) demonstrates excellent remodeling of the vessel with no residual stenosis and occlusion of the pseudoaneurysm.

artery to avoid occlusion of the arterial supply to the lower cranial nerves or embolization through anastomotic connections to the vertebral artery and spinal cord.[112]

ARTERIAL DISSECTION AND ANEURYSMS AT THE SKULL BASE

Aneurysms

Despite the protection from trauma afforded by the osseous anatomy of the carotid canal, the petrous and cavernous segments of the ICA are subject to aneurysm formation and traumatic dissection. Aneurysms affecting the petrous portion of the vessel are extremely uncommon.[113] Most petrous aneurysms are large and fusiform and thought to be congenital in origin, although other etiologies include trauma, radiation injury, and infection.[114–116] Symptoms associated with petrous ICA aneurysms include headache, nasal congestion, midface pain, and cranial neuropathies resulting in hearing loss and tinnitus.[113] Rupture occurs in approximately 25% of cases with subsequent otorhagia or epistaxis.[117] Unenhanced CT scan is less sensitive than MR imaging and may show expansion of the petrous carotid canal.[118] The typical patent aneurysmal lumen with rapid flow shows "flow void" on T1- and T2-weighted MR imaging.[119] CT angiography, MR angiography, and digital subtraction angiography remain the best ways to diagnose aneurysms in this location.

Large and giant petrous and cavernous aneurysms generally require therapy owing to increased risk of morbidity from stroke, hemorrhage and mass effect on surrounding structures such as cranial nerves. Therapy can be challenging, especially in giant, fusiform aneurysms. Balloon test occlusion of the carotid artery followed by endovascular occlusion can be performed if the artery is not considered salvageable. However, more recently, the availability of flow-diverting stents has been playing an important part in the treatment of these rare aneurysms, providing the ability to repair the vascular lumen and reconstruct the parent vessel.

Dissection

The extracranial segments of the carotid and vertebral arteries are much more likely to undergo dissection than their intracranial segments, although cervical ICA dissection can rarely extend into its intracranial segments and trauma at the skull base can result in intracranial ICA injury.[120] Cross-sectional imaging of arterial dissection demonstrates a narrowed lumen with crescent-shaped mural thickening, intimal flap, and dissecting aneurysm. Subacute intramural hematoma can be visualized as hyperintense on T1-weighted images with fat saturation and characteristically appears as a crescent-shaped hyperintensity around an eccentric "flow void" corresponding to the vessel lumen (**Fig. 4**). Time-of-flight MR angiography can also demonstrate subacute intramural hematoma because it does not suppress completely stationary tissues with short T1-weighted values.

A majority of arterial dissections are managed with conservative therapy that often involves anticoagulation or antiplatelet therapy and the prognosis of dissections resulting from blunt trauma is generally good. However, untreated, these lesions can result in serious morbidity and constitute an important cause of stroke in the young population. In selected instances, endovascular therapy can play a role. These include patients that suffer repeated transient ischemic attacks despite medical therapy and those with hemodynamically significant stenosis and/or growing dissecting aneurysms.[121]

SUMMARY

A wide range of congenital and acquired vascular entities may occur at the skull base. Although some are diagnosed incidentally on imaging and merit no treatment, others may require surgical or image-guided endovascular or percutaneous management. The complex anatomy of the skull base can make diagnosis of these entities challenging. A combination of CT and MR imaging as well as the judicious use of catheter angiography may be required for diagnosis and mapping of disease extent. Endovascular treatment plays an important part in many acquired vascular lesions, such as vascular neoplasms and traumatic dissections/aneurysms. Endovascular treatment is generally considered the gold standard for the treatment of vascular shunting abnormalities such as CCF and dAVFs.

REFERENCES

1. Davis WL, Harnsberger HR. MR angiography of an aberrant internal carotid artery. AJNR Am J Neuroradiol 1991;12(6):1225.
2. Lo WW, Solti-Bohman LG, McElveen JTJ. Aberrant carotid artery: radiologic diagnosis with emphasis on high-resolution computed tomography. Radiogr Rev Publ Radiol Soc N Am Inc 1985;5(6):985–93.
3. Morris P. Practical neuroangiography. Philadelphia: Lippincott Williams & Wilkins; 2013.
4. Madani G, Connor SEJ. Imaging in pulsatile tinnitus. Clin Radiol 2009;64(3):319–28.

5. Parmar H, Sitoh YY, Hui F. Normal variants of the intracranial circulation demonstrated by MR angiography at 3T. Eur J Radiol 2005;56(2):220–8.
6. SALTZMAN GF. Patent primitive trigeminal artery studied by cerebral angiography. Acta Radiol 1959;51(5):329–36.
7. Caldemeyer KS, Carrico JB, Mathews VP. The radiology and embryology of anomalous arteries of the head and neck. AJR Am J Roentgenol 1998; 170(1):197–203.
8. Oelerich M, Schuierer G. Primitive hypoglossal artery: demonstration with digital subtraction-, MR- and CT angiography. Eur Radiol 1997;7(9):1492–4.
9. Luh GY, Dean BL, Tomsick TA, et al. The persistent fetal carotid-vertebrobasilar anastomoses. AJR Am J Roentgenol 1999;172(5):1427–32.
10. Weissman JL, Hirsch BE. Imaging of tinnitus: a review. Radiology 2000;216(2):342–9.
11. Swartz J, Harnsberger H. Imaging of the temporal lobe. 3rd edition. Stuttgart (Germany): Georg Thieme Verlag; 1997.
12. Swartz JD, Harnsberger HR, Mukherji SK. The temporal bone. Contemporary diagnostic dilemmas. Radiol Clin North Am 1998;36(5):819–53, vi.
13. Weber AL, McKenna MJ. Radiologic evaluation of the jugular foramen. Anatomy, vascular variants, anomalies, and tumors. Neuroimaging Clin N Am 1994;4(3):579–98.
14. Rao AB, Koeller KK, Adair CF. From the archives of the AFIP. Paragangliomas of the head and neck: radiologic-pathologic correlation. Armed Forces Institute of Pathology. Radiographics 1999;19(6): 1605–32.
15. Borba LA, Al-Mefty O. Intravagal paragangliomas: report of four cases. Neurosurgery 1996;38(3): 569–75 [discussion: 575].
16. Kliewer KE, Wen DR, Cancilla PA, et al. Paragangliomas: assessment of prognosis by histologic, immunohistochemical, and ultrastructural techniques. Hum Pathol 1989;20(1):29–39.
17. Tasar M, Yetiser S. Glomus tumors: therapeutic role of selective embolization. J Craniofac Surg 2004; 15(3):497–505.
18. Parry DM, Li FP, Strong LC, et al. Carotid body tumors in humans: genetics and epidemiology. J Natl Cancer Inst 1982;68(4):573–8.
19. Zaslav AL, Myssiorek D, Mucia C, et al. Cytogenetic analysis of tissues from patients with familial paragangliomas of the head and neck. Head Neck 1995;17(2):102–7.
20. Barnes L, Taylor SR. Carotid body paragangliomas. A clinicopathologic and DNA analysis of 13 tumors. Arch Otolaryngol Head Neck Surg 1990; 116(4):447–53.
21. Zbaren P, Lehmann W. Carotid body paraganglioma with metastases. Laryngoscope 1985; 95(4):450–4.
22. Valavanis A, Schubiger O, Oguz M. High-resolution CT investigation of nonchromaffin paragangliomas of the temporal bone. AJNR Am J Neuroradiol 1983;4(3):516–9.
23. van Gils AP, van der Mey AG, Hoogma RP, et al. MRI screening of kindred at risk of developing paragangliomas: support for genomic imprinting in hereditary glomus tumours. Br J Cancer 1992;65(6): 903–7.
24. Vogl TJ, Juergens M, Balzer JO, et al. Glomus tumors of the skull base: combined use of MR angiography and spin-echo imaging. Radiology 1994; 192(1):103–10.
25. Vogl T, Bruning R, Schedel H, et al. Paragangliomas of the jugular bulb and carotid body: MR imaging with short sequences and Gd-DTPA enhancement. AJR Am J Roentgenol 1989;153(3): 583–7.
26. Moret J, Delvert JC, Bretonneau CH, et al. Vascularization of the ear: normal-variations-glomus tumors. J Neuroradiol 1982;9(3):209–60.
27. Gulya AJ. The glomus tumor and its biology. Laryngoscope 1993;103(11 Pt 2 Suppl 60):7–15.
28. Wright DJ, Pandya A, Noel F. Anaesthesia for carotid body tumour resection. A case report and review of the literature. Anaesthesia 1979;34(8):806–8.
29. Spector GJ, Druck NS, Gado M. Neurologic manifestations of glomus tumors in the head and neck. Arch Neurol 1976;33(4):270–4.
30. Jackson CG, Harris PF, Glasscock ME 3rd, et al. Diagnosis and management of paragangliomas of the skull base. Am J Surg 1990;159(4):389–93.
31. Belal AJ, Sanna M. Pathology as it related to ear surgery. I. Surgery of glomus tumours. J Laryngol Otol 1982;96(12):1079–97.
32. Myers EN, Newman J, Kaseff L, et al. Glomus jugulare tumor–a radiographic-histologic correlation. Laryngoscope 1971;81(11):1838–51.
33. Chakeres DW, LaMasters DL. Paragangliomas of the temporal bone: high-resolution CT studies. Radiology 1984;150(3):749–53.
34. Som PM, Curtin HD. Head and neck imaging, vol. 1. St Louis (MO): Mosby; 2003.
35. Som PM, Braun IF, Shapiro MD, et al. Tumors of the parapharyngeal space and upper neck: MR imaging characteristics. Radiology 1987;164(3):823–9.
36. Olsen WL, Dillon WP, Kelly WM, et al. MR imaging of paragangliomas. AJR Am J Roentgenol 1987; 148(1):201–4.
37. Tikkakoski T, Luotonen J, Leinonen S, et al. Preoperative embolization in the management of neck paragangliomas. Laryngoscope 1997;107(6):821–6.
38. Lasjaunias P, Berenstein A, Moret J. The significance of dural supply of central nervous system lesions. J Neuroradiol 1983;10(1):31–42.
39. Hesselink JR, Davis KR, Taveras JM. Selective arteriography of glomus tympanicum and jugulare

tumors: techniques, normal and pathologic arterial anatomy. AJNR Am J Neuroradiol 1981;2(4): 289–97.

40. Whiteman ML, Serafini AN, Telischi FF, et al. 111In octreotide scintigraphy in the evaluation of head and neck lesions. AJNR Am J Neuroradiol 1997; 18(6):1073–80.
41. Eldevik OP, Gabrielsen TO, Jacobsen EA. Imaging findings in schwannomas of the jugular foramen. AJNR Am J Neuroradiol 2000;21(6):1139–44.
42. Macdonald AJ, Salzman KL, Harnsberger HR, et al. Primary jugular foramen meningioma: imaging appearance and differentiating features. AJR Am J Roentgenol 2004;182(2):373–7.
43. Forbes JA, Brock AA, Ghiassi M, et al. Jugulotympanic paragangliomas: 75 years of evolution in understanding. Neurosurg Focus 2012; 33(2):E13.
44. Michael LM 2nd, Robertson JH. Glomus jugulare tumors: historical overview of the management of this disease. Neurosurg Focus 2004;17(2):E1.
45. Jackson RS, Myhill JA, Padhya TA, et al. The effects of preoperative embolization on carotid body paraganglioma surgery: a systematic review and meta-analysis. Otolaryngol Head Neck Surg 2015;153(6):943–50.
46. Harnsberger R, Hudgins P, Wiggins P. Diagnostic imaging: head and neck. Salt Lake City (UT): Amirsys; 2004.
47. Buetow P, Smirniotopoulous J, Wenig B. Pediatric sinonasal tumors. Appl Radiol 1993;22:21–8.
48. Paparella M, Shumrick D. Otolaryngology. Philadelphia: W B Saunders Co.; 1991.
49. Gemmete JJ, Ansari SA, McHugh J, et al. Embolization of vascular tumors of the head and neck. Neuroimaging Clin N Am 2009;19(2):181–98.
50. Fisch U. The infratemporal fossa approach for nasopharyngeal tumors. Laryngoscope 1983; 93(1):36–44.
51. Schick B, Kahle G. Radiological findings in angiofibroma. Acta Radiol 2000;41(6):585–93.
52. Momeni AK, Roberts CC, Chew FS. Imaging of chronic and exotic sinonasal disease: review. AJR Am J Roentgenol 2007;189(6 Suppl):S35–45.
53. Hurst RW, Rosenwasser R. Interventional neuroradiology. New York: Informa Health Care; 2007.
54. Davis KR. Embolization of epistaxis and juvenile nasopharyngeal angiofibromas. AJR Am J Roentgenol 1987;148(1):209–18.
55. Kania RE, Sauvaget E, Guichard JP, et al. Early postoperative CT scanning for juvenile nasopharyngeal angiofibroma: detection of residual disease. AJNR Am J Neuroradiol 2005;26(1):82–8.
56. Valavanis A. Preoperative embolization of the head and neck: indications, patient selection, goals, and precautions. AJNR Am J Neuroradiol 1986;7(5): 943–52.
57. Brugge KG, Brugge KT. Temporal and cervical tumors. In: Lasjaunias P, Berenstein A, editors. Surgical neuroangiography. Berlin: Springer-Verlag; 1987.
58. Robison JG, Shagets FW, Beckett WCJ, et al. A multidisciplinary approach to reducing morbidity and operative blood loss during resection of carotid body tumor. Surg Gynecol Obstet 1989; 168(2):166–70.
59. Murphy TP, Brackmann DE. Effects of preoperative embolization on glomus jugulare tumors. Laryngoscope 1989;99(12):1244–7.
60. Persky MS, Setton A, Niimi Y, et al. Combined endovascular and surgical treatment of head and neck paragangliomas–a team approach. Head Neck 2002;24(5):423–31.
61. Gandhi D, Gemmete JJ, Ansari SA, et al. Interventional neuroradiology of the head and neck. AJNR Am J Neuroradiol 2008;29(10):1806–15.
62. Moulin G, Chagnaud C, Gras R, et al. Juvenile nasopharyngeal angiofibroma: comparison of blood loss during removal in embolized group versus nonembolized group. Cardiovasc Intervent Radiol 1995;18(3):158–61.
63. Oka H, Kurata A, Kawano N, et al. Preoperative superselective embolization of skull-base meningiomas: indications and limitations. J Neurooncol 1998;40(1):67–71.
64. Hilal SK, Michelsen JW. Therapeutic percutaneous embolization for extra-axial vascular lesions of the head, neck, and spine. J Neurosurg 1975;43(3): 275–87.
65. LaMuraglia GM, Fabian RL, Brewster DC, et al. The current surgical management of carotid body paragangliomas. J Vasc Surg 1992;15(6):1038–44 [discussion: 1044–5].
66. Wang HH, Luo CB, Guo WY, et al. Preoperative embolization of hypervascular pediatric brain tumors: evaluation of technical safety and outcome. Childs Nerv Syst 2013;29(11):2043–9.
67. Alaraj A, Pytynia K, Carlson AP, et al. Combined preoperative onyx embolization and protective internal carotid artery covered stent placement for treatment of glomus vagale tumor: review of literature and illustrative case. Neurol Res 2012;34(6): 523–9.
68. Ladner TR, He L, Davis BJ, et al. Initial experience with dual-lumen balloon catheter injection for preoperative Onyx embolization of skull base paragangliomas. J Neurosurg 2016;124(6):1813–9.
69. Michelozzi C, Januel AC, Cuvinciuc V, et al. Arterial embolization with Onyx of head and neck paragangliomas. J Neurointerventional Surg 2016;8(6): 626–35.
70. Lasjaunias P, Moret J. Normal and non-pathological variations in the angiographic aspects of the arteries of the middle ear. Neuroradiology 1978;15(4):213–9.

71. Quadros RS, Gallas S, Delcourt C, et al. Preoperative embolization of a cervicodorsal paraganglioma by direct percutaneous injection of onyx and endovascular delivery of particles. AJNR Am J Neuroradiol 2006;27(9):1907–9.
72. Abud DG, Mounayer C, Benndorf G, et al. Intratumoral injection of cyanoacrylate glue in head and neck paragangliomas. AJNR Am J Neuroradiol 2004;25(9):1457–62.
73. Lasjaunias P, Menu Y, Bonnel D, et al. Non chromaffin paragangliomas of the head and neck. Diagnostic and therapeutic angiography in 19 cases explored from 1977 to 1980. J Neuroradiol 1981;8(4):281–99.
74. van der Mey AG, Maaswinkel-Mooy PD, Cornelisse CJ, et al. Genomic imprinting in hereditary glomus tumours: evidence for new genetic theory. Lancet Lond Engl 1989;2(8675):1291–4.
75. Berenstein A, Lasjaunias P. Dangerous vessels. In: Lasjaunias P, Berenstein A, editors. Surgical neuroangiography. Berlin: Springer-Verlag; 1987.
76. Halbach VV, Higashida RT, Hieshima GB, et al. Transvenous embolization of dural fistulas involving the cavernous sinus. AJNR Am J Neuroradiol 1989; 10(2):377–83.
77. Newton TH, Cronqvist S. Involvement of dural arteries in intracranial arteriovenous malformations. Radiology 1969;93(5):1071–8.
78. Chaudhary MY, Sachdev VP, Cho SH, et al. Dural arteriovenous malformation of the major venous sinuses: an acquired lesion. AJNR Am J Neuroradiol 1982;3(1):13–9.
79. Newton TH, Weidner W, Greitz T. Dural arteriovenous malformation in the posterior fossa. Radiology 1968;90(1):27–35.
80. Castaigne P, Bories J, Brunet P, et al. Meningeal arterio-venous fistulas with cortical venous drainage. Rev Neurol (Paris) 1976;132(3):169–81 [in French].
81. Lasjaunias P, Halimi P, Lopez-Ibor L, et al. Endovascular treatment of pure spontaneous dural vascular malformations. Review of 23 cases studied and treated between May 1980 and October 1983. Neurochirurgie 1984;30(4):207–23 [in French].
82. Gandhi D, Chen J, Pearl M, et al. Intracranial dural arteriovenous fistulas: classification, imaging findings, and treatment. AJNR Am J Neuroradiol 2012;33(6):1007–13.
83. Sarma D, ter Brugge K. Management of intracranial dural arteriovenous shunts in adults. Eur J Radiol 2003;46(3):206–20.
84. Lasjaunias P, Berenstein A. Endovascular treatment of craniofacial lesions. In: Lasjaunias P, Berenstein A, editors. Surgical neuroangiography. Berlin: Springer-Verlag; 1987. p. 312–35.
85. Kim MS, Han DH, Kwon OK, et al. Clinical characteristics of dural arteriovenous fistula. J Clin Neurosci 2002;9(2):147–55.
86. Cognard C, Gobin YP, Pierot L, et al. Cerebral dural arteriovenous fistulas: clinical and angiographic correlation with a revised classification of venous drainage. Radiology 1995;194(3):671–80.
87. Singh V, Smith WS, Lawton MT, et al. Risk factors for hemorrhagic presentation in patients with dural arteriovenous fistulae. Neurosurgery 2008;62(3): 628–35 [discussion: 628–35].
88. Awad IA, Little JR, Akarawi WP, et al. Intracranial dural arteriovenous malformations: factors predisposing to an aggressive neurological course. J Neurosurg 1990;72(6):839–50.
89. Peng T, Liu A, Jia J, et al. Risk factors for dural arteriovenous fistula intracranial hemorrhage. J Clin Neurosci 2014;21(5):769–72.
90. Borden JA, Wu JK, Shucart WA. A proposed classification for spinal and cranial dural arteriovenous fistulous malformations and implications for treatment. J Neurosurg 1995;82(2):166–79.
91. Barrow DL, Spector RH, Braun IF, et al. Classification and treatment of spontaneous carotid-cavernous sinus fistulas. J Neurosurg 1985;62(2): 248–56.
92. Kawaguchi S, Sakaki T, Morimoto T, et al. Surgery for dural arteriovenous fistula in superior sagittal sinus and transverse sigmoid sinus. J Clin Neurosci 2000;7(Suppl 1):47–9.
93. Roy D, Raymond J. The role of transvenous embolization in the treatment of intracranial dural arteriovenous fistulas. Neurosurgery 1997;40(6):1133–41 [discussion: 1141–4].
94. Castillo M. Neuroradiology companion: methods, guidelines, and imaging fundamentals. 4th edition. Philadelphia: Lippincott Williams & Wilkins; 2006.
95. Ahmadi J, Teal JS, Segall HD, et al. Computed tomography of carotid-cavernous fistula. AJNR Am J Neuroradiol 1983;4(2):131–6.
96. Halbach VV, Hieshima GB, Higashida RT, et al. Carotid cavernous fistulae: indications for urgent treatment. AJR Am J Roentgenol 1987;149(3):587–93.
97. Choi JW, Kim BM, Kim DJ, et al. Hypoglossal canal dural arteriovenous fistula: incidence and the relationship between symptoms and drainage pattern. J Neurosurg 2013;119(4):955–60.
98. Manabe S, Satoh K, Matsubara S, et al. Characteristics, diagnosis and treatment of hypoglossal canal dural arteriovenous fistula: report of nine cases. Neuroradiology 2008;50(8):715–21.
99. Ernst R, Bulas R, Tomsick T, et al. Three cases of dural arteriovenous fistula of the anterior condylar vein within the hypoglossal canal. AJNR Am J Neuroradiol 1999;20(10):2016–20.
100. Spittau B, Millan DS, El-Sherifi S, et al. Dural arteriovenous fistulas of the hypoglossal canal: systematic review on imaging anatomy, clinical findings, and endovascular management. J Neurosurg 2015;122(4):883–903.

101. McDougall CG, Halbach VV, Dowd CF, et al. Dural arteriovenous fistulas of the marginal sinus. AJNR Am J Neuroradiol 1997;18(8):1565–72.
102. Zhao J, Xu F, Ren J, et al. Dural arteriovenous fistulas at the craniocervical junction: a systematic review. J Neurointerventional Surg 2016;8(6):648–53.
103. Turner RD, Gonugunta V, Kelly ME, et al. Marginal sinus arteriovenous fistulas mimicking carotid cavernous fistulas: diagnostic and therapeutic considerations. AJNR Am J Neuroradiol 2007;28(10): 1915–8.
104. Blomquist MH, Barr JD, Hurst RW. Isolated unilateral hypoglossal neuropathy caused by dural arteriovenous fistula. AJNR Am J Neuroradiol 1998; 19(5):951–3.
105. Liu JK, Mahaney K, Barnwell SL, et al. Dural arteriovenous fistula of the anterior condylar confluence and hypoglossal canal mimicking a jugular foramen tumor. J Neurosurg 2008;109(2):335–40.
106. Ouanounou S, Tomsick TA, Heitsman C, et al. Cavernous sinus and inferior petrosal sinus flow signal on three-dimensional time-of-flight MR angiography. AJNR Am J Neuroradiol 1999;20(8):1476–81.
107. Gemmete JJ, Chaudhary N, Pandey A, et al. Treatment of carotid cavernous fistulas. Curr Treat Options Neurol 2010;12(1):43–53.
108. Venturi C, Bracco S, Cerase A, et al. Endovascular treatment of a cavernous sinus dural arteriovenous fistula by transvenous embolisation through the superior ophthalmic vein via cannulation of a frontal vein. Neuroradiology 2003;45(8):574–8.
109. Miller NR, Monsein LH, Debrun GM, et al. Treatment of carotid-cavernous sinus fistulas using a superior ophthalmic vein approach. J Neurosurg 1995;83(5):838–42.
110. Goldberg RA, Goldey SH, Duckwiler G, et al. Management of cavernous sinus-dural fistulas. Indications and techniques for primary embolization via the superior ophthalmic vein. Arch Ophthalmol 1996;114(6):707–14.
111. Satomi J, van Dijk JMC, Terbrugge KG, et al. Benign cranial dural arteriovenous fistulas: outcome of conservative management based on the natural history of the lesion. J Neurosurg 2002;97(4):767–70.
112. Lasjaunias P, editor. Craniofacial and upper cervical arteries. Baltimore (MD): Williams & Wilkins; 1981.
113. Morantz RA, Kirchner FR, Kishore P. Aneurysms of the petrous portion of the internal carotid artery. Surg Neurol 1976;6(6):313–8.
114. Vasama JP, Ramsay H, Markkola A. Petrous internal carotid artery pseudoaneurysm due to gunshot injury. Ann Otol Rhinol Laryngol 2001;110(5 Pt 1): 491–3.
115. Tanaka H, Patel U, Shrier DA, et al. Pseudoaneurysm of the petrous internal carotid artery after skull base infection and prevertebral abscess drainage. AJNR Am J Neuroradiol 1998;19(3):502–4.
116. Cheng KM, Chan CM, Cheung YL, et al. Endovascular treatment of radiation-induced petrous internal carotid artery aneurysm presenting with acute haemorrhage. A report of two cases. Acta Neurochir (Wien) 2001;143(4):351–5 [discussion: 355–6].
117. Costantino PD, Russell E, Reisch D, et al. Ruptured petrous carotid aneurysm presenting with otorrhagia and epistaxis. Am J Otol 1991;12(5):378–83.
118. Kelly WM, Harsh GR 4th. CT of petrous carotid aneurysms. AJNR Am J Neuroradiol 1985;6(5):830–2.
119. Patrick JT. Magnetic resonance imaging of petrous carotid aneurysms. J Neuroimaging 1996;6(3): 177–9.
120. Schievink WI. Spontaneous dissection of the carotid and vertebral arteries. N Engl J Med 2001; 344(12):898–906.
121. Jindal G, Fortes M, Miller T, et al. Endovascular stent repair of traumatic cervical internal carotid artery injuries. J Trauma Acute Care Surg 2013;75(5): 896–903.

Imaging of Cerebrospinal Fluid Rhinorrhea and Otorrhea

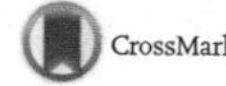

Mahati Reddy, MD, Kristen Baugnon, MD*

KEYWORDS

• CSF leak • Idiopathic intracranial hypertension (IIH) • Skull base fractures • Cisternogram

KEY POINTS

- Any clinically suspected cerebrospinal fluid (CSF) rhinorrhea or otorrhea should first be confirmed with testing for β2-transferrin, a protein specific to the CSF.
- High-resolution computed tomography (CT) imaging through the sinuses and mastoids should be the first step to diagnose the possible site of a CSF leak.
- CT cisternogram can be helpful to confirm the site of a leak in patients with multiple osseous defects on CT and an active leak.
- Magnetic resonance cisternogram is helpful in patients with intermittent leaks or suspected meningoencephaloceles.
- Morphologic features suggesting underlying idiopathic intracranial hypertension should be mentioned on imaging of suspected CSF leak, because this can alter the patient's management.

INTRODUCTION

A skull base cerebrospinal (CSF) leak or fistula is an abnormal communication of the sterile subarachnoid space with the sinonasal or tympanomastoid cavities, and presents clinically with clear rhinorrhea or otorrhea, caused by the presence of both an osseous and a dural defect. The flora of the sinonasal cavity and the middle ear create a conduit for the spread of infection that often results in meningitis, with an approximately 19% lifetime risk of meningitis in patients with persistent CSF rhinorrhea.[1] Despite advances in antibiotic therapy, mortality from bacterial meningitis in adults remains up to 33%, with severe morbidity among survivors, including seizure disorders, encephalopathy, and cranial nerve deficits.[2] The high risk of life-threatening complications underscores the importance of early detection, accurate diagnosis, and timely repair of CSF leaks. Endoscopic approaches to CSF leak repair are replacing open transcranial and transfacial methods because of similar rates of success, with significantly lower complication rates of wound infection, sepsis, and meningitis.[3,4] Especially in the setting of an endoscopic repair, a thorough radiologic investigation is imperative to determine the precise location of the fistula, define the dimensions of the osseous defect, and evaluate the subjective anatomy of the area. This process enables surgeons to plan the surgical approach, graft, and closure technique, and to avoid an open craniotomy.[5]

Not only is imaging essential in determining the site of a CSF leak but it can also aid in determining the underlying cause. CSF leaks can be traumatic or nontraumatic, with most nontraumatic leaks seen in the setting of idiopathic intracranial hypertension (IIH), also known as spontaneous leaks.[6,7] This article begins with a description of imaging

Disclosure: None.
Department of Radiology and Imaging Sciences, Emory University School of Medicine, Emory University Hospital, 1364 Clifton Road Northeast, Atlanta, GA 30322, USA
* Corresponding author.
E-mail address: kmlloyd@emory.edu

Radiol Clin N Am 55 (2017) 167–187
http://dx.doi.org/10.1016/j.rcl.2016.08.005
0033-8389/17/© 2016 Elsevier Inc. All rights reserved.

techniques used to diagnose and characterize the site of a CSF leak and then details the pathophysiology and associated imaging findings in traumatic and spontaneous leaks. In addition, it discusses some challenges in the diagnosis of initial and recurrent leaks with an emphasis on information that is most consequential to referring surgeons.

IMAGING PROTOCOLS

The first diagnostic study to evaluate a patient with CSF rhinorrhea or otorrhea and suspected CSF leak is testing a sample of the fluid for β2-transferrin, a protein specific to the CSF, because this is the most reliable confirmatory test for a CSF leak.[8] As discussed previously, rhinorrhea can be a sign of a defect along either the paranasal sinuses or mastoids. Frank otorrhea draining from the external auditory canal in the setting of a tegmen defect within the middle cranial fossa is rare, unless there is a perforation of the tympanic membrane (ie, in the setting of trauma), or a tympanostomy tube. Various methods of testing for β2-transferrin report sensitivities of 87% to 100% and specificities of 71% to 94%.[9] Patients with intermittent leaks may be able to collect an adequate volume of sample themselves over the course of a week, if necessary, without storage restrictions to prevent protein degradation.[10] Although not widely used in the United States, beta trace protein is another CSF marker, and some recent studies report that it has a higher sensitivity and specificity than β2-transferrin with lower cost and faster turnaround time.[9,11,12] Once the leak is confirmed, localization and characterization can be achieved with radiologic evaluation.

COMPUTED TOMOGRAPHY

High-resolution CT (HRCT) of the paranasal sinuses and mastoids should be the first line of imaging because computed tomography (CT) is the best modality to delineate osseous anatomy with the greatest spatial resolution to pinpoint a site of bony dehiscence. HRCT has a reported sensitivity of 88% to 95% in identifying the site of skull base defect after the presence of CSF leak is confirmed by β2-transferrin analysis.[13–16] In a single retrospective study at our institution, CT correctly predicted the site of leak in 100% of the cases when 0.625-mm axial images were available and multiplanar reformations could be generated.[17] In addition to excellent accuracy, HRCT provides unparalleled delineation of the remaining osseous sinonasal anatomy for surgeons to plan their operative approach and allows the use of an intraoperative image guidance system.[18] Patients should be scanned with multidetector row CT in the supine position with a field of view to include the paranasal sinuses and temporal bones. Continuous thin-section axial images of submillimeter (ie, 0.625 mm) collimation (volumetric) should be reconstructed in the bone algorithm, and sagittal and coronal reconstructions of the raw data should be performed.[17,19] One of the greatest strengths of HRCT in the evaluation of CSF leak is that an active leak does not need to be present at the time of imaging to be able to identify an osseous defect. However, if the patient has multiple osseous defects, it can be challenging to determine which defect is the definite source of the CSF leak, because the presence of an osseous defect is not always associated with a concomitant dural dehiscence. However, if only 1 osseous defect is identified and the location of the suspected leak on imaging corresponds with the clinical symptoms, no additional imaging is needed, and the patient can proceed to surgical repair.[20]

Computed Tomography Cisternography

Contrast-enhanced CT cisternography (CTC) is performed by instilling intrathecal nonionic myelographic iodinated contrast and scanning the sinuses in the prone and supine positions, with supine images also obtained before contrast injection for the purposes of comparison. In a positive study, there is extracranial fluid or soft tissue density adjacent to an osseous defect showing 50% or greater increase in Hounsfield units on the postcontrast scan compared with the precontrast scan, suggestive of interval contrast pooling. When introduced in 1977, CTC was considered the study of choice to evaluate CSF fistulae, but it is now selectively used as a problem-solving tool in specific scenarios, primarily in the setting of multiple osseous defects on CT, to determine the site of leak.[21,22] CTC has a wide range of reported sensitivities of 33% to 100% and specificity of approximately 94%.[8,13,23–25] The main limitation of CTC is that patients have to be actively leaking, or able to elicit a leak, at the time of examination. Low rates of sensitivity are predominantly attributed to imaging in the absence of an active leak, with other potential causes being obscuration of small leak in the setting of high-density contrast media adjacent to high-density bone and high viscosity of contrast media prohibiting leakage through a fistulous tract.[25,26] The disadvantages of CTC include high radiation dose related to multiple scans, inherent risk of a lumbar puncture, and potential adverse outcome from iodinated contrast.

Magnetic Resonance Cisternogram

Magnetic resonance (MR) cisternography (MRC) is performed by acquiring heavily T2-weighted (T2w) images to increase conspicuity of the contrast between CSF and the adjacent skull base. The spatial resolution of HRCT is far superior to that of MR imaging, but the advent of three-dimensional (3D)– fast spoiled gradient echo facilitated obtaining thin-slice images that can be reformatted into multiple planes, significantly improving MR imaging of the skull base. Nevertheless, MRC should continue to be used in conjunction with HRCT because MR imaging cannot provide the exquisite osseous detail of CT.[13,16,27] In a positive study, a CSF column is seen from the subarachnoid space communicating with the extracranial space with or without herniation of meninges and/or brain parenchyma. Sensitivity of these findings on MRC for identifying the site of leak is reported to be up to 94%.[28] The added benefit of MR imaging is improved soft tissue contrast that can characterize the contents of tissue herniating through an osseous defect in the setting of possible meningoencephaloceles.

Contrast-Enhanced Magnetic Resonance Cisternogram

Contrast-enhanced MRC is a technique in which intrathecal gadolinium is administered through a lumbar puncture and, subsequently, thin-section T1-weighted sequences are obtained in multiple planes. These sequences can be obtained immediately (1–2 hours after injection of contrast), and in a delayed fashion up to 24 hours after contrast administration if necessary. Similar to a CTC, a positive study shows leakage of contrast medium through dural disruption and adjacent osseous defect, and, similar to noncontrast MR imaging cisternogram, this study also requires HRCT for interpretation. Studies have shown enhanced sensitivity for detection of CSF leaks using this method compared with CT and standard MRC,[14,25,29] particularly in the setting of slow flow or intermittent leaks, a population that is difficult to diagnose with CTC, possibly in part due because of the ability to perform delayed imaging up to 24 hours later.[30] This technique has been reported to be up to 100% sensitive for high-flow leaks, and up to 60% to 70% sensitive for slow-flow leaks.[31] Additional potential benefits of this technique include the lack of ionizing radiation, the ability to assess for meningoceles at the time of the examination, and the ease of interpretation compared with CT cisternogram caused by the improved differentiation of contrast and bone. However, note that intrathecal administration of gadolinium is not yet approved by the US Food and Drug Administration (FDA), although it has been used safely at low doses (0.05 mmol) for several years throughout the world in selected patients.[29,32,33] Although long-term studies are still pending, a single study following 107 patients for an average of 4.2 years showed no long-term adverse effects related to the gadolinium administration.[34] However, given the invasive nature of the study, the known neurotoxicity of gadolinium in high doses, and current off-label use, selective use of this technique as a problem-solving tool is prudent,[8] particularly in patients with renal failure.[35] At our institution, this is included in the algorithm only in selected patients with normal renal function, inability to obtain fluid to test for β2-transferrin, and very high clinical suspicion, and is obtained only after thorough off-label use consent.

Radionuclide Cisternography

Radionuclide cisternography (RNC) is a nuclear medicine diagnostic examination in which a radiotracer (technetium-99 or indium-111) is injected intrathecally, then several pledgets are placed throughout the nasal cavity. After 24 to 48 hours, the radioactivity is measured in each pledget to confirm the presence of a CSF leak[8] and compared with baseline serum levels. A ratio of 2:1 or 3:1 is considered a positive study. Theoretically, some localization information could be obtained by corroborating locations of the radioactive pledgets to their precise location in the nasal cavity. However, anecdotal experience suggests that accurate localization is extremely limited, because the intranasal pledgets are not well tolerated by patients and often move, secretions can mix from side to side, and (as discussed previously) leaks within the middle ear may present with CSF in the nasal cavity through the eustachian tube. Additional disadvantages of RNC include the invasive nature of the study, high cost, and moderate accuracy.[8] In general, it is typically reserved only for rare problem-solving cases to confirm the presence or absence of a leak, and is not included in our standard imaging algorithm.

Fig. 1 shows our recommended imaging algorithm for patients with suspected skull base CSF leak. Our protocols for CT, CT, and MRC with and without intrathecal gadolinium are summarized in **Table 1**.

PATHOLOGY AND IMAGING FINDINGS

The imaging appearance of CSF leaks often depends on the underlying cause. As described

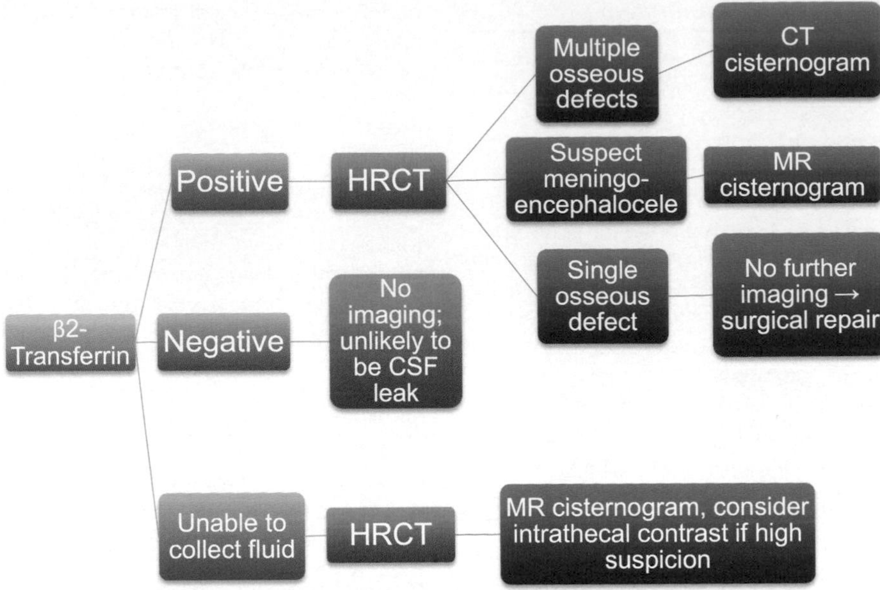

Fig. 1. Imaging algorithm for patient with suspected CSF leak.

earlier, CSF leaks can be classified as traumatic or nontraumatic, with the traumatic leaks resulting from either accidental or iatrogenic trauma, and the nontraumatic leaks are either secondary, caused by underlying tumor or congenital disorder, or spontaneous (without history of prior trauma, surgery, tumor, or congenital lesion).

Traumatic Leaks

Traumatic leaks, including both accidental and iatrogenic leaks, are still the most commonly encountered type of CSF leak, reportedly accounting for up to 80% to 90% of CSF leaks in older literature,[36] although spontaneous leaks are increasing in frequency, as discussed later.

Accidental trauma

Approximately 10% to 30% of skull base fractures are complicated by CSF leaks, particularly those that are comminuted and extend through the anterior cranial fossa, likely because of the tightly adherent dura in a region of inherently thin cribriform plates and ethmoid roofs. However, frontobasal fractures that extend through the posterior table of the frontal sinus, central skull base fractures extending through the sphenoid sinus, and temporal bone fractures extending through the tegmen can also result in CSF rhinorrhea or otorrhea.[37]

Imaging findings include a nondisplaced or comminuted fracture extending through the skull base, and often the presence of pneumocephalus (**Fig. 2**). Pneumocephalus in the traumatic setting should imply a skull base fracture and dural defect, and, if seen, careful attention to the areas described earlier should be undertaken to exclude the possibility of even a subtle or occult skull base fracture (**Fig. 3**).

Most patients (80%) present with CSF rhinorrhea or otorrhea in the first 48 hours, and 95% of patients present by the first 3 months after trauma.[38] The initial delay in presentation is likely caused by the resolution of hemorrhage initially sealing the defect, combined with increased activity as the patient heals and rehabilitates. However, a small subset of patients present in a very delayed fashion, months or years after the trauma, presumably due to atrophy of granulation tissue, or possibly because of bony fragments slowly eroding the dura over time. However, although CSF leaks are fairly common in the setting of complex skull base trauma, they rarely require treatment, because up to 85% of patients CSF leaks heal spontaneously with conservative management, including bed rest, avoiding Valsalva (ie, stool softeners), and occasionally lumbar drain placement for persistent leaks.[37,39] However, persistent leaks do necessitate repair; one study of 160 patients with traumatic leak showed a 1.3% chance of meningitis per day for the first 2 weeks after the trauma, which increased to 7.4% per week for the first month, 8.1% per month for the first 6 months, and 8.4% per year from then onward.[40] When patients require repair in the early posttraumatic period, the site of the leak is usually obvious and rarely a diagnostic dilemma, therefore

Table 1
Suggested imaging protocols for patients with suspected CSF leak

CT Paranasal Sinuses Without Contrast		
1	Scout	Tip of nose to back of mastoid
2	Axial bone thin	0.625 mm (or 0.6 mm)
3	Axial soft	2.5 mm (or 3 mm)
4	Coronal bone	0.625 mm (or 0.6 mm)
5	Sagittal bone	0.625 mm (or 0.6 mm)

CT Cisternogram (CT Paranasal Sinuses Without and with Intrathecal Contrast)		
1	Scout	Tip of nose to back of mastoid
2	Axial bone thin	Supine helical; 0.625 mm (or 0.6 mm)
3	Axial soft	2.5 mm (or 3 mm) reconstructed
4	Coronal bone	0.625 mm (or 0.6)
5	Sagittal bone	0.625 mm (or 0.6)
Patient to fluoroscopic suite for 5–7 mL of intrathecal iodinated myelographic contrast		
Before placing patient on CT table, head hanging/provocation techniques		
6	Scout	Tip of nose to back of mastoid
7	Coronal bone prone	Prone (detail, direct coronal); 0.625 mm
8	Axial bone thin	Supine; 0.625 mm
9	Axial soft postsupine	2.5 mm (reconstructed)
10	Coronal bone	0.625 or 0.6 mm (reconstructed from supine post data set)
11	Sagittal bone	0.625 or 0.6 mm (reconstructed from supine data set)

MR Cisternogram: MR Brain Without and with IV Contrast

#	Sequence	Plane	Comment
1	T1	Sagittal	Brain
2	T2 FLAIR	Axial	Brain
3	T1	Axial	Top of frontal sinus to tip of clivus (3 mm)
4	T1	Coronal	Tip of nose to back of mastoid (3 mm)
5	3D T2 SPACE	Coronal	Tip of nose to back of mastoid (1 mm)
6	T2	Coronal	Tip of nose to back of mastoid (3 mm)
Administer IV contrast			
7	T1 fat-saturated postcontrast	Axial	Top of frontal sinus to tip of clivus (3 mm)
8	T1 fat-saturated postcontrast	Coronal	Tip of nose to back of mastoid (3 mm)

Gadolinium-Enhanced MR Cisternogram (MR Brain Without and with Intrathecal Contrast)

#	Sequence	Plane	Comment
1	T1	Sagittal	Brain
2	T2 FLAIR	Axial	Brain
3	T2 SPACE	Coronal	Tip of nose to back of mastoid (1 mm)
4	T1 fat-saturated (VIBE)	Axial	Top of frontal sinus to tip of clivus (1 mm)
5	T1 fat-saturated (VIBE)	Coronal	Tip of nose to back of mastoid (1 mm)
6	MPRAGE	Coronal	Tip of nose to back of mastoid (1 mm)
Patient to fluoroscopic suite for administration of intrathecal contrast: 0.5 mL of gadopentetate Dimeglumine diluted in 5 mL of CSF, injected slowly, rescanned 1–2 h later, ± again in 4–24 h			
7	T1 fat-saturated (VIBE) postcontrast	Axial	Top of frontal sinus to tip of clivus (1 mm)
8	T1 fat-saturated (VIBE) postcontrast	Coronal	Tip of nose to back of mastoid (1 mm)
9	MPRAGE postcontrast	Coronal	Tip of nose to back of mastoid (1 mm)

Abbreviations: FLAIR, fluid-attenuated inversion recovery; IV, intravenous; MPRAGE, magnetization-prepared rapid gradient echo; SPACE, sampling perfection with application optimized contrasts using different flip angle evolutions, siemens 3D T2 TSE sequence; VIBE, volume interpolated breathhold examination, 3D spoiled turbo gradient echo with fat saturation.

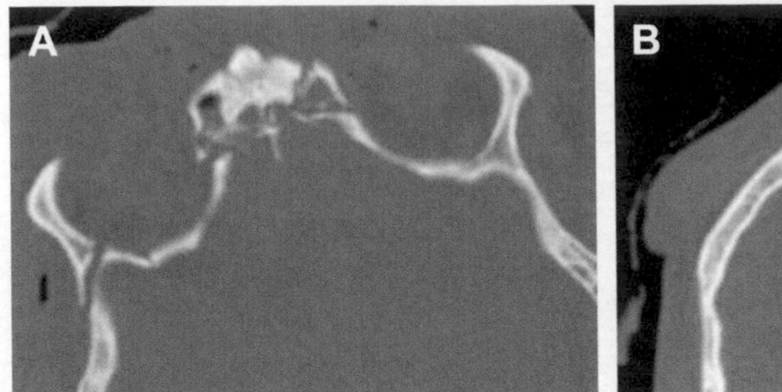

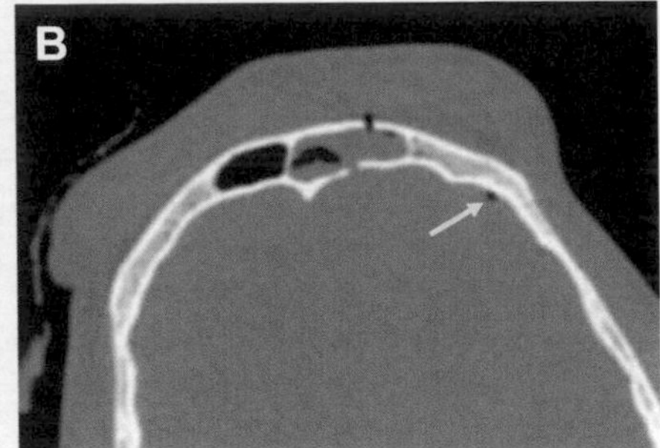

Fig. 2. (*A, B*) Axial CT images showing a comminuted complex frontobasal fracture extending through the frontal sinuses and anterior cranial fossa, resulting in traumatic CSF leak with pneumocephalus (*arrow in B*).

often only HRCT should be required preoperatively for surgical planning.[41] However, full radiologic evaluation and work-up can be necessary for those patients who present in a delayed fashion (**Fig. 4**).

Iatrogenic leaks

Iatrogenic CSF leaks can occur as a result of neurosurgical or otolaryngologic procedures along the skull base, and reportedly account for about 16% of cases of traumatic rhinorrhea.[42] Endoscopic endonasal approaches to skull base tumors, including pituitary or clival tumors, have significantly increased in frequency over the last decade, and CSF leaks are a known potential complication of this approach, reportedly occurring in up to 13.8% of patients in one study.[43] Most iatrogenic leaks occur in the first 2 postoperative weeks; resolve spontaneously or with lumbar drain placement; and, if they do require repair, typically only require HRCT for preoperative planning, because the site of the leak should be obvious (the site of the prior surgery) (**Fig. 5**). Postoperative changes with packing and blood products make CTC challenging in the early postoperative setting.

Postoperative CSF leaks can complicate craniotomies that inadvertently extend through the frontal sinus or mastoid air cells (**Fig. 6**), as well as those in which clinoidectomies are performed for exposure to the parasellar region, such as aneurysm clipping, if the patient's pneumatization of the sphenoid sinus extends into the clinoid process, which is a variant occurring in nearly one-third of the population (**Fig. 7**).[44] The risk of CSF leak after anterior clinoidectomy is reportedly up to 2% to 7%.[45] For this reason, any pneumatization of the clinoid process should be mentioned on preoperative CT angiography, particularly if the patient has a periclinoid aneurysm (**Fig. 8**).[46]

In addition, CSF leaks are a known potential complication of endoscopic sinus surgery, with the risk increasing in the setting of revision surgery or sinonasal polyposis, when the surgical

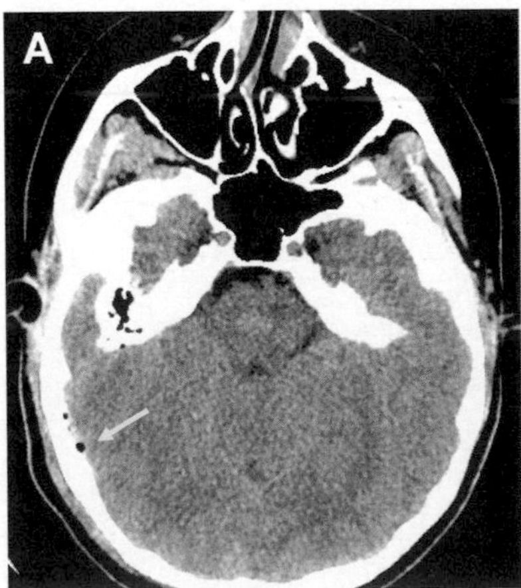

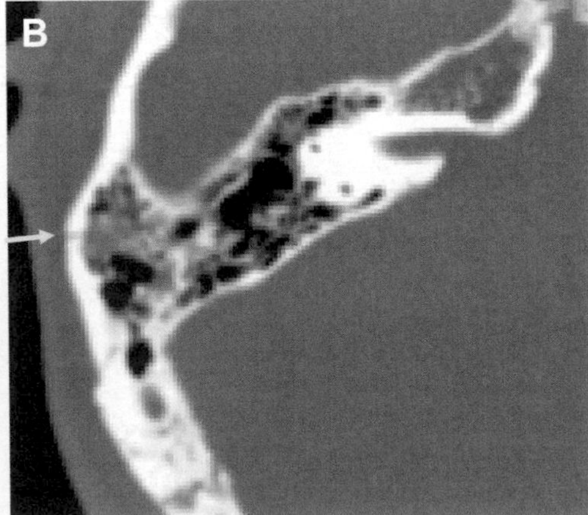

Fig. 3. (*A*) Axial CT image shows mild soft tissue swelling and subtle focus of pneumocephalus (*arrow*) along the right temporal lobe. (*B*) Temporal bone CT image with a subtle linear nondisplaced defect in the right mastoid air cells (*arrow*).

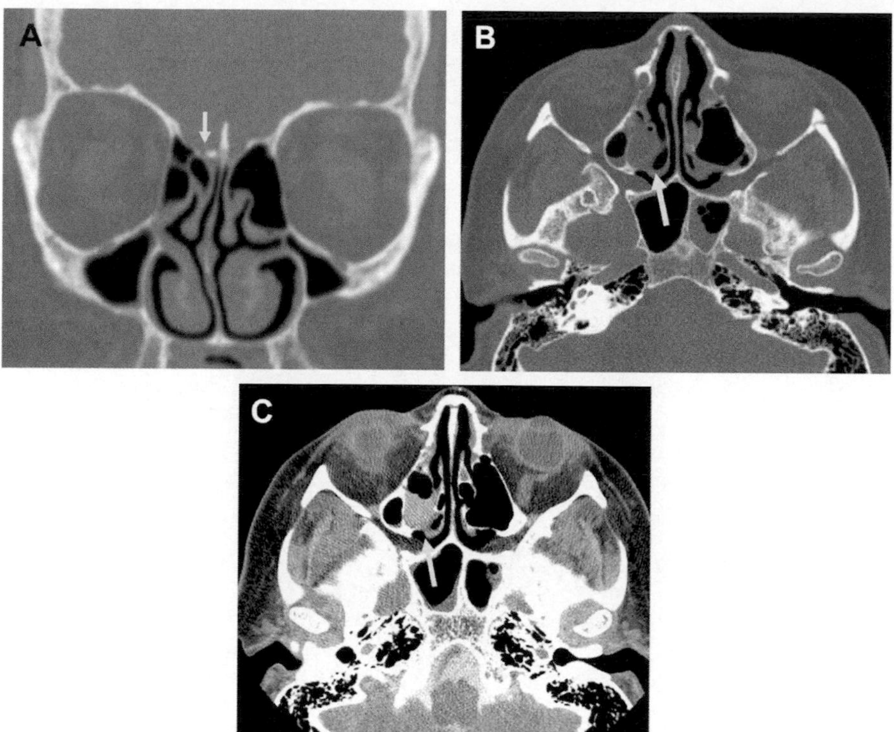

Fig. 4. A 42-year-old woman presenting with β2-transferrin–positive right-sided rhinorrhea. History of trauma 4 years previously. (*A*) Coronal CT bone window images show focal sclerosis along the right cribriform plate with dehiscence of the lateral lamella (*arrow*). The patient had an additional bony defect in the sphenoid sinus (not shown), and therefore underwent CTC. (*B*) Axial precontrast image shows opacification of a single right posterior ethmoid air cell (*arrow*) just posterior to the defect shown in *A*. (*C*) Postcontrast axial CT image (soft tissue window) shows increased density within the opacified cell, diagnostic of the site of the CSF leak (*arrow*).

landmarks are distorted. Using image guidance has been shown to reduce the risk significantly, is indicated in these complex settings, and has reduced the risk of CSF leak after endoscopic sinus surgery to reportedly only 0.5%.[42] Most of these iatrogenic leaks can be seen along the vertical insertion of the middle turbinate, at the thin cribriform plates and lateral lamella; however,

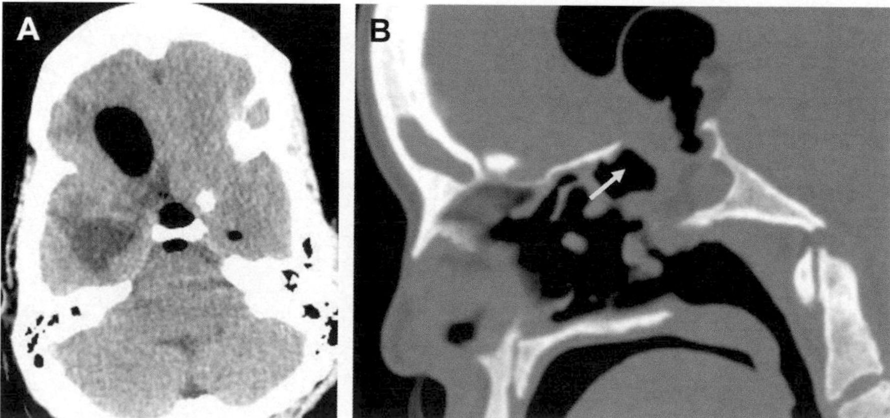

Fig. 5. A 22-year-old woman presents with headaches, lethargy, and rhinorrhea 3 weeks after transphenoidal approach for resection of craniopharyngioma. (*A*) Axial noncontrast head CT showing air within the suprasellar cistern, pneumocephalus within the prepontine cistern, and significant intraventricular air with hydrocephalus. (*B*) Sagittal reformat of preoperative sinus CT showing the large skull base defect and graft at the site of the prior surgery (*arrow*).

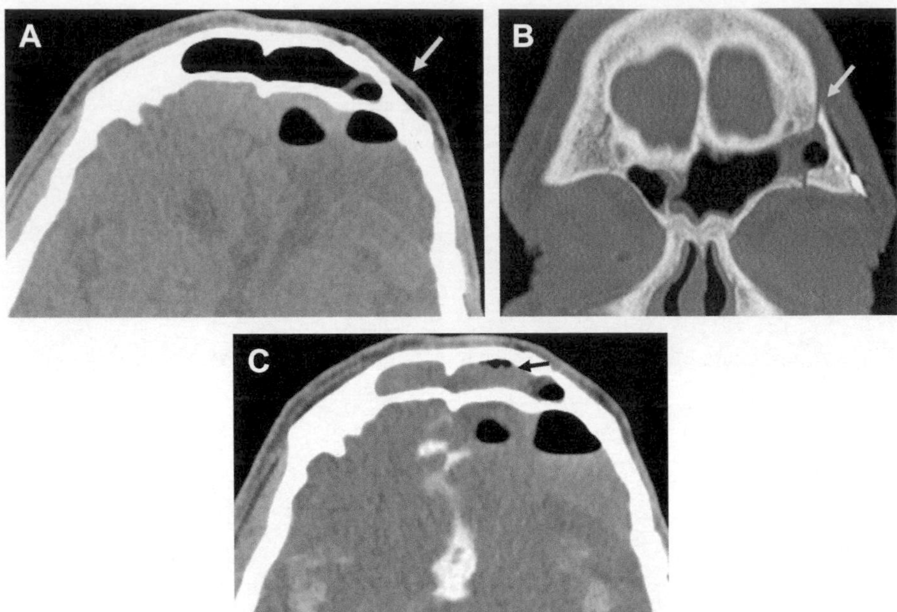

Fig. 6. A 59-year-old patient after craniotomy for sphenoid wing meningioma resection. (*A*) Axial precontrast CT cisternogram images showing a large air-filled and fluid-filled extra-axial collection, as well as an air bubble seen laterally in the left frontal sinus, and subcutaneous gas at the craniotomy site (*arrow*). (*B*) Coronal bone window reformatted precontrast images show the craniotomy extending through the lateral aspect of the frontal sinus (*arrow*). (*C*) Axial postcontrast CT cisternogram images showing contrast filling the frontal sinus with a fluid level, indicates an active leak (*black arrow*).

other common sites of injury include the posterior ethmoid roof, sphenoid sinus, and posterior table of the frontal sinus (**Fig. 9**).[47]

Nontraumatic Leaks

Secondary leaks

The least commonly encountered category of CSF leaks are those nontraumatic leaks in which a definite pathologic cause is identified. These leaks can be caused by erosion of the skull base by tumors (before or after radiation therapy), mucoceles, osteonecrosis, or other erosive processes (eg, Gorham-Stout disease) (**Fig. 10**). CSF leaks can also be caused by congenital lesions, which can occur with or without increased intracranial pressure. The congenital lesions reported to cause

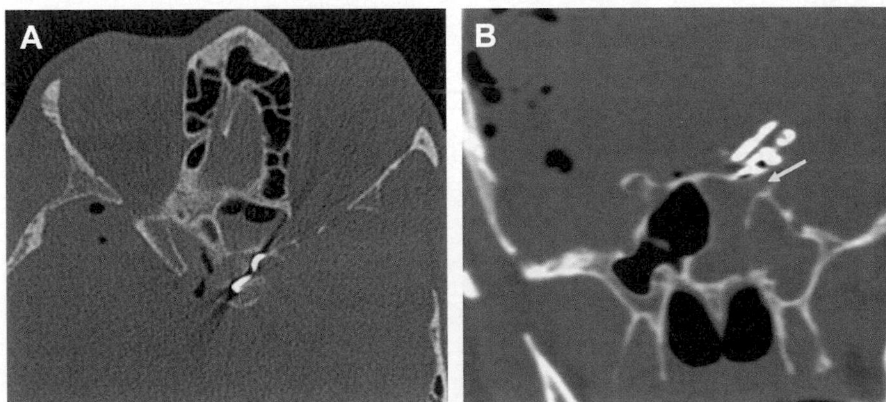

Fig. 7. A 48-year-old woman after craniotomy with clinoidectomy for periclinoid aneurysm clipping presenting with headache and rhinorrhea 1 week postoperatively. Axial (*A*) and coronal (*B*) bone window images of HRCT of the sinuses showing postoperative changes after clinoidectomy and aneurysm clipping with fluid level in the left sphenoid sinus and worsening pneumocephalus, indicating CSF leak. Note the fluid within the previously pneumatized optic strut adjacent to the aneurysm clip (*arrow in B*).

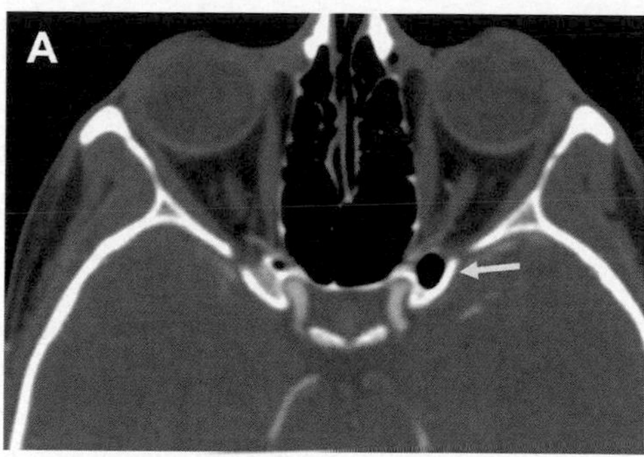

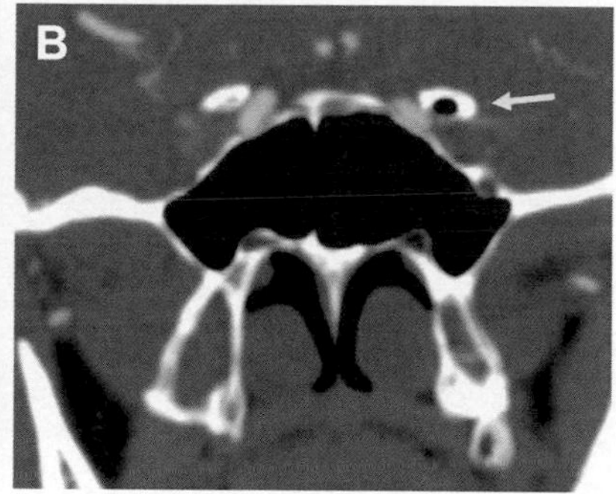

Fig. 8. Axial (*A*) and coronal (*B*) CT angiogram images performed to assess an aneurysm (not shown) showing a pneumatized left clinoid process (*arrow*). These processes should be mentioned in the report, particularly if ipsilateral to a periclinoid aneurysm.

CSF leak include congenital encephaloceles, persistent craniopharyngeal canal (with or without tumor) (**Fig. 11**), or congenital widening of the diaphragma sella (primary empty sella syndrome).[48]

Spontaneous leaks

Spontaneous leaks are those leaks without an underlying lesion, congenital abnormality, or history of trauma or surgery, and most of these are thought to be caused by underlying IIH. IIH is a headache syndrome classically seen in overweight women, with visual disturbance, papilledema, and sometimes tinnitus or hearing loss. Population studies in the United States performed in late 1980s showed an annual incidence of IIH of approximately 1 in 100,000 in the general population, which increased to 19 in 100,000 in overweight women aged in the range of 20 to 44 years.[49] There has also been an increased prevalence of this disease over the last few decades, likely caused by the epidemic of obesity in the United States, as well as increased awareness of IIH among health care professionals. There is a great deal of clinical and radiologic overlap between the findings of patients with IIH and spontaneous CSF leak, which has led to the proposed link between these 2 entities. It is proposed that, in patients with spontaneous CSF leak, increased intracranial pressure, possibly caused by increased intra-abdominal and intravenous pressures, leads to increased dural pulsations, which erode the skull base over time, ultimately leading to a dural tear and CSF leak.[7,50] In addition to these osteodural defects, this sustained increased pressure can also lead to the formation of prominent arachnoid pits at the skull base with areas of overlying dural thinning, as well as the formation of meningoceles and meningoencephaloceles. As such, spontaneous CSF leaks are emerging as a more frequent presentation of IIH,[51] and are becoming one of the most commonly encountered causes of CSF leak requiring imaging evaluation. Historically, nontraumatic spontaneous leaks have been reported to account for only approximately 4% of CSF leaks. However, more recent data suggest that spontaneous leaks may be more common than was previously considered, ranging from 20.8% to 40% of CSF leaks.[18,52,53]

Fig. 9. Coronal bone window CT images showing a large defect along the left cribriform plate, lateral lamella, and ethmoid roof (*arrow*), with adjacent polypoid nondependent soft tissue (concerning for meningoencephalocele).

Although the International Headache Society does not include imaging findings among the diagnostic criteria for IIH, neurologic imaging is required at the minimum to exclude hydrocephalus, mass, or structural or vascular lesion. Although not highly specific, there are many imaging findings that are suggestive of IIH, especially when seen in combination, and can help prompt additional work-up, including ophthalmologic evaluation and CSF opening pressures.[54] These indicative findings include empty sella, optic nerve sheath enlargement and/or tortuosity, optic nerve head protrusion with flattening of the posterior

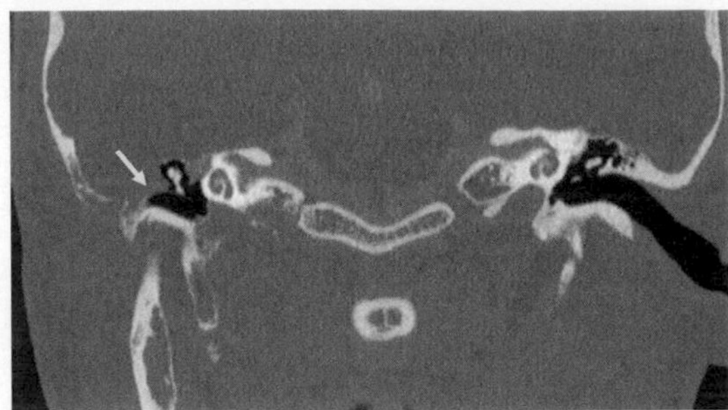

Fig. 10. A 22-year-old woman with a history of Gorham disease presenting with headaches and CSF rhinorrhea. Coronal bone window CT images from a CT cisternogram show osteolysis of the right temporal bone, involving the tegmen (*arrow*). The ipsilateral occipital bone and mandible were also involved.

globe, and optic nerve head edema with enhancement (**Fig. 12**). Findings at the skull base that can also be detected on the HRCT of the sinuses, in addition to the large empty sella include scalloping of the inner table of the calvarium, prominent arachnoid pits, multiple osseous defects along the skull base, and enlargement of the skull base foramina (**Fig. 13**).[51,55] The skull base should be interrogated carefully for meningoceles because they are significantly more common in patients with IIH, affecting up to 11% of all patients with IIH in some series,[56] but are seen in 50% to 100% of patients with spontaneous CSF leak in other series[51] (**Fig. 14**). Bilateral transverse sinus stenosis is also associated with IIH and is seen in these patients, although it is unclear whether this is the cause or result of the underlying disorder (**Fig. 15**). Another recently described finding seen in patients with IIH is low-lying cerebellar tonsils with inferiorly displaced brainstem and cerebellum, mimicking a Chiari 1 malformation.[57] The most common sites of spontaneous CSF leaks from IIH are the ethmoid roof/cribriform plate and lateral recess of the sphenoid.[58–60] Because these patients are prone to developing meningoceles and multiple skull base defects,[61] they often require multiple modalities of imaging for their work-up, including MR and CTC.

In the setting of an active CSF leak, patients with IIH may have pseudonormalized intracranial

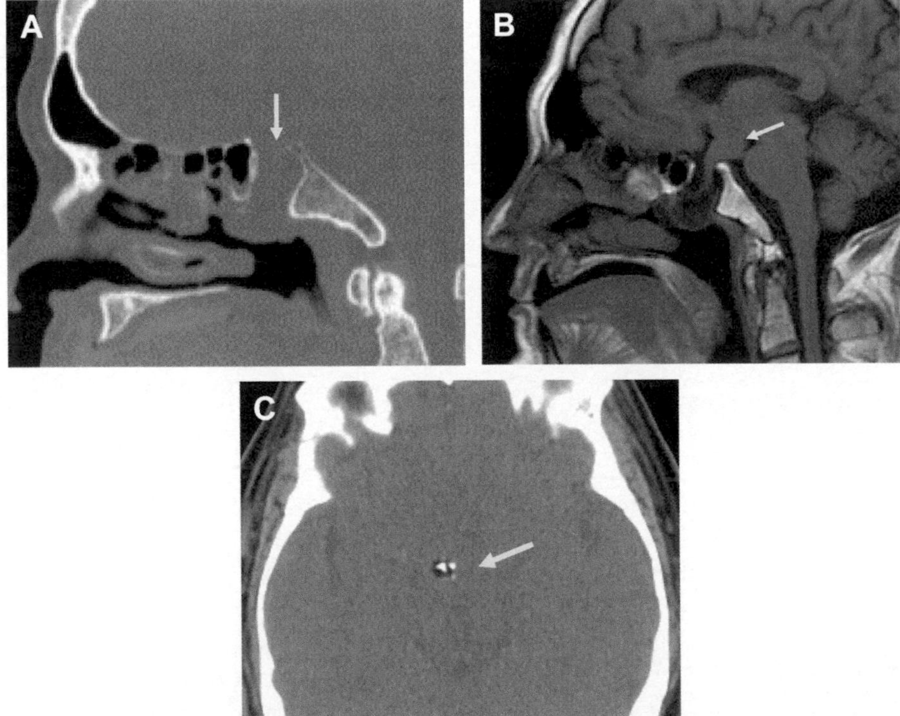

Fig. 11. A 49-year-old man presenting with recurrent meningitis. (*A*) Sagittal CT images show a large defect in the expected location of the craniopharyngeal canal (*arrow*), through which there is herniation of polypoid nondependent soft tissue into the nasopharynx. (*B*) Sagittal T1-weighted MR imaging through the midline shows a large cephalocele herniating through the defect, with herniation of the infundibulum. Note the soft tissue fullness in the expected location of the sella and suprasellar cistern (*arrow*). (*C*) Axial soft tissue window CT image showing fat and calcium in the large sellar/suprasellar mass compatible with a teratoma (*arrow*). This craniopharyngeal canal defect is type 3C,[69] presenting with recurrent meningitis caused by the large cephalocele.

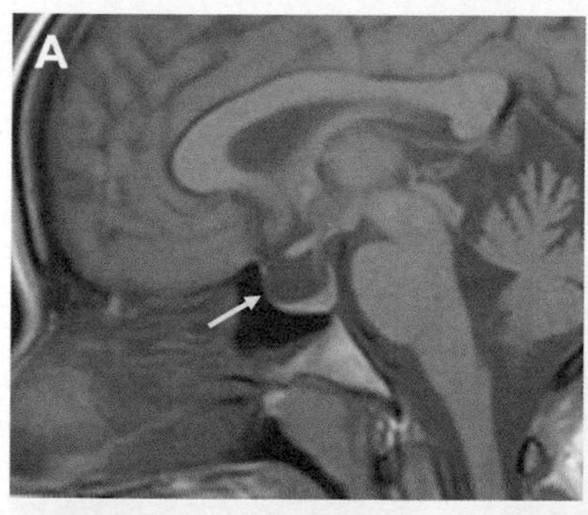

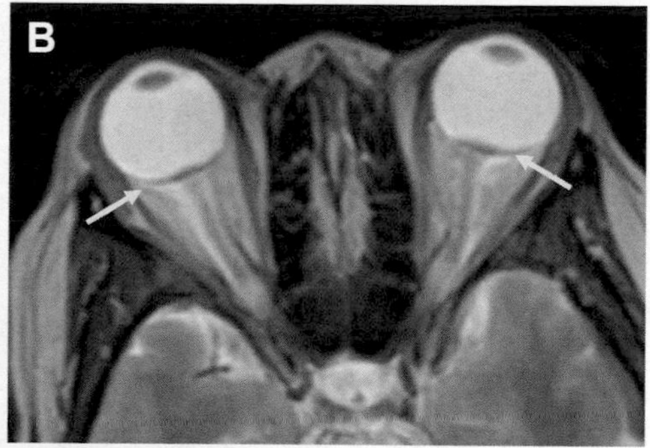

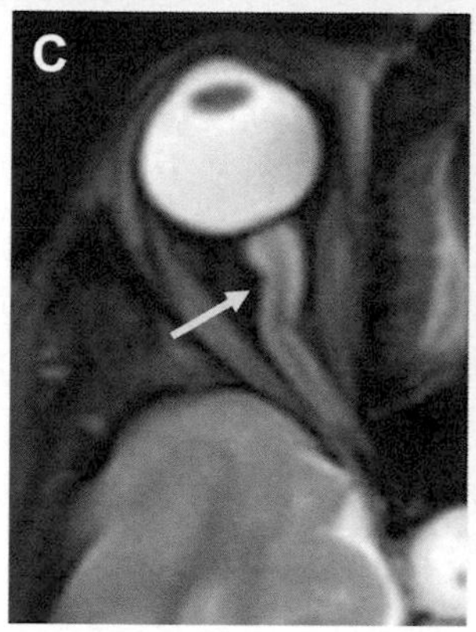

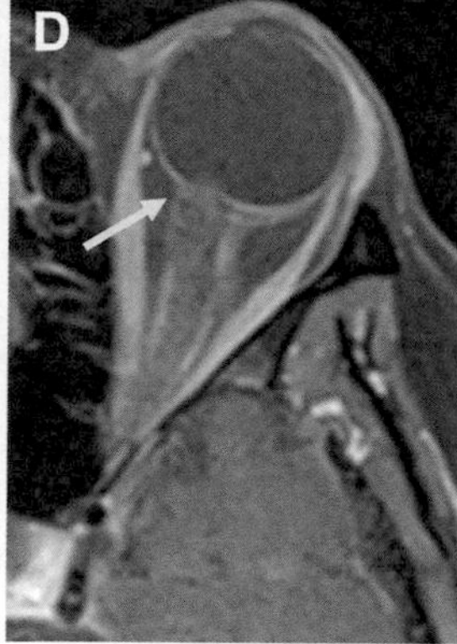

Fig. 12. Imaging findings of IIH. (*A*) Sagittal T1-weighted images showing a large partially empty sella (*arrow*). (*B, C*). Axial T2w images through the orbits showing optic nerve head protrusion with flattening of the posterior globes (*arrows in B*) and optic nerve sheath tortuosity (*arrow in C*). (*D*) Axial postcontrast fat-saturated images showing slight edema and enhancement of the optic nerve head (*arrow*).

pressure measurement caused by spontaneous decompression, therefore opening pressures may not be helpful at the time of diagnosis. However, the underlying diagnosis of IIH should be suggested if the characteristic imaging features described earlier are present in a patient with a CSF leak. Suggesting the diagnosis prospectively is helpful for the treating surgeon, because these patients have an overall worse prognosis, with increased tendency to recur after treatment, either at the site of initial repair, or frequently at another site of osseous thinning or dehiscence, particularly if their underlying IIH is not addressed. Recurrence rates after repair of idiopathic CSF leaks range from 25% to 87%.[38,51,62–65] In addition to considering surgical repair, patients with documented or suspected IIH may need to be managed medically via acetazolamide medication, weight reduction strategies, or even ventriculoperitoneal or lumbar-peritoneal shunting, as a last resort.[51]

DIAGNOSTIC CRITERIA

Clinical Diagnosis

As discussed earlier, the clinical diagnosis of CSF leak should be confirmed with β2-transferrin testing of the rhinorrhea or otorrhea, if possible. Endoscopic examination findings of CSF leak include the presence of clear watery rhinorrhea that pools and increases with Valsalva or provocative head-hanging maneuvers, as well as the possible presence of a blue pulsatile mass, if there is a large meningocele. However, the endoscopic visualization of the site of a leak depends on the variable degree of exposure of the skull base, and, in most circumstances, examination is normal. If the site of a leak is in question, and the patient is presenting with CSF rhinorrhea, one other possible technique for clinical diagnosis is the intrathecal administration of sodium fluorescein, a green dye, in an effort to localize the site of the leak on nasal endoscopy. This fluorescein may be administered preoperatively (often at the time of perioperative lumbar drain placement), to aid the surgeons in diagnosing the leak intraoperatively and/or confirm watertight closure on repair. However, the false-negative rate of this technique reportedly ranges from 15% to 44%, and the intrathecal use of fluorescein is currently not FDA approved, so this technique is typically reserved for problem-solving cases only.[66]

Imaging Diagnosis

Imaging is essential to localize the site of the leak and aid in preoperative planning. Specific criteria

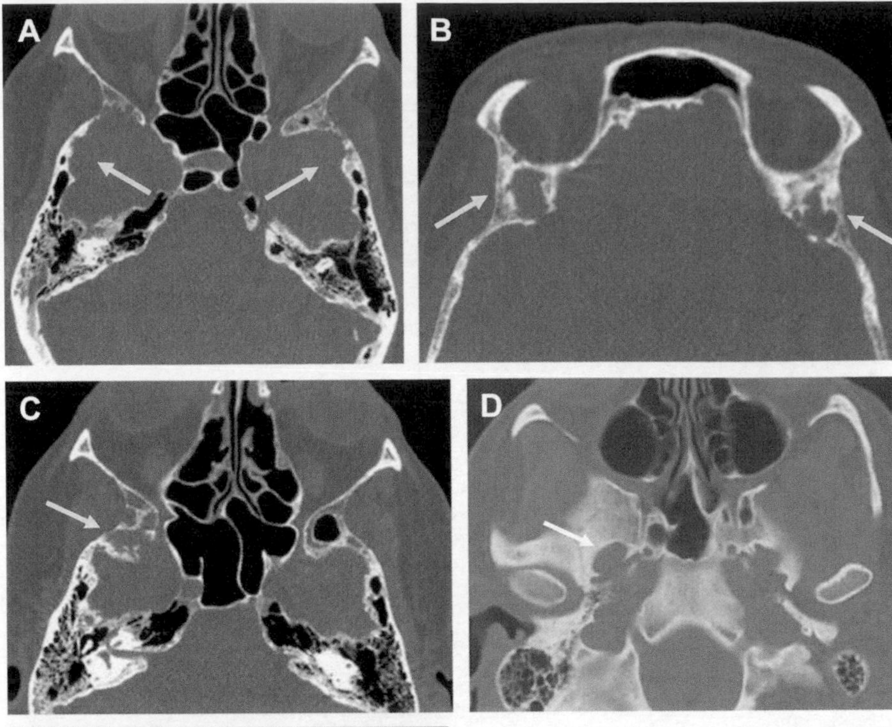

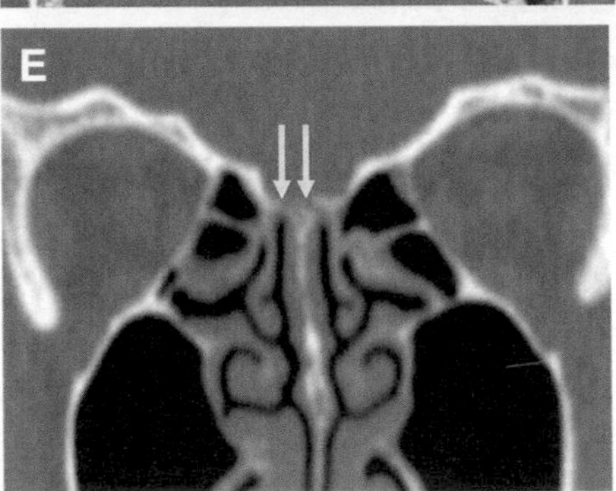

Fig. 13. CT findings in the setting of IIH. Axial and coronal CT bone window images of a patient with IIH. (*A*) Scalloping of the inner table of the calvarium (*arrows*). (*B, C*) Prominent arachnoid pits, in their common location along the sphenoid wing (*arrows*). (*D*) Enlarged neural foramina, as seen in this enlarged foramen ovale on the right (*arrow*). (*E*) Multiple osseous defects: bilateral defects along the cribriform plates (*arrows*).

for diagnosing a CSF leak on each of the previously described modalities is as follows:

- CT (**Fig. 16**):
  - Presence of osseous defects in the skull base, particularly if there is adjacent fluid layering dependently within or adjacent to the bony defect in the sinuses or mastoids
  - Polypoid nondependent soft tissue in the sinonasal cavity, or along the tegmen, adjacent to an osseous defect (suspicious for meningoencephalocele)[20]
    - Particularly nondependent unilateral soft tissue in the olfactory recess in isolation should be suspicious for small meningocele[67]
- CTC (**Fig. 17**):
  - Presence of osseous defects in the skull base, plus
  - Increased density or pooling of high-density soft tissue in the sinuses or mastoids adjacent to the defect
    - Can measure region of interest (ROI) and compare on the precontrast and postcontrast images: a 2-fold increase in attenuation is diagnostic of a leak[20]
    - Other findings include contrast washout intracranially ipsilateral to a high-flow leak, soufflé effect with increasing density of contrast dependently, and movement of contrast with changes in patient position, confirming an active leak

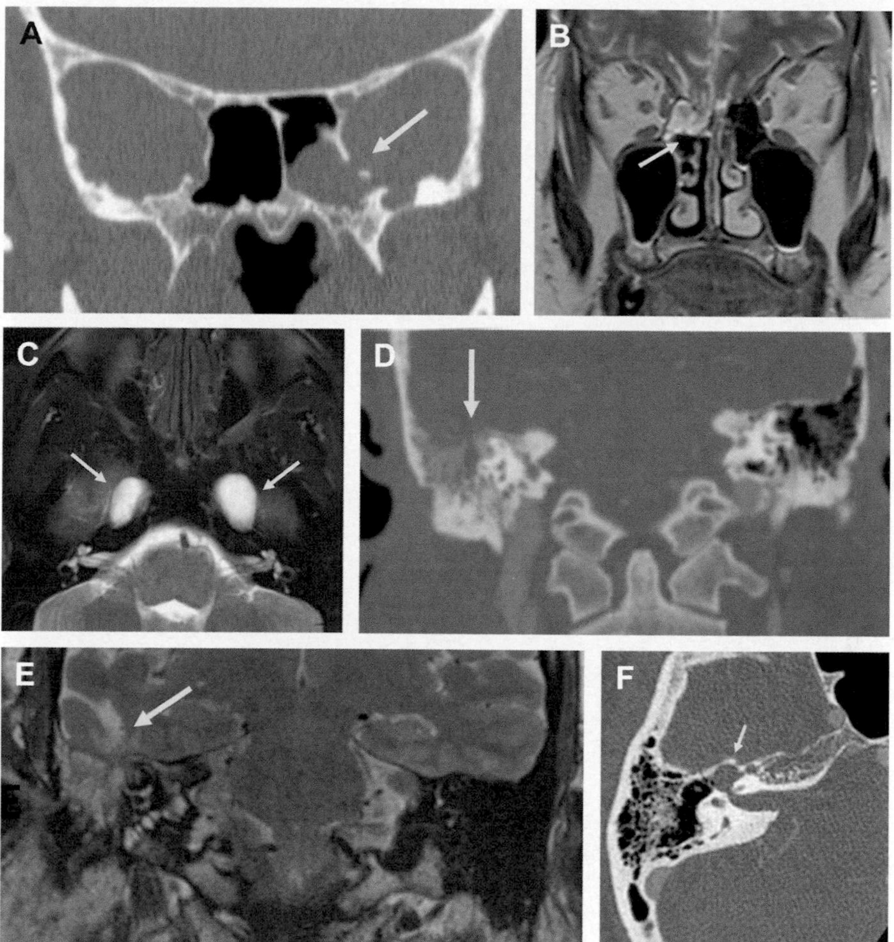

Fig. 14. Images showing the typical appearances and locations of meningoceles in the setting of IIH. (*A*) CT showing polypoid nondependent soft tissue adjacent to bony defect in the lateral recess of the sphenoid sinus (*arrow*), adjacent to foramen rotundum. (*B*) Coronal T2w MR imaging showing herniation of right frontal lobe and CSF into the right ethmoid sinuses (*arrow*). (*C*) Axial T2w images showing bilateral Meckel cave meningoceles (*arrow*). (*D, E*) Coronal CT and T2w images showing a meningocele along the tegmen mastoideum (*arrow*). Note the downward tethering of temporal lobe parenchyma and adjacent traction gliosis of the temporal lobe on MR imaging (*arrow in E*). (*F*) Polypoid soft tissue and enlargement of the geniculate ganglion (*arrow*), as commonly seen in facial meningoceles in patients with IIH.

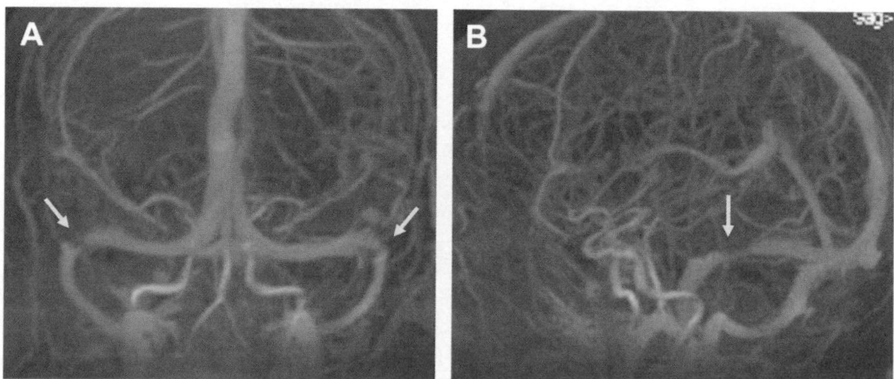

Fig. 15. A 28-year-old woman with IIH. (*A, B*) Maximal intensity projection reformatted images from MR venography show bilateral high-grade stenosis in the distal transverse sinuses (*arrows*).

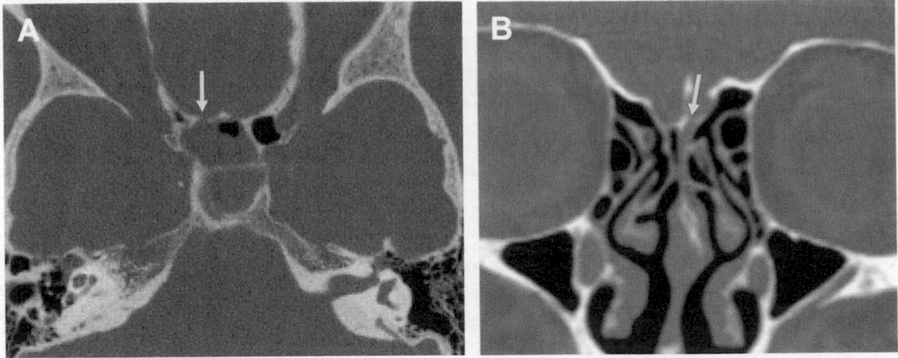

Fig. 16. CT findings of site of CSF leak include osseous defect along the skull base, particularly with fluid/opacification within the adjacent nasal cavity or sinus. (*A*) Axial CT showing linear defect in the planum sphenoidale and fluid level in the sphenoid sinus (*arrow*). (*B*) Coronal CT showing polypoid nondependent soft tissue in the left olfactory recess, suspicious for meningocele (*arrow*).

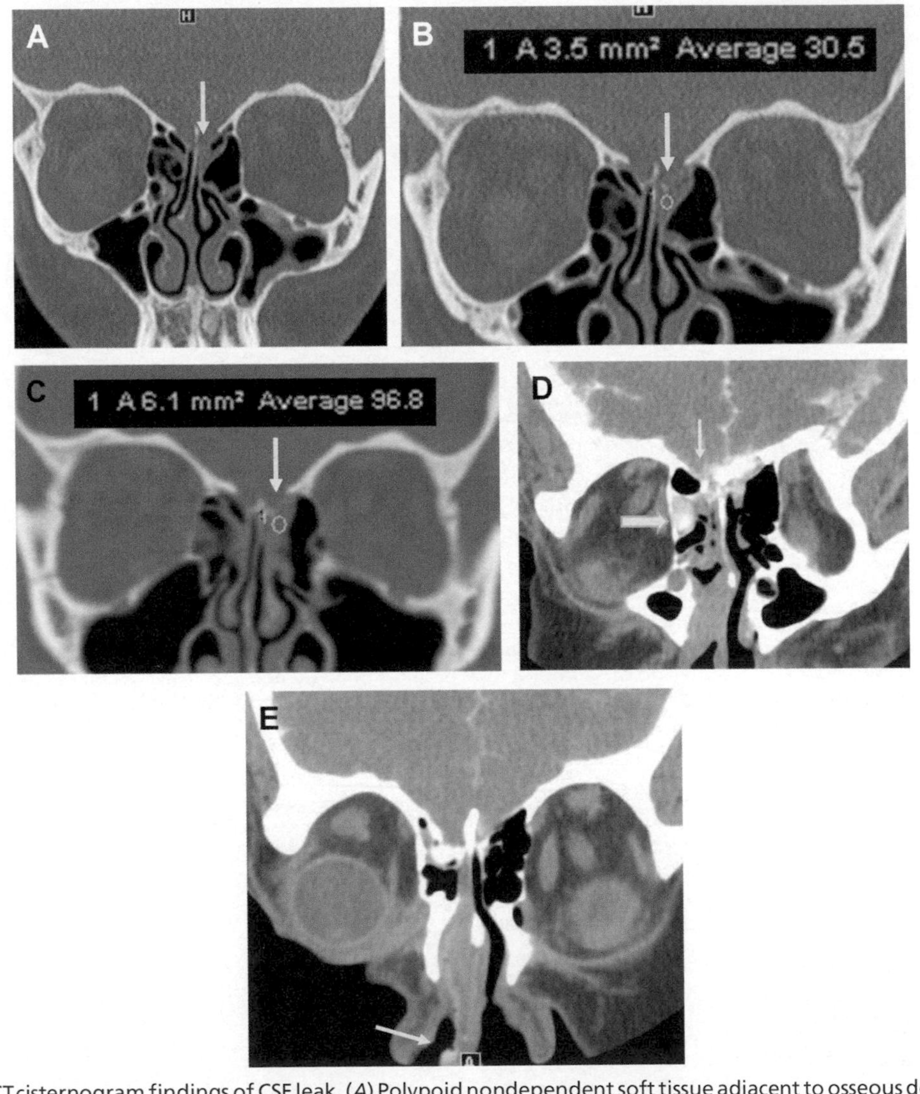

Fig. 17. CT cisternogram findings of CSF leak. (*A*) Polypoid nondependent soft tissue adjacent to osseous defect in the left olfactory recess, which increases in attenuation from the precontrast (*B*) to the postcontrast (*C*) cisternogram images (*arrows*), confirming the site of leak. (*D, E*) Direct coronal imaging of another patient in the prone position, showing rapid washout of the CSF intracranially on the side of the leak compared with the other side (*arrow in D*), as well as the soufflé effect of layering of the dense contrast dependently in a patient with active leak along the right ethmoid roof into the ethmoid sinuses (*thick arrow in D*). Note also the movement of contrast with changes in patient position, as seen in this patient with contrast trickling anteriorly out of the nose in the prone position (*arrow in E*).

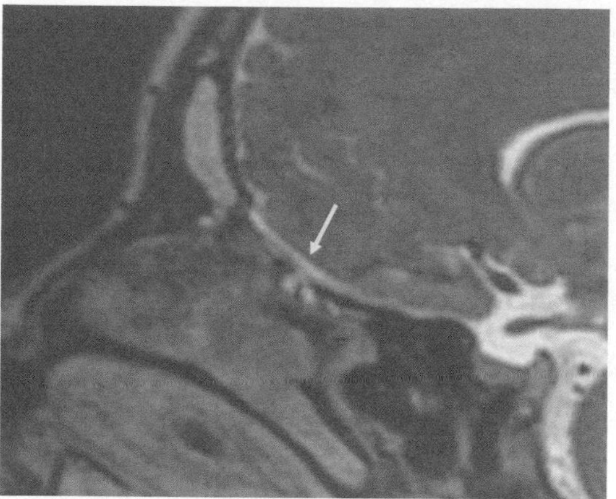

Fig. 18. MR cisternogram findings of CSF leak. Sagittal T2 SPACE sequence image showing a continuous column of CSF extending inferiorly through a defect in the cribriform plate. Note the multiple linear tracts in this complex meningocele along the cribriform plate (*arrow*).

- MRC (**Fig. 18**):
  - Continuous column of T2 hyperintense CSF extending from the subarachnoid space into the sinonasal cavity or mastoid/petrous air cells (isointense to CSF on all sequences) through an area of osseous defect (confirmed on prior CT)[14]
    - May or may not contain herniated brain contents
- Contrast-enhanced MRC (**Fig. 19**):
  - Continuous column of T1 hyperintense gadolinium contrast extending from the subarachnoid space into the sinonasal cavity or mastoid/petrous air cells through an area of osseous defect (confirmed on CT)[32]
    - Helpful to obtain precontrast T1-weighted images for comparison

Differential Diagnosis

There is not much of a differential diagnosis in the setting of a suspected CSF leak. The patient is either leaking CSF or not, and because rhinorrhea or otorrhea could also have benign inflammatory causes, testing the fluid for β2-transferrin is imperative and confirmatory.

However, a differential diagnosis does exist for a suspected meningocele. Polypoid nondependent soft tissue in the sinonasal cavity on CT with an adjacent bony defect could be caused by sinonasal polyposis or sinonasal neoplasm, thus MR imaging is often necessary to differentiate these entities (**Fig. 20**). In addition, occasionally a skull base cholesteatoma eroding through the tegmen tympani can appear similar to a meningocele extending inferiorly on CT and even routine MR imaging sequences (T2 hyperintense, T1 hypointense, and possibly even peripherally enhancing), but diffusion-weighted sequences should be able to differentiate between those entities, because cholesteatoma should show restricted diffusion (**Fig. 21**).[68] In addition, spontaneous lateral sphenoid cephaloceles along the greater wing of the sphenoid bone or in the clivus can mimic other skull base neoplasms, such as chordoma or chondrosarcoma (**Fig. 22**), and meningoceles in the region of the geniculate ganglion can mimic other facial nerve tumors such as hemangioma (see **Fig. 14**).[55] Looking for other morphologic features suggestive of IIH can be helpful, and contrast-enhanced MR imaging confirms the diagnosis. The absence of central enhancement, isointensity to CSF on all sequences, and tethering and/or

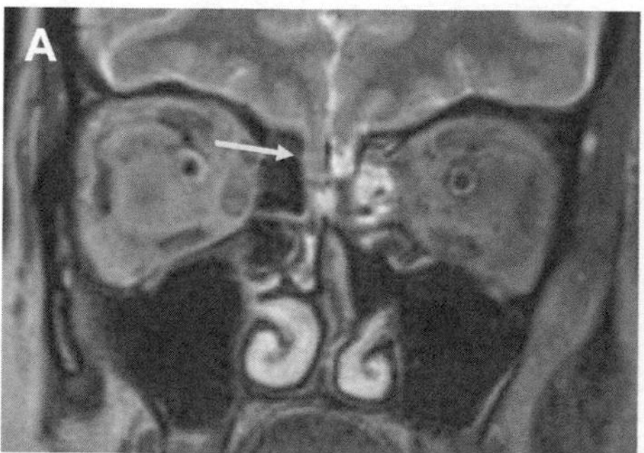

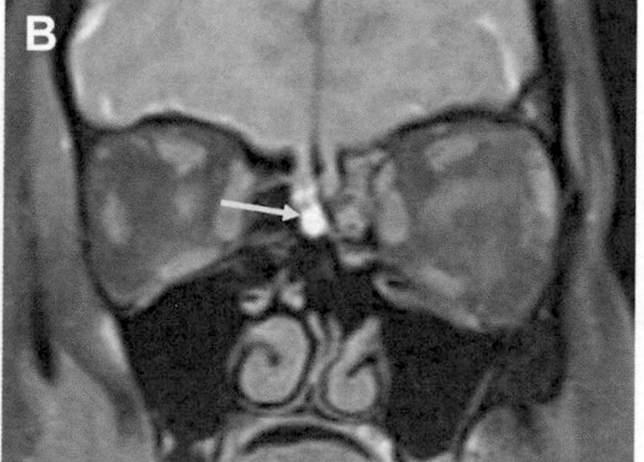

Fig. 19. Contrast-enhanced MR cisternogram findings of CSF leak. (*A*) Coronal T2w MR images showing T2 hyperintense soft tissue along the superior nasal septum on the right and within the left ethmoid air cells in a patient with intermittent leak and osseous defects adjacent to both sites. However, the right side is most suspicious for meningocele, because there is also tethering/low-lying gyrus rectus on that side (*arrow*). (*B*) Coronal T1-weighted (T1w) fat-saturated images from contrast-enhanced MR cisternogram with intrathecal gadolinium, showing filling of a meningocele along the superior nasal septum on the right (*arrow*), confirming the site of the leak.

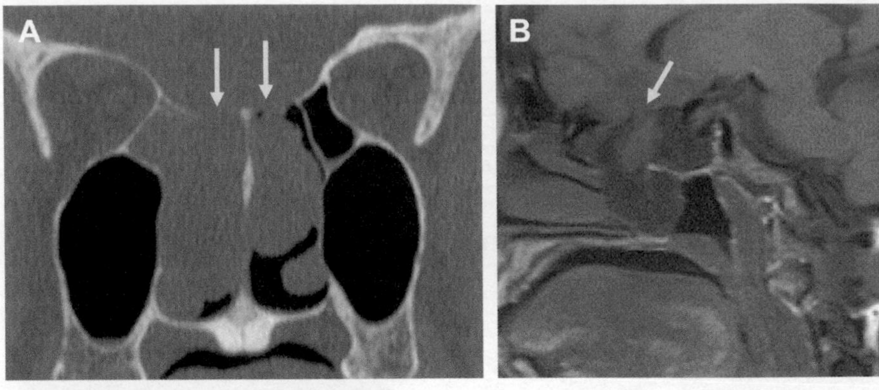

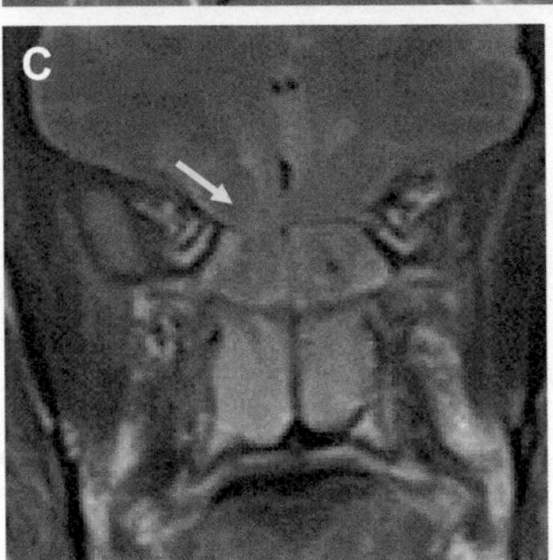

Fig. 20. Meningoceles mimicking sinonasal polyposis. (*A*) Coronal CT sinus image of a patient imaged for headache shows bilateral polypoid masses in the nasal cavity, with the appearance of sinonasal polyposis. However, note the defects along the adjacent posterior ethmoid roof (*arrows*). MR imaging was therefore recommended. Sagittal T1w (*B*) and Coronal T2w MR images (*C*) showing herniation of gliotic brain tissue and CSF into the nasal cavity, compatible with bilateral meningoencephaloceles (*arrows*).

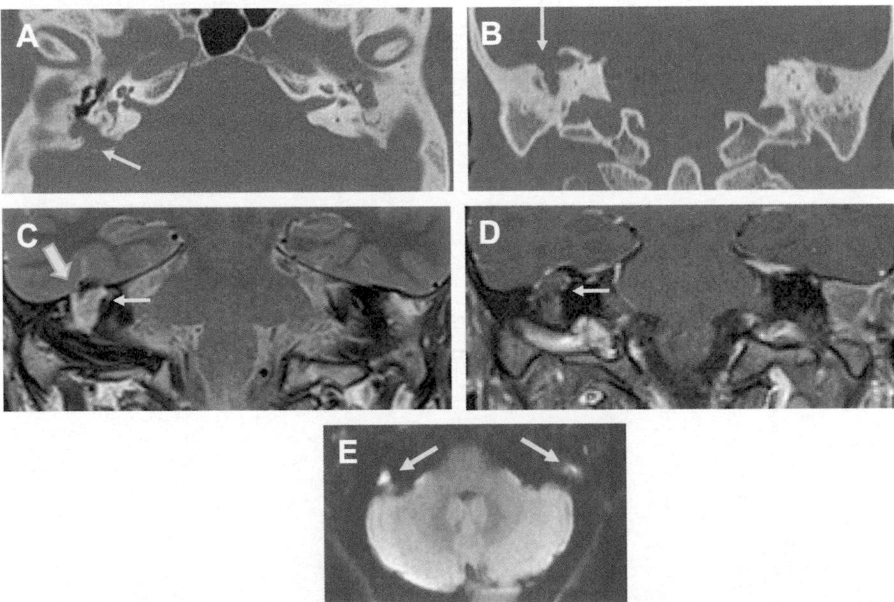

Fig. 21. Cholesteatoma mimicking meningocele. A 21-year-old man with bilateral hearing loss. (*A*, *B*). Axial and coronal temporal bone CT shows right-sided soft tissue mass with erosion of the tegmen posteriorly (*arrows*). Note also the sclerotic underpneumatized mastoid and the left-sided middle ear and mastoid soft tissue mass. (*C*, *D*) Coronal T2w and T1w postcontrast fat-saturated sequences showing the right-sided mass to be T2 hyperintense and T1 hypointense with peripheral enhancement (*arrows*). Note the thinning of the tegmen, but without inferior herniation or tethering of brain parenchyma (*thick arrow in C*). (*E*) Axial diffusion-weighted sequences showing diffusion restriction within the mastoid and middle ear masses bilaterally, compatible with cholesteatoma (*arrows*).

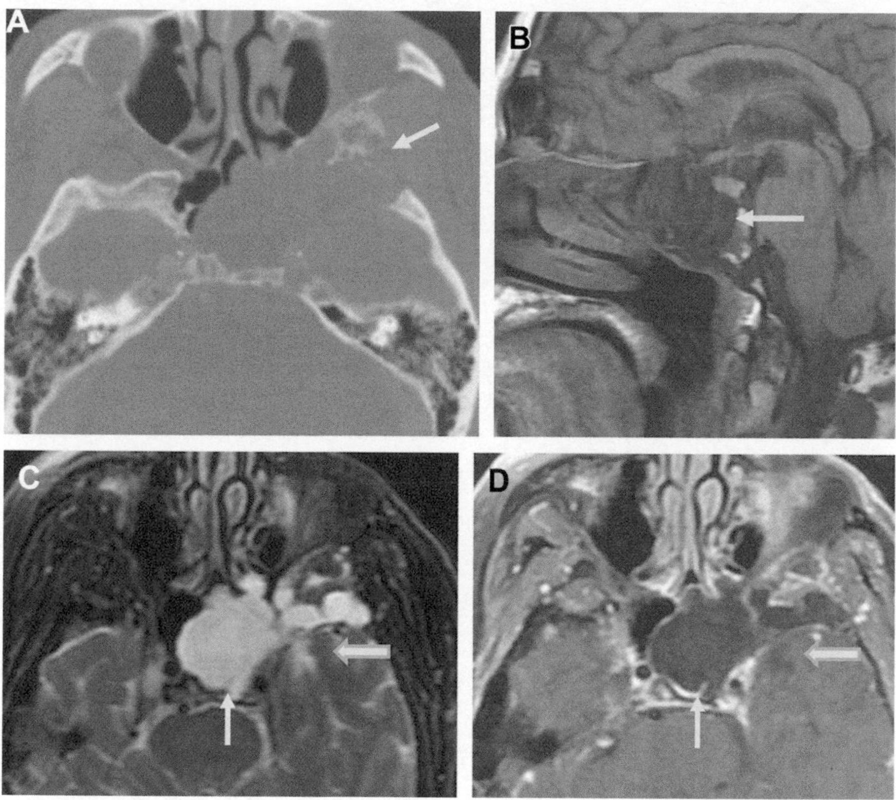

Fig. 22. Sphenoid wing meningocele mimicking skull base neoplasm (ie, chordoma). (*A*) Axial CT images show expansile lucent mass replacing the left sphenoid wing and clivus, eroding the middle cranial fossa. Note the scalloped appearance often seen with arachnoid pits and meningoceles in the sphenoid wing (*arrow*). Sagittal T1w (*B*), axial T2w (*C*), and axial T1w fat-saturated postcontrast (*D*) MR images show the lesion to be isointense to CSF on all sequences, without central enhancement, compatible with meningoencephalocele (*arrows*). Note the tethering and gliosis of the adjacent left temporal lobe (*thick arrows in C, D*).

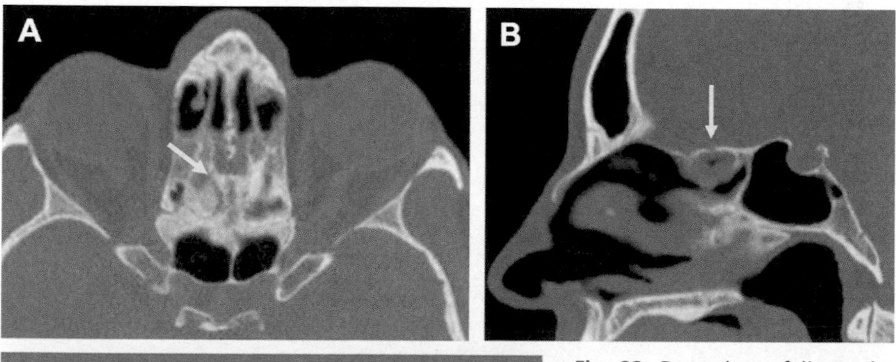

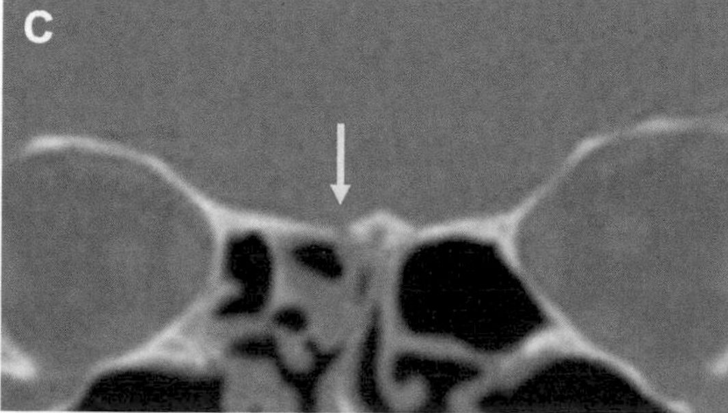

Fig. 23. Detection of linear lucencies and site of CSF leak on CT can be challenging. Reformatting in multiple planes can help to determine the site of leak and show its size and trajectory in multiple dimensions, as in this case of a right ethmoid roof defect, difficult to clearly identify in the axial plane (*A*), but confirmed on the sagittal (*B*) and coronal (*C*) reformats (*arrows*).

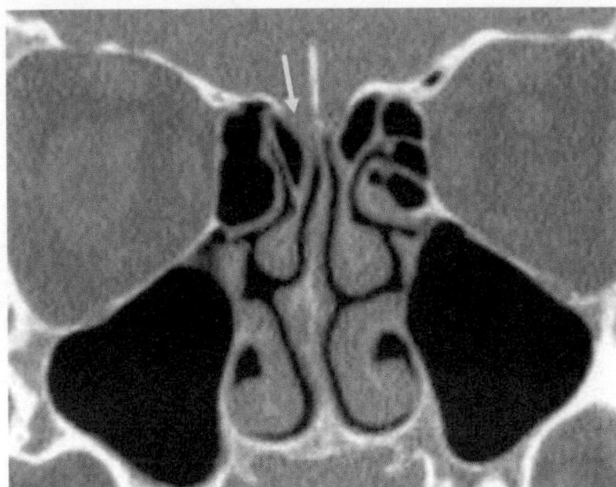

Fig. 24. Patient with right-sided CSF rhinorrhea, positive β2-transferrin, with subtle lucency along the right cribriform plate and lateral lamella, associated with soft tissue in the right olfactory recess (*arrow*), which was proved to be the site of the leak intraoperatively.

gliosis of adjacent brain parenchyma, when present, should all suggest a meningocele.

PITFALLS

There are numerous pitfalls and challenges in the complex work-up and evaluation of patients with CSF rhinorrhea and otorrhea. Some of the more frequently encountered include:

- Patients may present with pneumocephalus, middle ear effusion, or meningitis without rhinorrhea, therefore fluid cannot be tested for β2-transferrin. In this case, a combination of HRCT and MR cisternogram can be helpful to determine a site of a leak, with or without the administration of intrathecal gadolinium.
- Detecting osseous defects on CT can be challenging. Reviewing images on a 3D workstation independently in multiple planes, magnifying views, and optimizing the window and level settings are all techniques that help to minimize this challenge (**Fig. 23**).
- Inherent thinning and irregularity of the cribriform plates is seemingly present throughout the population, even in patients without CSF leaks. However, at our institution, we mention all focal defects in patients with proven leaks, particularly if there is adjacent soft tissue in the olfactory recess (**Fig. 24**).
- Particularly in the setting of IIH, the presence of multiple osseous defects and/or meningoceles complicates determining which site is currently leaking. CT or MR cisternograms can be helpful in this setting, but occasionally these are negative if the patient is not leaking at the time of imaging. In these cases, the surgeons often stage the repairs, and address the site that is considered most suspicious first.
- CTC in the postoperative setting, particularly in the setting of a recurrent leak, is challenging, because osteoneogenesis, inspissated secretions, and postoperative graft/granulation tissue are all increased in density. Thus, it is imperative to review precontrast and postcontrast images side by side. Soft tissue algorithm images can be helpful in assessing density differences (**Fig. 25**).
- Drawing ROIs in the mastoid air cells or other small variant cells on CTC can be difficult. Magnifying the images can help, but occasionally it is impossible.
- Occasionally, particularly in the setting of IIH, meningoceles can present with a canal-like appearance, with linear tracts extending through the bone. It is important to delineate the entire course of the meningocele to minimize the potential for recurrence, which can be done via a combination of thin section T2w MR cisternograms and CT (**Fig. 26**).

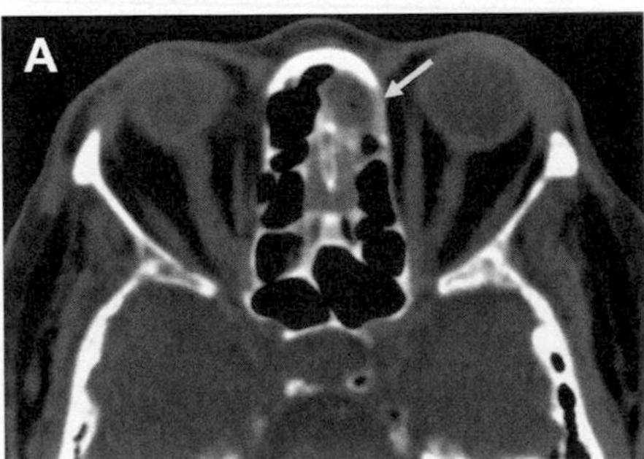

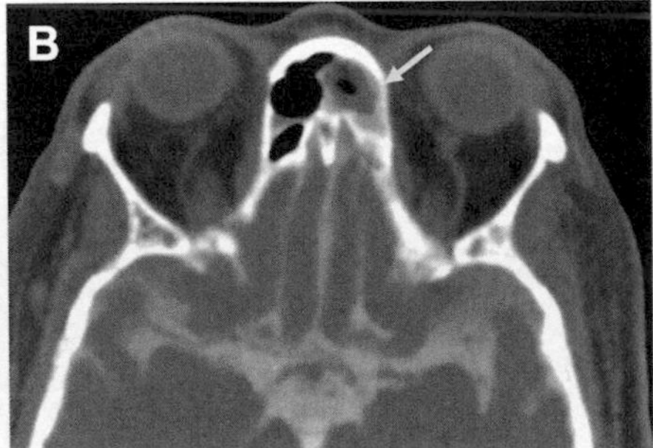

Fig. 25. Pitfall: CT cisternogram in the postoperative setting can be challenging because of underlying osteoneogenesis, as in this patient with recurrent leak after repair of a left frontal sinus meningocele. Comparing the precontrast (*A*) and postcontrast (*B*) images shows only peripheral osteoneogenesis in the left frontal sinus (*arrows*), without definite leak at the postoperative site. Optimizing window and level settings on soft tissue windows is often helpful.

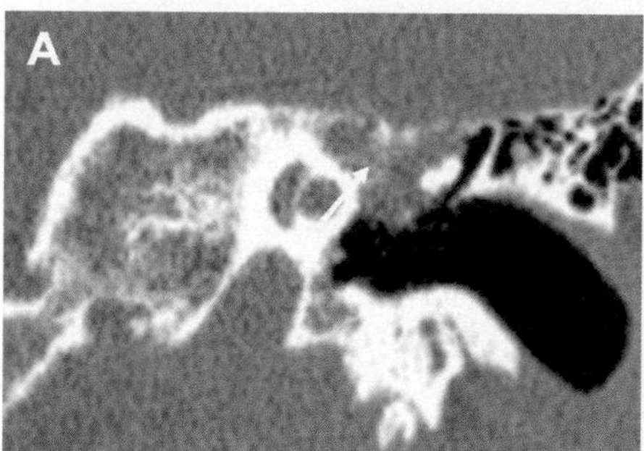

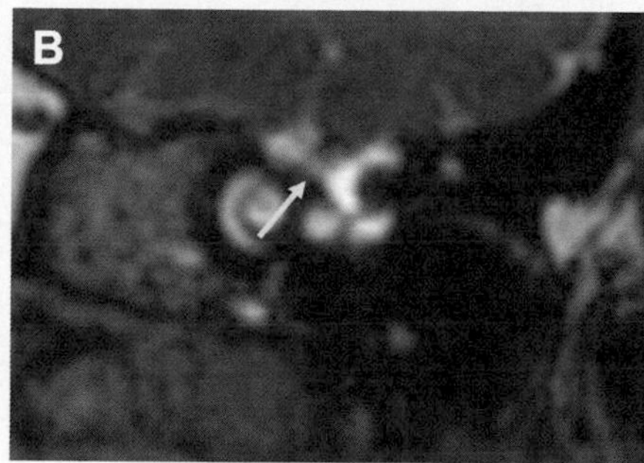

Fig. 26. Pitfall: meningoceles can be multifocal and present with a canal-like appearance, particularly in the setting of IIH, with linear tracts connecting different areas of meningoceles, as in this patient with a meningocele in the left middle ear, medial to ossicles seen on Coronal temporal bone CT (A) and T2w MRI images (B). This meningocele communicated via a tract to the region of the geniculate ganglion (*arrows*), a finding that was confirmed intraoperatively. Identifying the entire course of the meningocele is important to minimize the potential for recurrence postoperatively.

- Performing lumbar punctures for cisternography on obese patients (commonly encountered in IIH) may be technically challenging. A standard-length 89-mm (3.5-inch) spinal needle is used to access the thecal sac in most patients. In obese patients, 127-mm (5-inch) and 178-mm (7-inch) needles may be needed; however, these can become difficult to steer. In these cases, clinicians can use an 18-gauge 89-mm needle to guide the longer needle using a coaxial technique.

WHAT SURGEONS WANT TO KNOW

All of the following information should be included in the imaging reports of these patients, if possible:

- Location and size of defects measured in multiple planes; scrutinize entire skull base, including sinuses and mastoids.
- Anatomy of sinonasal cavity (ie, nasal septal deviation, perforation, variants) for surgical planning/approach.
- Presence of associated meningoencephaloceles (may need MR cisternogram).
- Presence of imaging features suggestive of underlying IIH.
- Sites that are actively leaking.
- Entire course of meningocele tract (heavily T2w images and CT).
- Opening pressure, if performing cisternography. However, keep in mind that it is common for the opening pressure to be normal or only borderline increased in patients with IIH in the setting of an ongoing leak.

SUMMARY

The work-up of CSF rhinorrhea and otorrhea can be complex, often requiring a time-intensive and labor-intensive thorough investigation of the skull base on multiple modalities. It is important to have an algorithm for the approach to this challenging clinical problem, to be aware of potential pitfalls in imaging these patients, and to focus on what surgeons need to know to guide appropriate surgical planning.

REFERENCES

1. Daudia A, Biswas D, Jones NS. Risk of meningitis with cerebrospinal fluid rhinorrhea. Ann Otol Rhinol Laryngol 2007;116(12):902–5.
2. Miner JR, Heegaard W, Mapes A, et al. Presentation, time to antibiotics, and mortality of patients with bacterial meningitis at an urban county medical center. J Emerg Med 2001;21(4):387–92.
3. Komotar RJ, Starke RM, Raper D, et al. Endoscopic endonasal versus open repair of anterior skull base CSF leak, meningocele, and encephalocele: a systematic review of outcomes. J Neurol Surg A Cent Eur Neurosurg 2013;74(4):239–50.
4. Sharma S, Kumar G, Bal J, et al. Endoscopic repair of cerebrospinal fluid rhinorrhoea. Eur Ann Otorhinolaryngol Head Neck Dis 2016;133(3):187–90.
5. Locatelli D, Rampa F, Acchiardi I, et al. Endoscopic endonasal approaches for repair of cerebrospinal fluid leaks: nine-year experience. Neurosurgery 2006;58(4):ONS-246–56.
6. Ommaya AK, Di Chiro G, Baldwin M, et al. Non-traumatic cerebrospinal fluid rhinorrhea. J Neurol Neurosurg Psychiatr 1968;31(3):214–25.
7. Schlosser RJ, Wilensky EM, Grady MS, et al. Elevated intracranial pressures in spontaneous cerebrospinal fluid leaks. Am J Rhinol 2003;17:191–5.
8. Oakley GM, Alt JA, Schlosser RJ, et al. Diagnosis of cerebrospinal fluid rhinorrhea: an evidence-based review with recommendations. Int Forum Allergy Rhinol 2016;6:8–16.

9. McCudden CR, Senior BA, Hainsworth S, et al. Evaluation of high resolution gel β2-transferrin for detection of cerebrospinal fluid leak. Clin Chem Lab Med 2013;51(2):311–5.
10. Bleier BS, Debnath I, O'Connell BP, et al. Preliminary study on the stability of beta-2 transferrin in extracorporeal cerebrospinal fluid. Otolaryngol Head Neck Surg 2011;144(1):101–3.
11. Schnabel C, Di Martino E, Gilsbach JM, et al. Comparison of β2-transferrin and β-trace protein for detection of cerebrospinal fluid in nasal and ear fluids. Clin Chem 2004;50(3):661–3.
12. Arrer E, Meco C, Oberascher G, et al. β-Trace protein as a marker for cerebrospinal fluid rhinorrhea. Clin Chem 2002;48(6):939–41.
13. Mostafa BE, Khafagi A. Combined HRCT and MRI in the detection of CSF rhinorrhea. Skull Base 2004; 14(3):157–61.
14. Algin O, Hakyemez B, Gokalp G, et al. The contribution of 3D-CISS and contrast-enhanced MR cisternography in detecting cerebrospinal fluid leak in patients with rhinorrhoea. Br J Radiol 2014; 83(987):225–32.
15. Zapalac JS, Marple BF, Schwade ND. Skull base cerebrospinal fluid fistulas: a comprehensive diagnostic algorithm. Otolaryngol Head Neck Surg 2002;126(6):669–76.
16. Shetty PG, Shroff MM, Sahani DV, et al. Evaluation of high-resolution CT and MR cisternography in the diagnosis of cerebrospinal fluid fistula. AJNR Am J Neuroradiol 1998;19(4):633–9.
17. La Fata V, McLean N, Wise S, et al. CSF leaks: correlation of high-resolution CT and multiplanar reformations with intraoperative endoscopic findings. AJNR Am J Neuroradiol 2008;29(3):536–41.
18. Zuckerman JD, DelGaudio JM. Utility of preoperative high-resolution CT and intraoperative image guidance in identification of cerebrospinal fluid leaks for endoscopic repair. Am J Rhinol 2008;22(2):151–4.
19. Schuknecht B, Simmen D, Briner H, et al. Nontraumatic skull base defects with spontaneous CSF rhinorrhea and arachnoid herniation: imaging findings and correlation with endoscopic sinus surgery in 27 patients. AJNR Am J Neuroradiol 2008;29(3):542–9.
20. Lloyd KM, DelGaudio JM, Hudgins PA. Imaging of skull base cerebrospinal fluid leaks in adults. Radiology 2008;248(3):725–36.
21. Drayer BP, Wilkins RH, Boehnke M, et al. Cerebrospinal fluid rhinorrhea demonstrated by metrizamide CT cisternography. AJR Am J Roentgenol 1977; 129(1):149–51.
22. Vimala LR, Jasper A, Irodi A. Non-invasive and minimally invasive imaging evaluation of CSF rhinorrhoea - a retrospective study with review of literature. Pol J Radiol 2016;81:80–5.
23. Stone JA, Castillo M, Neelon B, et al. Evaluation of CSF leaks: high-resolution CT compared with contrast-enhanced CT and radionuclide cisternography. AJNR Am J Neuroradiol 1999;20(4):706–12.
24. Tahir MZ, Khan MB, Bashir MU, et al. Cerebrospinal fluid rhinorrhea: an institutional perspective from Pakistan. Surg Neurol Int 2011;2:174.
25. Goel G, Ravishankar S, Jayakumar P, et al. Intrathecal gadolinium-enhanced magnetic resonance cisternography in cerebrospinal fluid rhinorrhea: road ahead? J Neurotrauma 2007;24(10):1570–5.
26. Chow JM, Goodman D, Mafee MF. Evaluation of CSF rhinorrhea by computerized tomography with metrizamide. Otolaryngol Head Neck Surg 1989;100(2): 99–105.
27. Tuntiyatorn L, Laothammatas J. Evaluation of MR cisternography in diagnosis of cerebrospinal fluid fistula. J Med Assoc Thai 2004;87(12):1471–6.
28. Rajeswaran R, Chandrasekharan A, Mohanty S, et al. Role of MR cisternography in the diagnosis of cerebrospinal fluid rhinorrhoea with diagnostic nasal endoscopy and surgical correlation. Indian J Radiol Imaging 2006;16(3):315.
29. Ragheb AS, Mohammed FF, El-Anwar MW. Cerebrospinal fluid rhinorrhea: diagnostic role of gadolinium enhanced MR cisternography. The Egyptian Journal of Radiology and Nuclear Medicine 2014;45(3):841–7.
30. Delgaudio JM, Baugnon KL, Wise SK, et al. Magnetic resonance cisternogram with intrathecal gadolinium with delayed imaging for difficult to diagnose cerebrospinal fluid leaks of the anterior skull base. Int Forum Allergy Rhinol 2015;5(4):333–8.
31. Selcuk H, Albayram S, Ozer H, et al. Intrathecal gadolinium-enhanced MR cisternography in the evaluation of CSF leakage. AJNR Am J Neuroradiol 2010;31(1):71–5.
32. Aydin K, Terzibasioglu E, Sencer S, et al. Localization of cerebrospinal fluid leaks by gadolinium-enhanced magnetic resonance cisternography: a 5-year single-center experience. Neurosurgery 2008;62(3):584–9.
33. Arbeláez A, Medina E, Rodríguez M, et al. Intrathecal administration of gadopentetate dimeglumine for MR cisternography of nasoethmoidal CSF fistula. AJR Am J Roentgenol 2007;188(6):W560–4.
34. Vanhee A, Dedeken P, Casselman J, et al. MRI with intrathecal gadolinium to detect a CSF leak: feasibility and long term safety from an open label single centre cohort study. Neurology 2016;86(16 Suppl P4):113.
35. Dillon WP. Intrathecal gadolinium: its time has come? AJNR Am J Neuroradiol 2008;29:3–4.
36. Zlab MK, Moore GF, Daly DT, et al. Cerebrospinal fluid rhinorrhea: a review of the literature. Ear Nose Throat J 1992;71(7):314–7.
37. Baugnon KL, Hudgins PA. Skull base fractures and their complications. Neuroimaging Clin N Am 2014; 24(3):439–65.
38. Schlosser RJ, Bolger WE. Nasal cerebrospinal fluid leaks: critical review and surgical considerations. Laryngoscope 2004;114:255–65.

39. Bell RB, Dierks EJ, Homer L, et al. Management of cerebrospinal fluid leak associated with craniomaxillofacial trauma. J Oral Maxillofac Surg 2004;62(6):676–84.
40. Eljamel MS, Foy PM. Acute traumatic CSF fistulae: the risk of intracranial infection. Br J Neurosurg 1990;4:381–5.
41. Lloyd MN, Kimber PM, Burrows EH. Post-traumatic CSF rhinorrhea: modern HRCT is all that is required for the effective demonstration of the site of leakage. Clin Radiol 1994;49:100–3.
42. Platt MP, Parnes SM. Management of unexpected cerebrospinal fluid leak during endoscopic sinus surgery. Curr Opin Otolaryngol Head Neck Surg 2009;17:28–32.
43. Naunheim MR, Sedaghat AR, Lin DT, et al. Immediate and delayed complications following endoscopic skull base surgery. J Neurol Surg B Skull Base 2015;76(5):390–6.
44. Ota N, Tanikawa R, Miyazaki T, et al. Surgical microanatomy of the anterior clinoid process for paraclinoid aneurysm surgery and efficient modification of extradural anterior clinoidectomy. World Neurosurg 2015;83(4):635–43.
45. Spektor S, Dotan S, Mizrahi CJ. Safety of drilling for clinoidectomy and optic canal unroofing in anterior skull base surgery. Acta Neurochir 2013;155(6):1017–24.
46. Batier HH, Welch BG. Respecting the clinoid: an application of preoperative computed tomography angiography. World Neurosurg 2015;83(6):1022–3.
47. Bumm K, Heupel J, Bozzato A, et al. Localization and infliction pattern of iatrogenic skull base defects following endoscopic sinus surgery at a teaching hospital. Auris Nasus Larynx 2009;36:671–6.
48. Yadav YR, Parihar V, Janakiram N, et al. Endoscopic management of cerebrospinal fluid rhinorrhea. Asian J Neurosurg 2016;11(3):183–93.
49. Durcan PJ, Corbett JJ, Wall M. The incidence of pseudotumor cerebri: population studies in Iowa and Louisiana. Arch Neurol 1988;45(8):875–7.
50. O'Connell B, Stevens S, Xiao C, et al. Lateral skull base attenuation in patients with anterior cranial fossa spontaneous cerebrospinal fluid leaks. Otolaryngol Head Neck Surg 2016;154(6):1138–44.
51. Wang EW, Vandergrift WA, Schlosser RJ. Spontaneous CSF leaks. Otolaryngol Clin North Am 2011;44(4):845–56.
52. Tabaee A, Kassenoff TL, Kacker A, et al. The efficacy of computer assisted surgery in the endoscopic management of cerebrospinal fluid rhinorrhea. Otolaryngol Head Neck Surg 2005;133(6):936–43.
53. Banks CA, Palmer JN, Chiu AG, et al. Endoscopic closure of CSF rhinorrhea: 193 cases over 21 years. Otolaryngol Head Neck Surg 2009;140(6):826–33.
54. Bidot S, Saindane AM, Peragallo JH, et al. Brain imaging in idiopathic intracranial hypertension. J Neuroophthalmol 2015;35(4):400–11.
55. Settecase F, Harnsberger HR, Michel MA, et al. Spontaneous lateral sphenoid cephaloceles: anatomic factors contributing to pathogenesis and proposed classification. AJNR Am J Neuroradiol 2014;35:784–9.
56. Bialer OY, Rueda MP, Bruce BB, et al. Meningoceles in idiopathic intracranial hypertension. AJR Am J Roentgenol 2014;202(3):608.
57. Aiken AH, Hoots J, Saindane A, et al. Incidence of cerebellar tonsillar ectopia in idiopathic intracranial hypertension: a mimic of the Chiari I malformation. AJNR Am J Neuroradiol 2012;33(10):1901–6.
58. Mishara S, Mathew G, Paul R, et al. Endoscopic repair of CSF rhinorrhea: an institutional experience. Iran J Otorhinolaryngol 2016;28(84):39–43.
59. Clark D, Bullock P, Hui T, et al. Benign intracranial hypertension: a cause of CSF rhinorrhoea. J Neurol Neurosurg Psychiatr 1994;57(7):847–9.
60. Shetty PG, Shroff MM, Fatterpekar GM, et al. A retrospective analysis of spontaneous sphenoid sinus fistula: MR and CT findings. AJNR Am J Neuroradiol 2000;21(2):337–42.
61. Schlosser RJ, Bolger WE. Management of multiple spontaneous nasal meningoencephaloceles. Laryngoscope 2002;112(6).980–5.
62. Hubbard JL, McDonald TJ, Pearson BW, et al. Spontaneous cerebrospinal fluid rhinorrhea: evolving concepts in diagnosis and surgical management based on the Mayo Clinic experience from 1970 through 1981. Neurosurgery 1985;16:314–21.
63. Schick B, Ibing R, Brors D, et al. Long term study of endonasal duraplasty and review of the literature. Ann Otol Rhinol Laryngol 2001;110:142–7.
64. Gassner HG, Ponikau JU, Sherris DA, et al. CSF rhinorrhea: 95 consecutive surgical cases with long term follow-up at the Mayo Clinic. Am J Rhinol 1999;13:439–47.
65. Chaaban MR, Illing E, Riley KO, et al. Spontaneous cerebrospinal fluid leak repair: a five year prospective evaluation. Laryngoscope 2014;124(1):70–5.
66. Keerl R, Weber RK, Draf W, et al. Use of sodium fluorescein solution for detection of cerebrospinal fluid fistulas: an analysis of 420 administrations and reported complications in Europe and the United States. Laryngoscope 2004;114:266–72.
67. Manes RP, Ryan MW, Marple BF. A novel finding on CT in the diagnosis and localization of CSF leaks without a clear bony defect. Int Forum Allergy Rhinol 2012;2(5):402–4.
68. Schwartz KM, Lane JI, Bolster BD Jr, et al. The utility of diffusion weighted imaging for cholesteatoma evaluation. AJNR Am J Neuroradiol 2011;32:430–6.
69. Abele TA, Salzman KL, Harnsberger HR, et al. Craniopharyngeal canal and its spectrum of pathology. Am J Neuroradiol 2014;35(4):772–7.

Advanced Imaging Techniques of the Skull Base

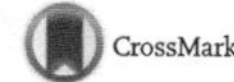

Elliot Dickerson, MD, Ashok Srinivasan, MBBS*

KEYWORDS

• MR perfusion • CT perfusion • Diffusion-weighted imaging • Head and neck imaging
• Head and neck squamous cell carcinoma

KEY POINTS

- Magnetic resonance (MR) diffusion-weighted imaging is helpful in staging head and neck squamous cell cancer, especially possible sites of nodal metastasis. Major challenges to diffusion-weighted imaging are susceptibility artifact in the neck as well as variability in acquisition parameters between different scanners.
- MR perfusion is helpful in staging as well as predicting response to radio/chemotherapy: higher K^{trans} before therapy is associated with a better response to chemoradiation.
- CT perfusion is helpful in staging as well as in predicting response to radio/chemotherapy: higher blood volume before therapy is associated with a better response to chemoradiation.

INTRODUCTION

Since the advent of computed tomography (CT) and MR imaging, cross-sectional imaging has played a crucial role in the evaluation of the skull base in patients presenting with symptoms that can be localized to this region. Although conventional imaging can depict the anatomy of this region with exquisite detail, it often falls short in its ability to characterize tissue physiology and abnormality; this is especially seen in the posttherapy setting where benign posttreatment changes and recurrent tumors can both show intense postcontrast enhancement and similar features on conventional imaging.

Advanced imaging includes a variety of CT, MR imaging, and nuclear medicine–based techniques that can evaluate tissue physiology and, along with conventional imaging, provide a more accurate assessment of the skull base. In this article, the technical details and clinical applications of different advanced imaging techniques are described with a primary focus on diffusion-weighted imaging.

DIFFUSION-WEIGHTED IMAGING

- Take-home points
  - Technical
    - An MR sequence with 2 equal, opposed gradients to dephase and rephase spins over a narrow slice; protons with restricted diffusion will remain in place and susceptible to rephasing and producing signal
    - Diffusion images are mathematically transformed into apparent diffusion coefficient (ADC) maps
    - Major problems in head and neck:
      - Susceptibility
      - Motion artifact

Disclosure Statement: The authors have nothing to disclose.
Department of Radiology, University of Michigan Health System, 1500 East Medical Center Drive B2-A209D, Ann Arbor, MI 48109-5030, USA
* Corresponding author.
E-mail address: ashoks@umich.edu

Radiol Clin N Am 55 (2017) 189–200
http://dx.doi.org/10.1016/j.rcl.2016.08.004
0033-8389/17/© 2016 Elsevier Inc. All rights reserved.

- Lack of standardization in ADC values between scanners and vendors
- Clinical
  - Tumor often restricts diffusion
  - Major applications in head and neck squamous cell carcinoma:
    - Initial staging
    - Differentiating recurrent tumor from treatment effect
    - Developing frontiers: monitoring response to therapy

Technical Background

DWI describes the rate of Brownian motion of water molecules in tissue. Pure water will demonstrate a high degree of diffusion, but barriers such as cell membranes and attachment of water to cellular macromolecules (proteins, and so forth) restrict diffusion. Clinical DWI identifies regions of diffusion restriction such as the damaged, swollen cells of a brain infarct where water shifts from the extracellular spaces to become bound within cellular walls (acute stroke imaging) or in oncologic imaging due to the tendency of many malignancies to restrict diffusion due to a proliferation of closely packed cellular walls[1] (**Fig. 1**).

Although DWI imaging is well established for intracranial processes such as acute stroke, DWI of the skull base and neck presents several important challenges: susceptibility artifact arises from several sources, including air/tissue interfaces as the many irregular surfaces of the neck and metal in some patients (cervical spinal hardware, dental fillings, and so forth).[2] Compared with the intracranial compartment, the neck is heavily affected by physiologic movements, including breathing and swallowing. Approaches being developed to minimize susceptibility artifact include parallel imaging and readout-segmented DWI, which fills k space over multiple excitations rather than the single-shot methods in traditional DWI.[3] Another important challenge is limited reproducibility of diffusion thresholds between scanners and institutions; the values of derived ADC maps will depend to some degree on the b values chosen to generate the map, MR imaging magnetic field strength, subtle mathematical differences in how b values are transformed to an ADC map, and the strengths of the phasing and dephasing gradients.

Although ADC maps ostensibly describe the objective physical parameter of rate of diffusion, one problem highlighted by systematic reviews[4–6] is the variance between ADCs from different institutions and even different MR imaging scanners

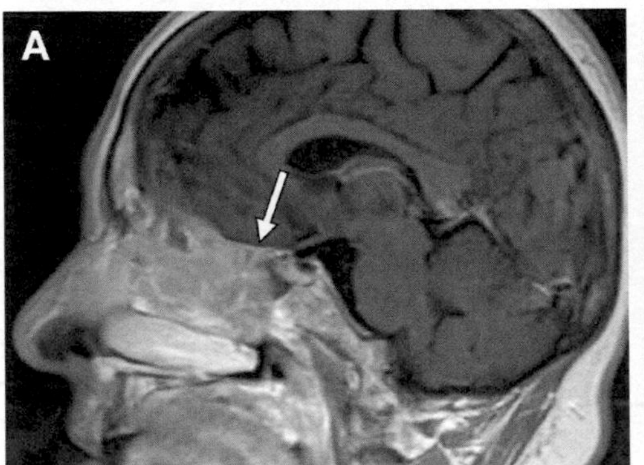

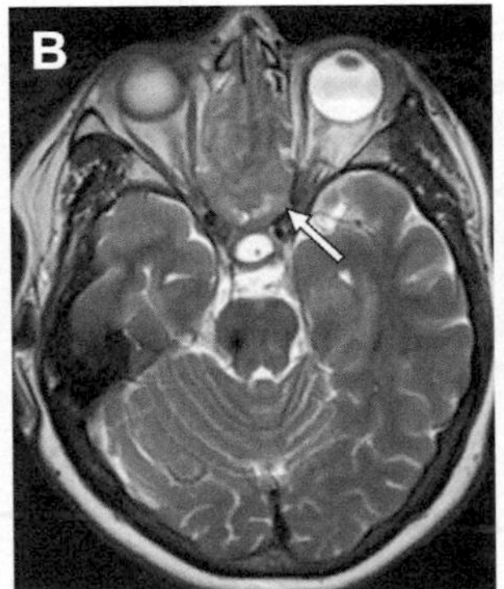

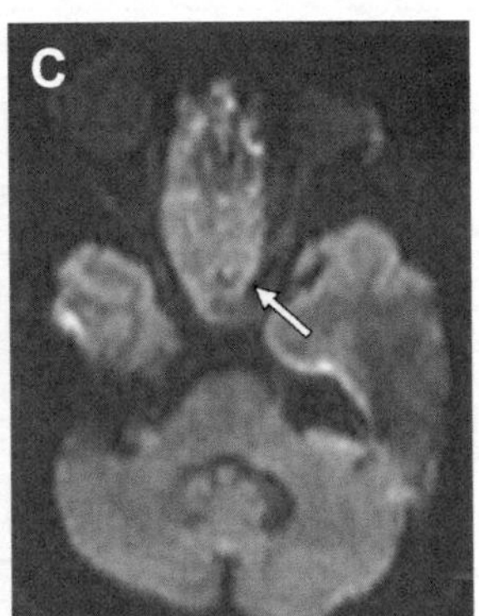

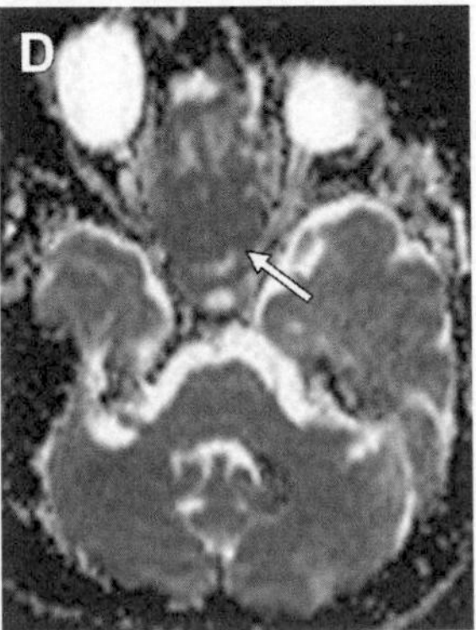

Fig. 1. A 48-year-old woman with nasal lymphoma. Sagittal T1 postcontrast (*A*) and axial T2 images (*B*) demonstrate an avidly enhancing, T2 hypointense mass (*arrows*) filling the ethmoid sinuses with destruction of the osseous walls of the ethmoid sinuses. Note the hyperintensity of this mass relative to the brain on a diffusion-weighted (high b value, B-900) image (*arrow*) (*C*) and hypointensity on the ADC map (*D*). The brain serves as a useful internal control in DWI; the brain generally restricts diffusion to a greater extent than most physiologic tissues in the head and neck. This patient's densely cellular tumor (nasal lymphoma) restricted water diffusion to a greater extent than the brain and well above other skull base and neck soft tissues at this level.

due to different technical parameters in acquisition and calculation of ADC maps, especially because the vast majority of publications on ADC in head and neck squamous cell cancer (HNSCC) used post hoc thresholds rather than a priori–defined thresholds to differentiate benign and malignant lesions. Therefore, the need of the hour is standardizing numbers using normal tissues to create ratios that can be used for clinical application irrespective of the strength of magnet, b values, or vendor.

Clinical Applications

Head and neck squamous cell cancer

The most extensively explored application of DWI in skull base imaging is in HNSCC (**Fig. 2**). Situations where DWI now has repeatedly demonstrated applicability include initial staging of HNSCC, differentiating HNSCC recurrence from benign posttreatment changes, and identifying sites of primary tumor when a primary site is unknown. Within the limitations of ADC reproducibility discussed above, published ADC thresholds (ADC values greater than this threshold suggest benignity, values less than this threshold suggest malignancy) vary from 1.22 to 1.61×10^{-3} mm^2/s in the setting of detecting primary tumor,[5,7–10] from 0.94 to 1.00×10^{-3} mm^2/s in detecting nodal staging,[11–14] and from 1.16 to 1.46×10^{-3} mm^2/s in differentiating disease recurrence.[15–19]

Reported test performance characteristics of DWI in initial staging of known HNSCC report good diagnostic performance of DWI with sensitivity between 73% and 92% and specificity between 84% and 96%.[4,5] For differentiating recurrence from therapy-related changes, systematic reviews report a sensitivity of 67% to 100% and specificity between 86% and 100% (mean 93%).[5]

Promising applications of DWI in HNSCC include detecting invasion of cartilage structures,[20] predicting tumor grade,[21] predicting response to neoadjuvant therapy,[22] and describing response to treatment effects, although understanding the published literature describing response to treatment effects is greatly complicated by heterogeneity in when scanning is performed before and after therapy and treatments provided.[23–25] Generally, tumors that are responding to treatment will show increasing ADC values (presumably as more areas of viable tumor are replaced by necrosis with higher ADC),[1,13,23,25–27] and the necrotic component of tumors will have higher ADC values than viable regions.[28] Somewhat paradoxically, tumors with lower ADC values before therapy tend to respond better to therapy; this may reflect the portion of the tumor replaced with necrosis.[22,25]

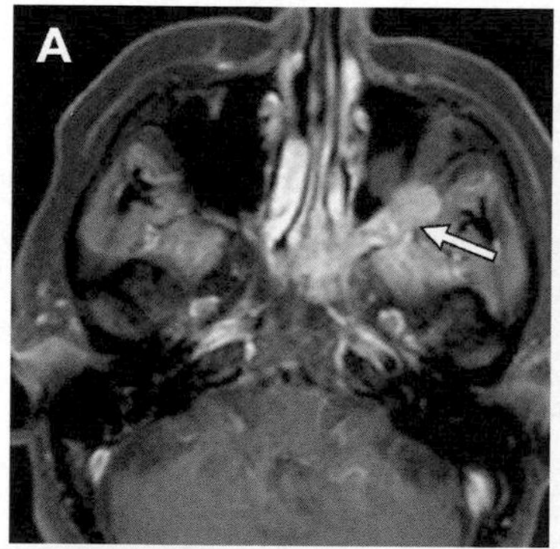

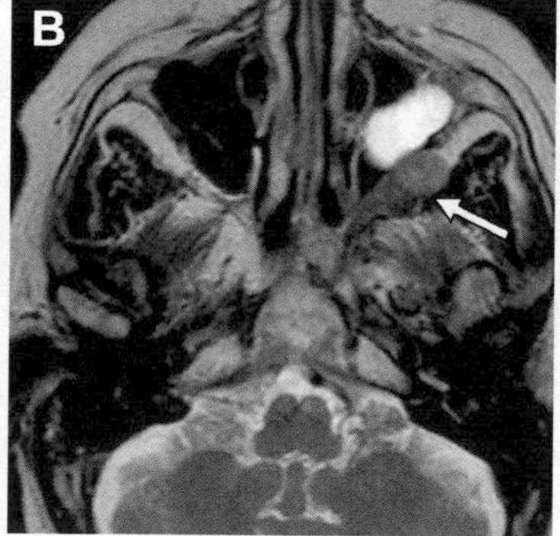

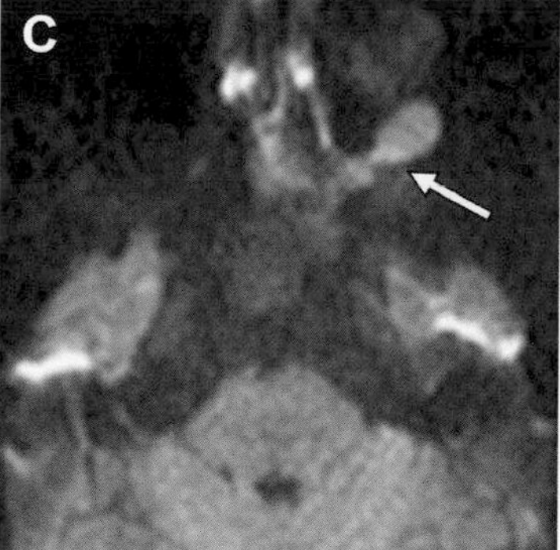

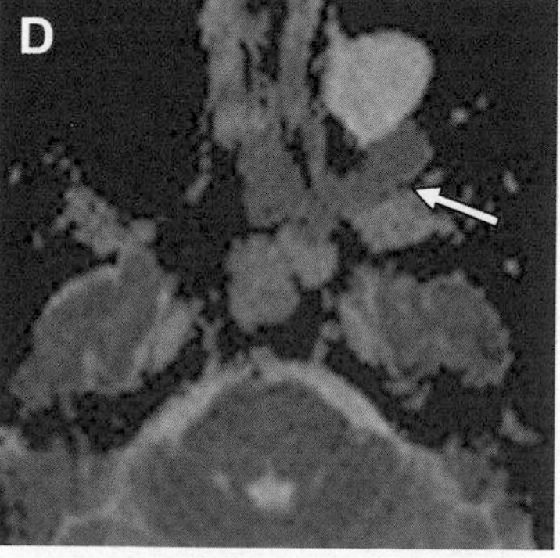

Fig. 2. A 62-year-old woman with squamous cell carcinoma of the nasal cavity. Axial T1 postcontrast (*A*), axial T2 (*B*) shows an enhancing, dumbbell-shaped mass based in the nasal cavity extending into the pterygopalatine fossa. Diffusion-weighted B-900 images (*C*) and ADC maps (*D*) help to define perineural extension to the pterygopalatine fossa (*arrows*).

Other applications of diffusion-weighted imaging

Promising application of DWI outside of HNSCC includes differentiating malignant and benign thyroid lesions,[29] predicting the malignancy and/or histopathology of parotid gland tumors,[30,31] and functional assessment of salivary glands.[32]

MAGNETIC RESONANCE PERFUSION

- Take-home points
  - Technical
    - Describes rate and level of blood flow (BF) to tissues through several techniques: most commonly susceptibility artifact from contrast (dynamic susceptibility contrast-enhanced, DSC) followed by contrast enhancement (dynamic contrast-enhanced, DCE) and arterial spin labeling (ASL)
  - Clinical
    - Helps to characterize possible metastatic lymph nodes
    - Predicting HNSCC response to radio/chemotherapy: more perfusion is associated with a better response (perhaps availability of oxygen and/or chemotherapy)
    - After radio/chemotherapy treatment, loss of excess perfusion suggests better patient outcomes

Technical Background

MR perfusion is a functional imaging technique that aims to describe the delivery of blood and blood-borne contents to tissues. The 3 most common techniques in clinical use are DSC, DCE, and ASL. Briefly, DSC technique uses gadolinium with rapidly acquired echoplanar sequences that quantify the T2* contrast from susceptibility artifact caused by injected gadolinium contrast, whereas DCE technique uses the T1-shortening effect of injected gadolinium contrast. ASL is a technique performed less frequently in clinical practice that uses blood radiofrequency pulses to tag blood as an endogenous tracer.[33]

The diversity of the different techniques of performing MR perfusion gives rise to a diversity of perfusion parameters measured. Generally, DSC best describes the speed and quantity in which a bolus of contrast is delivered to tissue; these are summarized as BF, blood volume (BV) (**Figs. 3** and **4**), and the time required for the bolus to pass through the tissue (mean transit time). DCE reflects the process of tissue gadolinium enhancement with excellent time resolution; this is a process that involves the contrast available to the tissue in the bloodstream as well as the degree of "leakiness" of capillaries within the tissue so DCE best measures a parameter called the transfer constant (k^{trans}) (**Fig. 5**). Arterial spin labeling most reliably measures cerebral BF. In clinical practice, multiple techniques such as both DCE and DSC may be used through split boluses of gadolinium contrast to paint a complete picture of the perfusion characteristics of a lesion.[33] Among the 3 techniques, DCE perfusion has been studied the most for head and neck applications due to the significant susceptibility artifact arising from the DSC technique near the skull base and air–soft tissue interfaces and the relatively prolonged acquisitions with the ASL method.

Clinical Applications

Perfusion MR has been studied in several intracranial applications, which include predicting glioma grade, differentiating recurrent tumor from radiation necrosis, and differentiating tumor progression from pseudoprogression.[34] Studies investigating head and neck applications including the skull base are more limited and have been most promising in predicting treatment response in HNSCC.[35–42]

Generally, higher pretherapy perfusion values of k^{trans} or BV have been found to predict better response to therapy, although this is a complex relationship based on the plethora of techniques available for MR perfusion as well as time points for performing the MR perfusion examination, most commonly either before treatment or in the early period following initial treatment.

Multiple groups have found that increased tumor BV,[35] permeability (k^{trans}),[36–38,41,42] or BF[40,43] is associated with improved local control or disease-free survival of HNSCC. This trend of improved control with increased perfusion is hypothesized to reflect the better delivery of chemotherapy agents to the tumor and/or the availability of oxygen to form free radicals during radiation treatment. Research frontiers include using MR perfusion to identify portions of tumors or nodal metastases that have been insufficiently treated by prior radiation therapy[39] and distinguishing benign from malignant causes of masses or metastases.[44]

COMPUTED TOMOGRAPHIC PERFUSION

- Take-home points
  - Technical
    - Describes rate and level of BF to tissues by tracking attenuation from iodine

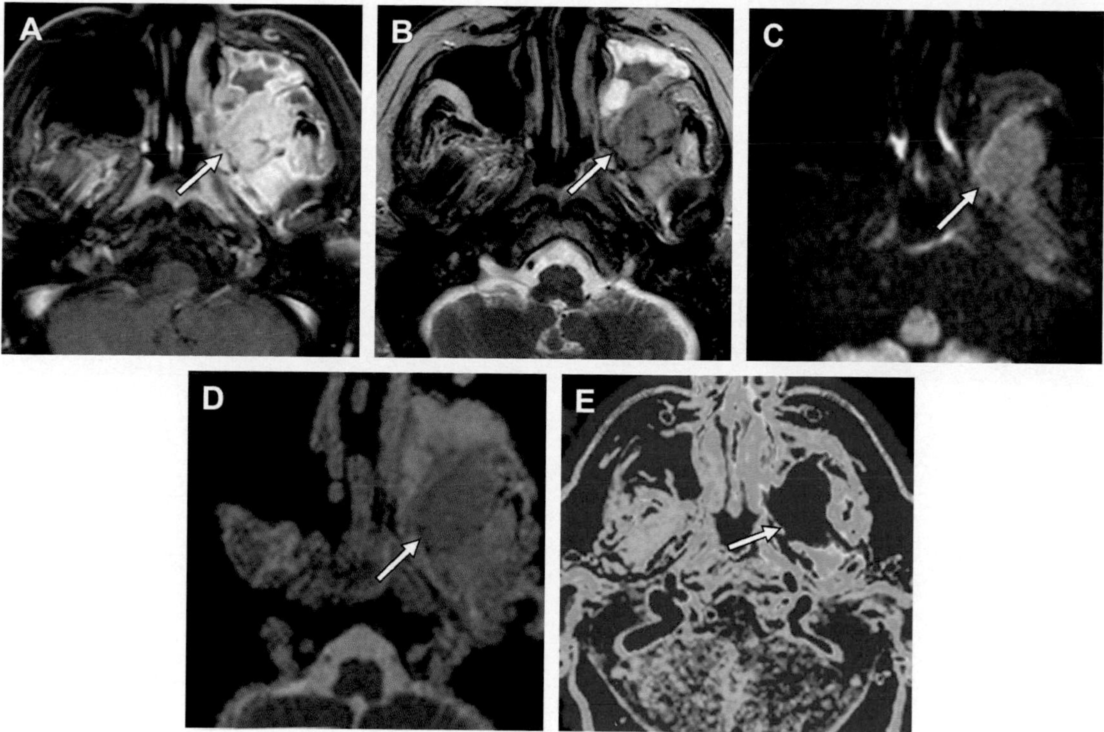

Fig. 3. A 56-year-old man with adenocarcinoma of the left maxillary sinus. Axial T1 postcontrast (*A*) and axial T2 (*B*) images show an enhancing, T2 isointense mass centered in the left maxillary sinus (*arrows*). It is easier to appreciate the margins of the tumor and its extent on DWI (*C*) and ADC map (*D*) as the surrounding normal structures do not demonstrate any significant signal on DWI. MR perfusion BV map (*E*) demonstrates greatly increased BV in the body of the tumor that also well demonstrates posterior extent (*arrows*) and improves differentiation from the reactive mucosal thickening of the left maxillary sinus, which could be confused for tumor involvement on T2 and postcontrast images.

contrast over time (comparable to DCE MR imaging perfusion)

- Clinical
  - Helps to characterize possible metastatic lymph nodes
  - Predicting HNSCC response to radio/chemotherapy: more perfusion is associated with a *better* response (perhaps availability of oxygen and/or chemotherapy)
  - After radio/chemotherapy treatment, loss of excess perfusion suggests better patient outcomes

Technical Background

Similar to MR perfusion, CT perfusion aims to describe the delivery of blood and blood-borne products to tissues. CT perfusion monitors the increase and washout of tissue attenuation over time as iodinated contrast material is delivered to the tissue by blood, analogous to DCE MR perfusion imaging, and uses deconvolution analysis of attenuation-time curves to generate estimates of parameters such as BF, BV, transit times, and permeability.

As CT perfusion inherently requires repeated scanning of the same anatomy to describe dynamic changes over time, this involves more radiation deposition compared with a conventional CT scan covering the same anatomy. Attempts to reduce radiation dose in CT perfusion parallel attempts to reduce dose reduction efforts in other applications of CT, such as advanced reconstruction models, reducing scanning peak vilovoltage (with the coincidental effect of increasing the attenuation effect of iodinated contrasts),[45] and limiting the size of regions scanned to a minimum (such as single-slice scanning of a tumor site rather than the entire neck).[46]

Clinical Applications

As in MR perfusion, most of the extant literature focuses on the application of CT perfusion to HNSCC. The results in later discussion parallel findings from MR perfusion as discussed above. In fact, MR and CT perfusion values correlate

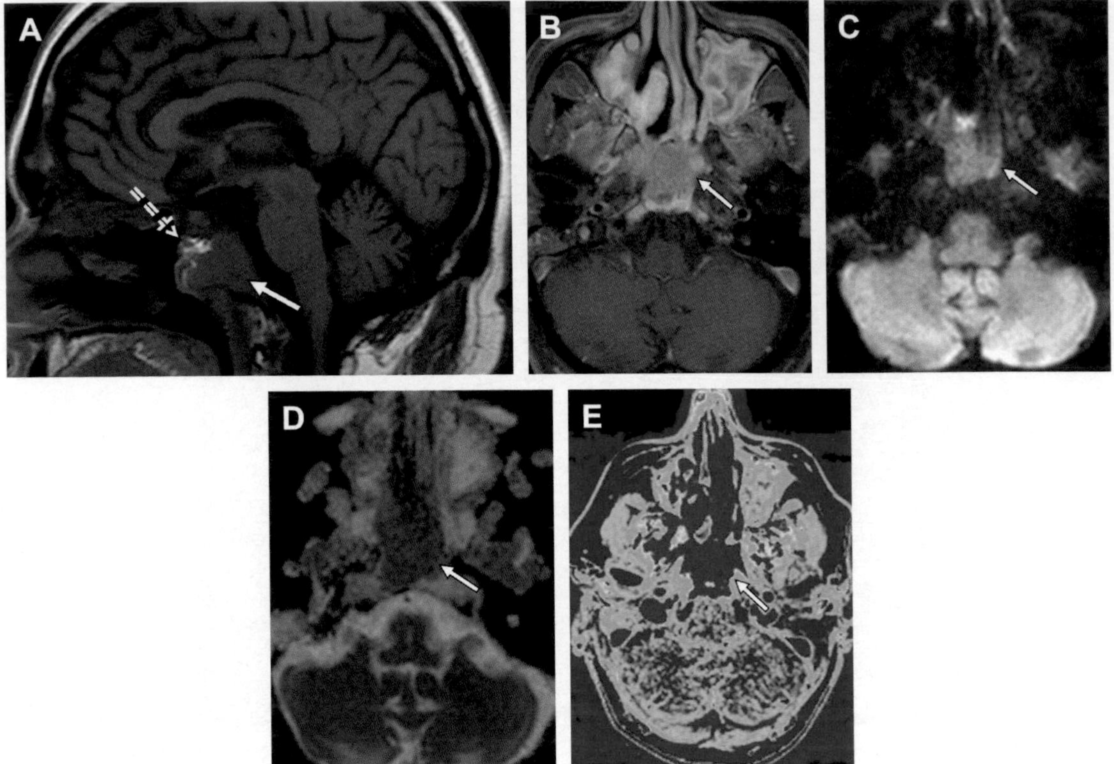

Fig. 4. A 60-year-old man with posttreatment recurrent squamous cell carcinoma of the sphenoid sinus. Sagittal T1 precontrast (*A*) and axial T1 postcontrast (*B*) images of an enhancing, expansile mass centered in the sphenoid sinus (*arrows*) displacing the T1 bright residual fat packing anteriorly (*dashed arrow*). DWI (*C*) and ADC maps (*D*) demonstrate that this mass has greater diffusion restriction than brain at the same level (*arrows*). Significantly increased BV is seen in the mass on the MR perfusion map (*arrow*) (*E*). Both the DWI and the MR perfusion maps are strongly suggestive of recurrent tumor rather than posttreatment changes.

well (although CT-derived values tend to be lower in absolute terms, especially as perfusion values increase[47]) so there is likely significant overlap in the applicability between literature on CT and MR perfusion.

Several studies of CT perfusion in HNSCC have consistently established that HNSCC tends to demonstrate higher perfusion parameters than most normal tissues.[48–51] Accordingly, CT perfusion has utility both in identifying primary sites of tumor and in adding information about potential metastatic involvement of lymph nodes not fully characterized by morphologic criteria alone[52] or the extent of primary tumor (**Figs. 6** and **7**).

A significant application of CT perfusion is in predicting how HNSCC will respond to chemoradiotherapy. As with MR perfusion, multiple studies have found increased perfusion parameters (namely BF and permeability) in tumors that respond *well* (ie, longer survival after treatment) to radiation and chemotherapy.[49,53–55] The tendency of hyperperfused tumors to respond well to chemoradiation has been hypothesized to reflect increased availability of oxygen to produce oxygen free-radicals from radiation therapy and to increase drug delivery from chemotherapy. Although tumors with high perfusion parameters *before* treatment appear to respond better to chemotherapy and radiation, there is a trend toward better patient outcomes with larger decreases in perfusion parameters *following* treatment[48,55,56] (**Fig. 8**).

MAGNETIC RESONANCE SPECTROSCOPY

- Take-home points
  - Technical
    - MR spectroscopy (MRS) focuses on chemical information with minimal spatial information
    - Attempts to quantify differences in metabolites present at low concentrations relative to water and fat: choline (Cho), creatine (Cr)
    - Usually ^{1}H nuclei, research on other atomic nuclei

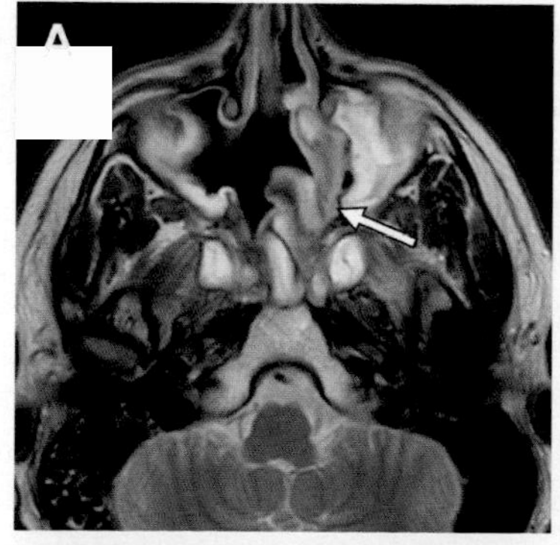

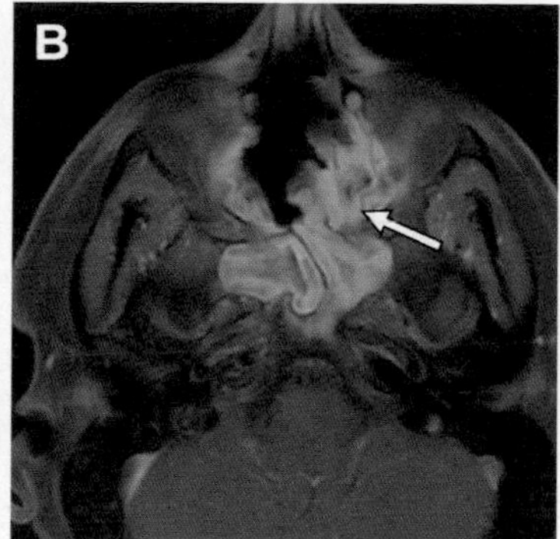

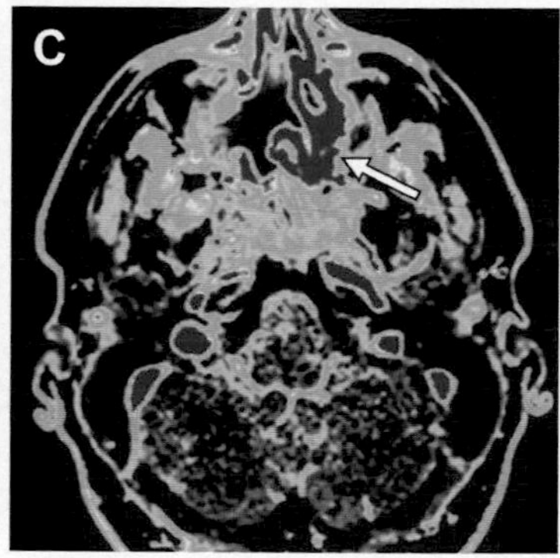

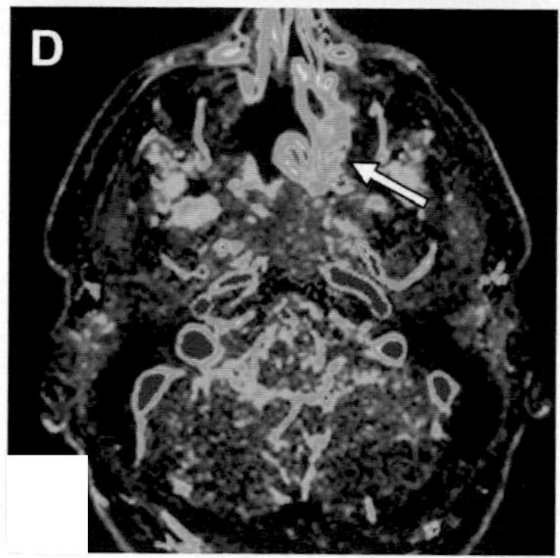

Fig. 5. A 58-year-old man with recurrence of maxillary sinus squamous cell carcinoma. Differentiation of tumor recurrence (*arrows*) from adjacent benign mucosal thickening can be challenging on axial T2 (*A*) and T1 postcontrast (*B*) images, but becomes significantly easier on BV (*C*) and ktrans (*D*) maps that demonstrate distinctively different color between malignant tumor tissue and benign tissues.

- Clinical
  - Multiple studies have demonstrated an increased Cho- (cell wall component) to-Cr ratio in malignant versus lymph nodes
  - Research frontiers: predicting and following response to radio/chemotherapy

Technical Background

Rather than contributing the anatomic information contained in conventional MR imaging, MRS focuses on evaluating different metabolites, such as Cho, Cr, amino acids, and lactate, in a prescribed voxel of interest because different types of tissue contain varying concentrations of these metabolites. MRS typically focuses on the signal

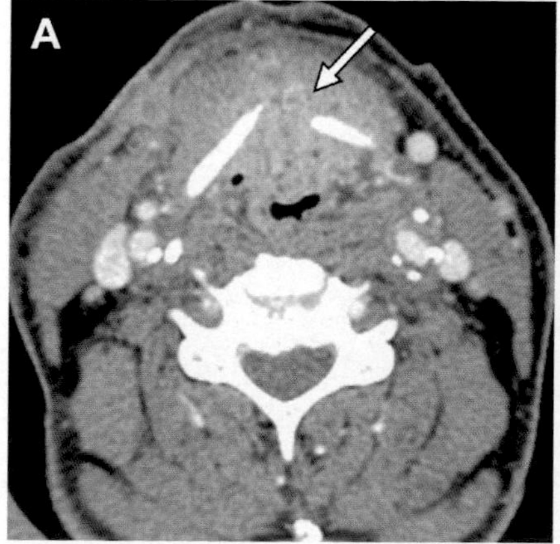

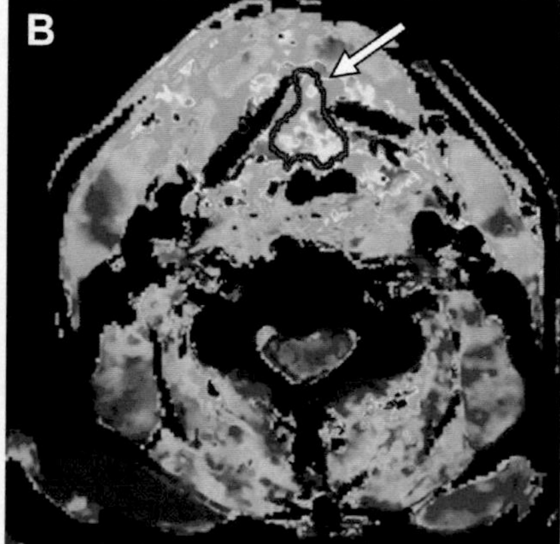

Fig. 6. A 55-year-old man with laryngeal squamous cell carcinoma with extralaryngeal spread. The contrast between the tumor (*arrow*) and surrounding soft tissues on conventional postcontrast axial CT (*A*) is improved on the BF CT perfusion image (*B*) that shows extension of hyperperfused tissue external to the left thyroid cartilage (*arrow*) consistent with extralaryngeal spread.

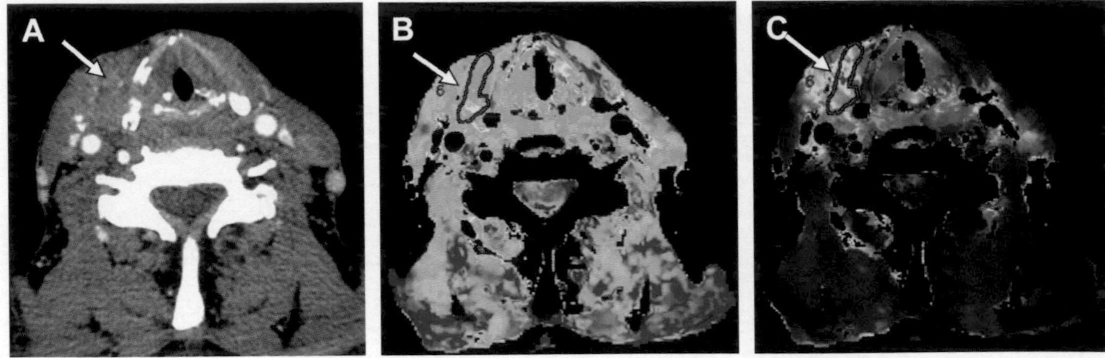

Fig. 7. A 60-year-old man with laryngeal squamous cell carcinoma with extralaryngeal spread. There is minimal contrast on axial postcontrast CT (*A*) between tumor and background soft tissue, but the hyperperfused tumor extension external to the larynx (*arrows*) is well seen on BV (*B*) and BF (*C*) maps (*arrows*).

of ^{1}H nuclei, although MRS has been applied to other atomic nuclei such as ^{31}P.[57]

Disadvantages of MRS include considerable added scan time (especially when multiple voxels of MRS data are obtained to produce maps of MRS spectra) and several added technical challenges such as improving B_0 magnetic field homogeneity through shimming as well as ensuring adequate water and lipid suppression to focus on the MRS signal from the metabolites present in

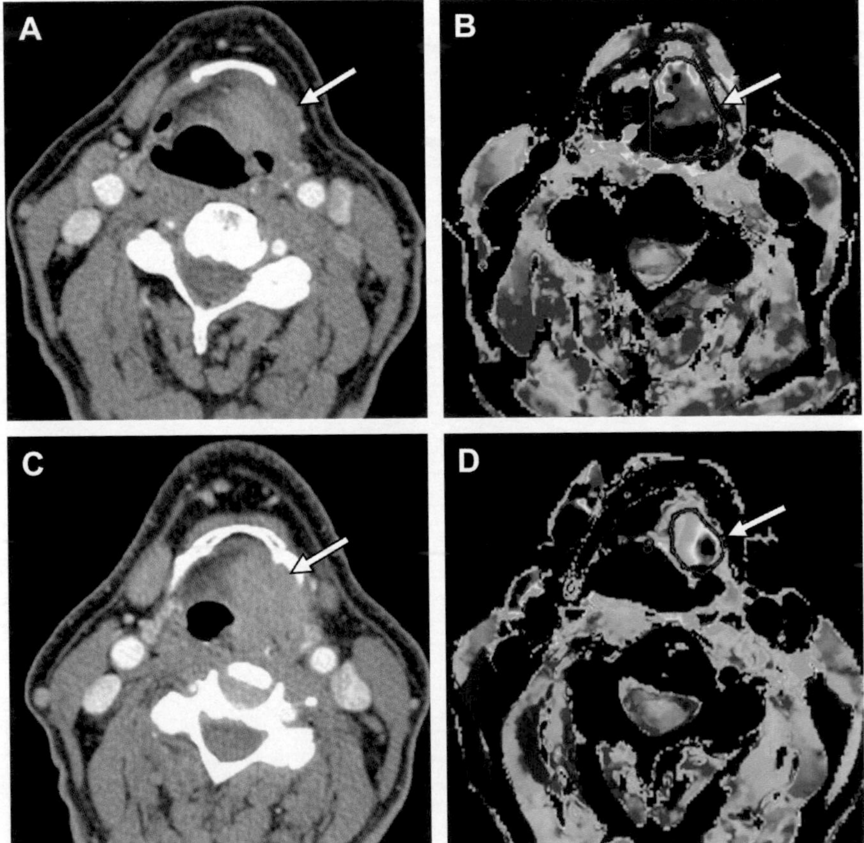

Fig. 8. A 70-year-old man with laryngeal squamous cell carcinoma (*arrows*) both before (axial CT with contrast [*A*] and BV maps [*B*]) and after one round of chemotherapy treatment (axial CT with contrast [*C*] and BV maps [*D*]). Note both dramatic decrease in the size and the degree and extent of hyperperfusion on BV maps (average BV in region of interest circling tumor dropped from 7.31 to 5.33 mL/100 g) following treatment. This decrease in perfusion parameters predicts a good response to radiochemotherapy in HNSCC.

concentrations much lower than the water and lipid prevalent throughout much of the body. The latter problem with lipid suppression is especially pertinent to skull base and neck imaging, where normal fat is abundant and intermixed with other soft tissues.

Clinical Applications

Clinical applications for MRS include identification and characterization of malignancy. The increased membrane turnover associated with actively dividing and tightly packed cell walls in malignancy leads to increased concentration of Cho relative to other metabolites such as Cr, which are relatively constant in both malignant and normal cells. Accordingly, a Cho/Cr ratio can be used to help differentiate malignant from benign lesions such as infection.[58–62]

More recent research efforts have attempted to use MRS of tumors before or shortly after starting therapy to predict response to therapy with mixed results at predicting clinically important outcomes such as disease progression.[63–65]

Several ex vivo studies of tissue samples with MRS have suggested tantalizing possibilities for future in vivo studies and applications of MRS. These possibilities include accurate prediction of the histologic grade of HNSCC tumors and surrounding tissue[66] or predicting which patients would experience treatment failure over a 3-year period from 58 explanted tumors.[67] However, similar results in in vivo uses will require substantial technologic improvements to MRS.

OTHER TECHNIQUES

PET/MR imaging

PET/CT is now a routine component of clinical practice for staging head and neck cancers at many institutions with a substantial evidence base.[68] PET/CT benefits from the added characterization of ^{18}F-fludeoxyglucose metabolism localized by CT. Fused PET/MR imaging holds the promise of adding substantially more anatomic information or even the advanced MR imaging information discussed elsewhere in this publication to further increase sensitivity and specificity for head and neck cancer staging.[69,70]

Ultrasmall Superparamagnetic Iron Oxide–enhanced MR Imaging

Healthy lymph node tissue shows avid uptake of several compounds, including ultrasmall superparamagnetic iron oxide (USPIO) particles, which in turn leads to susceptibility artifact, causing nodes to appear markedly hypointense on MR imaging. Conversely, lymph nodes replaced by metastatic tumor cells will not have marked signal loss from USPIO uptake, which makes USPIO-MR a technique with good diagnostic performance for staging metastatic HNSCC in some studies.[71,72] However, clinical performance of this technique is substantially limited by logistical challenges, including a long delay between contrast injection and imaging (usually 24 hours). In addition, there are currently no clinically approved USPIO contrast agents marketed in many nations, including the United States.[73]

REFERENCES

1. Hamstra DA, Lee KC, Moffat BA, et al. Diffusion magnetic resonance imaging: an imaging treatment response biomarker to chemoradiotherapy in a mouse model of squamous cell cancer of the head and neck. Transl Oncol 2008;1:187–94.
2. Thoeny HC, De Keyzer F, King AD. Diffusion-weighted MR imaging in the head and neck. Radiology 2012;263:19–32.
3. Iima M, Yamamoto A, Brion V, et al. Reduced-distortion diffusion MRI of the craniovertebral junction. AJNR Am J Neuroradiol 2012;33:1321–5.
4. Zhou M, Lu B, Lv G, et al. Differential diagnosis between metastatic and non-metastatic lymph nodes using DW-MRI: a meta-analysis of diagnostic accuracy studies. J Cancer Res Clin Oncol 2015;141:1119–30. Springer Berlin Heidelberg.
5. Driessen JP, van Kempen PMW, van der Heijden GJ, et al. Diffusion-weighted imaging in head and neck squamous cell carcinomas: a systematic review. Eisele DW, editor. Head Neck 2015;37:440–8.
6. Wu LM, Xu JR, Hua J, et al. Value of diffusion-weighted MR imaging performed with quantitative apparent diffusion coefficient values for cervical lymphadenopathy. J Magn Reson Imaging 2013;38:663–70.
7. Sakamoto J, Yoshino N, Okochi K, et al. Tissue characterization of head and neck lesions using diffusion-weighted MR imaging with SPLICE. Eur J Radiol 2009;69:260–8.
8. Srinivasan A, Dvorak R, Perni K, et al. Differentiation of benign and malignant pathology in the head and neck using 3T apparent diffusion coefficient values: early experience. AJNR Am J Neuroradiol 2008;29:40–4.
9. Wang J, Takashima S, Takayama F, et al. Head and neck lesions: characterization with diffusion-weighted echo-planar MR imaging. Radiology 2001;220:621–30.
10. Shang D-S, Ruan L-X, Zhou S-H, et al. Differentiating laryngeal carcinomas from precursor lesions by diffusion-weighted magnetic resonance imaging at 3.0 T: a preliminary study. PLoS One 2013;8:e68622.
11. de Bondt RBJ, Hoeberigs MC, Nelemans PJ, et al. Diagnostic accuracy and additional value of

diffusion-weighted imaging for discrimination of malignant cervical lymph nodes in head and neck squamous cell carcinoma. Neuroradiology 2009; 51:183–92.
12. Dirix P, Vandecaveye V, De Keyzer F, et al. Diffusion-weighted MRI for nodal staging of head and neck squamous cell carcinoma: impact on radiotherapy planning. Int J Radiat Oncol 2010;76:761–6.
13. Vandecaveye V, Dirix P, De Keyzer F, et al. Predictive value of diffusion-weighted magnetic resonance imaging during chemoradiotherapy for head and neck squamous cell carcinoma. Eur Radiol 2010;20: 1703–14.
14. Barchetti F, Pranno N, Giraldi G, et al. The role of 3 Tesla diffusion-weighted imaging in the differential diagnosis of benign versus malignant cervical lymph nodes in patients with head and neck squamous cell carcinoma. Biomed Res Int 2014;2014:532095.
15. Gouhar GK, El-Hariri MA. Feasibility of diffusion weighted MR imaging in differentiating recurrent laryngeal carcinoma from radionecrosis. Egypt J Radiol Nucl Med 2011;42(2):169–75.
16. Abdel Razek AAK, Kandeel a Y, Soliman N, et al. Role of diffusion-weighted echo-planar MR imaging in differentiation of residual or recurrent head and neck tumors and posttreatment changes. AJNR Am J Neuroradiol 2007;28:1146–52.
17. Vandecaveye V, De Keyzer F, Nuyts S, et al. Detection of head and neck squamous cell carcinoma with diffusion weighted MRI after (chemo)radiotherapy: correlation between radiologic and histopathologic findings. Int J Radiat Oncol Biol Phys 2007;67:960–71.
18. Tshering Vogel DW, Zbaeren P, Geretschlaeger A, et al. Diffusion-weighted MR imaging including biexponential fitting for the detection of recurrent or residual tumour after (chemo)radiotherapy for laryngeal and hypopharyngeal cancers. Eur Radiol 2013; 23:562–9.
19. Hwang I, Choi SH, Kim YJ, et al. Differentiation of recurrent tumor and posttreatment changes in head and neck squamous cell carcinoma: application of high b-value diffusion-weighted imaging. AJNR Am J Neuroradiol 2013;34:2343–8.
20. Taha MS, Hassan O, Amir M, et al. Diffusion-weighted MRI in diagnosing thyroid cartilage invasion in laryngeal carcinoma. Eur Arch Otorhinolaryngol 2014;271:2511–6.
21. Yun TJ, Kim J, Kim KH, et al. Head and neck squamous cell carcinoma: differentiation of histologic grade with standard- and high-b-value diffusion-weighted MRI. Head Neck 2013;35:626–31.
22. Kato H, Kanematsu M, Tanaka O, et al. Head and neck squamous cell carcinoma: usefulness of diffusion-weighted MR imaging in the prediction of a neoadjuvant therapeutic effect. Eur Radiol 2009; 19:103–9.
23. King AD, Mo FKF, Yu K-H, et al. Squamous cell carcinoma of the head and neck: diffusion-weighted MR imaging for prediction and monitoring of treatment response. Eur Radiol 2010;20:2213–20.
24. Schouten CS, Hoekstra OS, Leemans CR, et al. Response evaluation after chemoradiotherapy for advanced staged oropharyngeal squamous cell carcinoma: a nationwide survey in the Netherlands. Eur Arch Otorhinolaryngol 2014;272:3507–13.
25. Kim S, Loevner L, Quon H, et al. Diffusion-weighted magnetic resonance imaging for predicting and detecting early response to chemoradiation therapy of squamous cell carcinomas of the head and neck. Clin Cancer Res 2009;15:986–94.
26. Galbán CJ, Mukherji SK, Chenevert TL, et al. A feasibility study of parametric response map analysis of diffusion-weighted magnetic resonance imaging scans of head and neck cancer patients for providing early detection of therapeutic efficacy. Transl Oncol 2009;2:184–90.
27. Berrak S, Chawla S, Kim S, et al. Diffusion weighted imaging in predicting progression free survival in patients with squamous cell carcinomas of the head and neck treated with induction chemotherapy. Acad Radiol 2011;18:1225–32. Elsevier Ltd.
28. Razek AAKA, Megahed AS, Denewer A, et al. Role of diffusion-weighted magnetic resonance imaging in differentiation between the viable and necrotic parts of head and neck tumors. Acta Radiol 2008; 49:364–70.
29. Shi HF, Feng Q, Qiang JW, et al. Utility of diffusion-weighted imaging in differentiating malignant from benign thyroid nodules with magnetic resonance imaging and pathologic correlation. J Comput Assist Tomogr 2013;37:505–10.
30. Habermann CR, Arndt C, Graessner J, et al. Diffusion-weighted echo-planar MR imaging of primary parotid gland tumors: is a prediction of different histologic subtypes possible? AJNR Am J Neuroradiol 2009;30:591–6.
31. Eida S, Sumi M, Sakihama N, et al. Apparent diffusion coefficient mapping of salivary gland tumors: prediction of the benignancy and malignancy. AJNR Am J Neuroradiol 2007;28:116–21.
32. Dirix P, De Keyzer F, Vandecaveye V, et al. Diffusion-weighted magnetic resonance imaging to evaluate major salivary gland function before and after radiotherapy. Int J Radiat Oncol 2008;71:1365–71.
33. Essig M, Shiroishi MS, Nguyen TB, et al. Perfusion MRI: the five most frequently asked technical questions. Am J Roentgenol 2013;200:24–34.
34. Essig M, Nguyen TB, Shiroishi MS, et al. Perfusion MRI: the five most frequently asked clinical questions. Am J Roentgenol 2013;201:W495–510.
35. Cao Y, Popovtzer A, Li D, et al. Early prediction of outcome in advanced head-and-neck cancer based on tumor blood volume alterations during therapy: a

prospective study. Int J Radiat Oncol Biol Phys 2008;72:1287–90.
36. Kim S, Loevner LA, Quon H, et al. Prediction of response to chemoradiation therapy in squamous cell carcinomas of the head and neck using dynamic contrast-enhanced MR imaging. AJNR Am J Neuroradiol 2010;31:262–8.
37. Chawla S, Kim S, Loevner LA, et al. Prediction of disease-free survival in patients with squamous cell carcinomas of the head and neck using dynamic contrast-enhanced MR imaging. AJNR Am J Neuroradiol 2011;32:778–84.
38. Chikui T, Kitamoto E, Kawano S, et al. Pharmacokinetic analysis based on dynamic contrast-enhanced MRI for evaluating tumor response to preoperative therapy for oral cancer. J Magn Reson Imaging 2012;36:589–97.
39. Wang P, Popovtzer A, Eisbruch A, et al. An approach to identify, from DCE MRI, significant subvolumes of tumors related to outcomes in advanced head-and-neck cancer. Med Phys 2012;39:5277.
40. Agrawal S, Awasthi R, Singh A, et al. An exploratory study into the role of dynamic contrast-enhanced (DCE) MRI metrics as predictors of response in head and neck cancers. Clin Radiol 2012;67:e1–5. The Royal College of Radiologists.
41. Ng S-H, Lin C-Y, Chan S-C, et al. Dynamic contrast-enhanced MR imaging predicts local control in oropharyngeal or hypopharyngeal squamous cell carcinoma treated with chemoradiotherapy. PLoS One 2013;8:e72230.
42. Chawla S, Kim S, Dougherty L, et al. Pretreatment diffusion-weighted and dynamic contrast-enhanced MRI for prediction of local treatment response in squamous cell carcinomas of the head and neck. Am J Roentgenol 2013;200:35–43.
43. Fujima N, Yoshida D, Sakashita T, et al. Usefulness of pseudocontinuous arterial spin-labeling for the assessment of patients with head and neck squamous cell carcinoma by measuring tumor blood flow in the pretreatment and early treatment period. AJNR Am J Neuroradiol 2016;37(2):342–8.
44. Razek AAKA, Elsorogy LG, Soliman NY, et al. Dynamic susceptibility contrast perfusion MR imaging in distinguishing malignant from benign head and neck tumors: a pilot study. Eur J Radiol 2011;77:73–9. Elsevier Ireland Ltd.
45. Ash L, Teknos TN, Gandhi D, et al. Head and neck squamous cell carcinoma: CT perfusion can help noninvasively predict intratumoral microvessel density. Radiology 2009;251:422–8.
46. Tawfik AM, Nour-Eldin N-E, Naguib NN, et al. CT perfusion measurements of head and neck carcinoma from single section with largest tumor dimensions or average of multiple sections: agreement between the two methods and effect on intra- and inter-observer agreement. Eur J Radiol 2012; 81(10):2692–6. Elsevier Ireland Ltd.
47. Bisdas S, Medov L, Baghi M, et al. A comparison of tumour perfusion assessed by deconvolution-based analysis of dynamic contrast-enhanced CT and MR imaging in patients with squamous cell carcinoma of the upper aerodigestive tract. Eur Radiol 2008; 18:843–50.
48. Petralia G, Preda L, Giugliano G, et al. Perfusion computed tomography for monitoring induction chemotherapy in patients with squamous cell carcinoma of the upper aerodigestive tract: correlation between changes in tumor perfusion and tumor volume. J Comput Assist Tomogr 2009;33:552–9.
49. Bisdas S, Nguyen SA, Anand SK, et al. Outcome prediction after surgery and chemoradiation of squamous cell carcinoma in the oral cavity, oropharynx, and hypopharynx: use of baseline perfusion CT microcirculatory parameters vs. tumor volume. Int J Radiat Oncol Biol Phys 2009;73: 1313–8.
50. Bisdas S, Baghi M, Smolarz A, et al. Quantitative measurements of perfusion and permeability of oropharyngeal and oral cavity cancer, recurrent disease, and associated lymph nodes using first-pass contrast-enhanced computed tomography studies. Invest Radiol 2007;42:172–9.
51. Gandhi D, Hoeffner EG, Carlos RC, et al. Computed tomography perfusion of squamous cell carcinoma of the upper aerodigestive tract. Initial results. J Comput Assist Tomogr 2003;27:687–93.
52. Veit-Haibach P, Schmid D, Strobel K, et al. Combined PET/CT-perfusion in patients with head and neck cancers. Eur Radiol 2013;23:163–73.
53. Bisdas S, Rumboldt Z, Surlan-Popovic K, et al. Perfusion CT in squamous cell carcinoma of the upper aerodigestive tract: long-term predictive value of baseline perfusion CT measurements. AJNR Am J Neuroradiol 2010;31:576–81.
54. Zima A, Carlos R, Gandhi D, et al. Can pretreatment CT perfusion predict response of advanced squamous cell carcinoma of the upper aerodigestive tract treated with induction chemotherapy? AJNR Am J Neuroradiol 2007;28:328–34.
55. Rana L, Sharma S, Sood S, et al. Volumetric CT perfusion assessment of treatment response in head and neck squamous cell carcinoma: comparison of CT perfusion parameters before and after chemoradiation therapy. Eur J Radiol Open 2015;2:46–54. Elsevier Ltd.
56. Šurlan-Popovič KŠ, Bisdas S, Rumboldt Z, et al. Changes in perfusion CT of advanced squamous cell carcinoma of the head and neck treated during the course of concomitant chemoradiotherapy. AJNR Am J Neuroradiol 2010;31:570–5.
57. Abdel Razek AAK, Poptani H. MR spectroscopy of head and neck cancer. Eur J Radiol 2013;82:982–9. Elsevier Ireland Ltd.

58. Mukherji SK, Schiro S, Castillo M, et al. Proton MR spectroscopy of squamous cell carcinoma of the extracranial head and neck: in vitro and in vivo studies. AJNR Am J Neuroradiol 1995;18:1057–72.
59. Yu Q, Yang J, Wang P. Malignant tumors and chronic infections in the masticator space: preliminary assessment with in vivo single-voxel 1H-MR spectroscopy. AJNR Am J Neuroradiol 2008;29:716–9.
60. Mukherji SK, Schiro S, Castillo M, et al. Proton MR spectroscopy of squamous cell carcinoma of the upper aerodigestive tract: in vitro characteristics. AJNR Am J Neuroradiol 1996;17:1485–90.
61. Fahmy DM, El-Hawarey G, El-Serougy L, et al. Hydrogen MR spectroscopy of neck masses. Egypt J Radiol Nucl Med 2012;43(3):421–7.
62. Kendi T, Arikan OK, Koç C. MR spectroscopy in a cervical abscess. Neuroradiology 2003;45:631–3.
63. Abdel Razek AAK, Poptani H, Bezabeh T, et al. Pretreatment and early intratreatment prediction of clinicopathologic response of head and neck cancer to chemoradiotherapy using 1H-MRS. Eur J Radiol 2008;14:421–7. Elsevier B.V.
64. King AD, Yeung DKW, Yu KH, et al. Pretreatment and early intratreatment prediction of clinicopathologic response of head and neck cancer to chemoradiotherapy using 1H-MRS. J Magn Reson Imaging 2010;32:199–203.
65. Jansen JFA, Schöder H, Lee NY, et al. Tumor metabolism and perfusion in head and neck squamous cell carcinoma: pretreatment multimodality imaging with 1H magnetic resonance spectroscopy, dynamic contrast-enhanced MRI, and [18F]FDG-PET. Int J Radiat Oncol 2012;82:299–307.
66. Srivastava S, Roy R, Gupta V, et al. Proton HR-MAS MR spectroscopy of oral squamous cell carcinoma tissues: an ex vivo study to identify malignancy induced metabolic fingerprints. Metabolomics 2011;7:278–88.
67. Bezabeh T, Odlum O, Nason R, et al. Prediction of treatment response in head and neck cancer by magnetic resonance spectroscopy. Cancer 2005;26:2108–13.
68. Furukawa M, Anzai Y. Diagnosis of cervical lymph node metastasis in head and neck cancer: evidence-based neuroimaging. Evidence-based neuroimaging diagnosis treat. New York: Springer New York; 2013. p. 693–718.
69. Varoquaux A, Rager O, Dulguerov P, et al. Diffusion-weighted and PET/MR imaging after radiation therapy for malignant head and neck tumors. Radiographics 2015;35:1502–27.
70. Queiroz MA, Hullner M, Kuhn F, et al. Use of diffusion-weighted imaging (DWI) in PET/MRI for head and neck cancer evaluation. Eur J Nucl Med Mol Imaging 2014;41:2212–21.
71. Anzai Y, Piccoli CW, Outwater EK, et al. Evaluation of neck and body metastases to nodes with ferumoxtran 10-enhanced MR imaging: phase III safety and efficacy study. Radiology 2003;228:777–88.
72. Mack MG, Mack MG, Balzer JO, et al. Superparamagnetic iron oxide-enhanced MR imaging of head and neck lymph nodes. Radiology 2002;222:239–44.
73. Weissleder R, Nahrendorf M, Pittet MJ. Imaging macrophages with nanoparticles. Nat Mater 2014;13:125–38. Nature Publishing Group.

Index

Note: Page numbers of article titles are in **boldface** type.

Radiol Clin N Am 55 (2017) 201–207
http://dx.doi.org/10.1016/S0033-8389(16)30170-1
0033-8389/17

D

U

V

Moving?

Make sure your subscription moves with you!

To notify us of your new address, find your **Clinics Account Number** (located on your mailing label above your name), and contact customer service at:

Email: journalscustomerservice-usa@elsevier.com

800-654-2452 (subscribers in the U.S. & Canada)
314-447-8871 (subscribers outside of the U.S. & Canada)

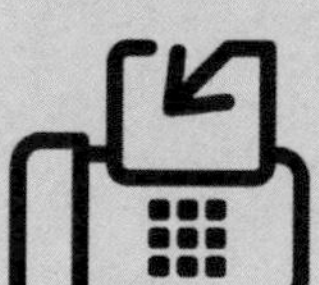

Fax number: 314-447-8029

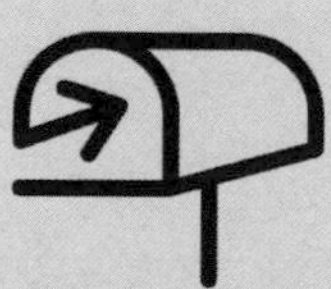

Elsevier Health Sciences Division
Subscription Customer Service
3251 Riverport Lane
Maryland Heights, MO 63043

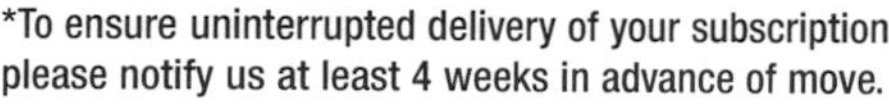

*To ensure uninterrupted delivery of your subscription, please notify us at least 4 weeks in advance of move.

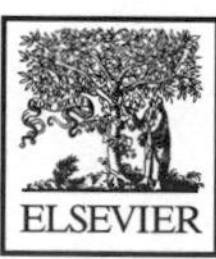